Practical Endocrinology and Diabetes in Children

Practical Endocrinology and Diabetes in Children

Third edition

Joseph E. Raine MD, FRCPCH, DCH

Consultant Paediatrician
Whittington Hospital
London, UK

Malcolm D. C. Donaldson MD, FRCP, DCH

Senior Lecturer in Child Health and Consultant Paediatric Endocrinologist
Royal Hospital for Sick Children
Yorkhill
Glasgow, UK

John W. Gregory MBChB, MD, FRCP, DCH, FRCPCH

Professor in Paediatric Endocrinology
Department of Child Health
School of Medicine
Cardiff University
Cardiff, UK

Guy Van Vliet MD

Professeur de Pédiatrie
Université de Montréal
Chef, Service d'Endocrinologie
Hôpital Sainte-Justine
Montréal, Québec, Canada

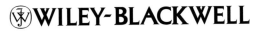

WILEY-BLACKWELL

A John Wiley & Sons, Ltd., Publication

This edition first published 2011, © 2006, 2001 by Joseph E. Raine, Malcolm D.C. Donaldson, John W. Gregory, Guy Van Vliet

Blackwell Publishing was acquired by John Wiley & Sons in February 2007. Blackwell's publishing program has been merged with Wiley's global Scientific, Technical and Medical business to form Wiley-Blackwell.

Registered office: John Wiley & Sons Ltd, The Atrium, Southern Gate, Chichester, West Sussex, PO19 8SQ, UK

Editorial offices: 9600 Garsington Road, Oxford, OX4 2DQ, UK
                       The Atrium, Southern Gate, Chichester, West Sussex, PO19 8SQ, UK
                       111 River Street, Hoboken, NJ 07030-5774, USA

For details of our global editorial offices, for customer services and for information about how to apply for permission to reuse the copyright material in this book please see our website at www.wiley.com/wiley-blackwell

The right of the author to be identified as the author of this work has been asserted in accordance with the Copyright, Designs and Patents Act 1988.

Library of Congress Cataloging-in-Publication Data

Raine, Joseph E., author.
   Practical endocrinology and diabetes in children / Joseph E. Raine / Malcolm D. C. Donaldson / John W. Gregory / Guy Van Vliet - Third edition.
       p. ; cm.
   Includes bibliographical references and index.
       ISBN 978-1-4051-9634-5 (hardback : alk. paper)   1. Diabetes in children.   2. Pediatric endocrinology.   I. Donaldson, Malcolm D. C., author.   II. Gregory, John W., author.   III. Van Vliet, Guy, author.   IV. Practical endocrinology and diabetes in children. Revision of (work):   V. Title.
   [DNLM: 1. Endocrine System Diseases.   2. Child.   3. Diabetes Mellitus. WS 330]
   RJ420.D5D52 2011
   618.92′462–dc22

                                                                            2010052326

A catalogue record for this book is available from the British Library.

This book is published in the following electronic formats: ePDF 9781444342109; Wiley Online Library 9781444342116

Set in 9.25/11.5pt Minion by Aptara® Inc., New Delhi, India
Printed and bound in Singapore by Markono Print Media Pte Ltd

1   2011

P008939

Contents

Preface to the Third Edition

There are few books that bridge the gap between the large detailed endocrine reference book and the short review of aspects of paediatric endocrinology. The aim of this book is to provide a practical, concise and up-to-date account of paediatric endocrinology and diabetes in a readable and user-friendly format.

Given the importance of diabetes in clinical practice, particular emphasis has been placed on its management. The management of emergencies has been highlighted in the text by providing a grey background to those sections. At the end of the chapters, there are guidelines on which conditions should be discussed with a specialist centre, an outline of controversial areas and sections on transition, potential pitfalls and future developments. We have also listed, at the end of the chapters, 'Significant guidelines/consensus statements' and 'Useful sources of information for patients and their families'. There is also an appendix with growth charts at the end of the book.

At the end of each chapter, there are 4–5 interesting cases which illustrate diagnostic difficulties. These should also help those studying for postgraduate exams many of which include such 'grey cases'.

The book is aimed primarily at paediatricians in general hospitals and at junior paediatric staff with an interest in paediatric endocrinology and/or diabetes. However, we hope that the book will also be useful to medical students, nurses working in paediatric endocrinology wards and to diabetes nurse specialists.

This edition has been extensively revised and updated and incorporates a new editor, Guy Van Vliet, Professor of Pediatrics at the University of Montreal. Professor Van Vliet has helped to provide a North American perspective for the book that we hope will increase its relevance and international appeal.

JER, MDCD, JWG, GVV
January 2011

Acknowledgements

The authors would like to thank Dr David Levy, Consultant Diabetologist, Whipps Cross Hospital, London; Dr Jill Challener, Consultant Paediatrician Hinchingbrooke Hospital, Cambridgeshire; Dr Joanna Walker, Consultant Paediatrician, St Mary's Hospital, Portsmouth; Dr Faisal Ahmed, Consultant Paediatric Endocrinologist, Mr Stuart O'Toole, Consultant Paediatric Surgeon and Ms Wendy Paterson, Auxologist, Royal Hospital For Sick Children, Glasgow; Professor Robert Fraser, MRC Blood Pressure Unit, Western Infirmary, Glasgow; Dr Helen Lyall, Consultant Gynaecologist and Dr Mike Wallace, Consultant Clinical Scientist, Biochemistry Department, Glasgow Royal Infirmary, Sam Hope, Insulin Pump Trainer, Animas; Dr Céline Huot, Paediatric Endocrinologist, Hôpital Sainte-Justine, Dr Mark Vanderpump, Consultant Endocrinologist, Royal Free Hospital, London; Ms Heulwen Morgan, Consultant Gynaecologist and Dr Karen Anthony, Consultant Endocrinologist, Whittington Hospital, London for their help and advice with different sections of the book.

Abbreviations

ACTH	adrenocorticotrophic hormone	GP	general practitioner
ACR	albumin creatinine ratio	HbA1c	glycosylated haemoglobin
AFP	alpha-foetoprotein	hCG	human chorionic gonadotrophin
AHO	Albright's hereditary osteodystrophy	HDL	high-density lipoprotein
AMH	anti-Müllerian hormone	hGH	human growth hormone
ATP	adenosine triphosphate	17-OHP	17-hydroxyprogesterone
AVP	arginine vasopressin	IGF-1	insulin-like growth factor 1
BMI	body mass index	IGFBPs	IGF binding proteins
BP	blood pressure	IUGR	intrauterine growth retardation
CAH	congenital adrenal hyperplasia	IV	intravenous
CAIS	complete androgen insensitivity syndrome	K	potassium
cAMP	cyclic adenosine monophosphate	LH	luteinizing hormone
cGy	centigray units	MDI	multiple daily injections
CNS	central nervous system	MEN	multiple endocrine neoplasia
CRP	C reactive protein	MPH	mid-parental height
CSII	continuous subcutaneous insulin infusion	MRI	magnetic resonance imaging
CT	computerized tomography	PAIS	partial androgen insensitivity syndrome
DDAVP	desamino-D-arginine vasopressin or desmopressin	PCOS	polycystic ovary syndrome
		PCR	polymerase chain reaction
DEXA	dual energy X-ray absorptiometry	PHV	peak height velocity
DHEAS	dehydroepiandrosterone-sulfate	PTH	parathyroid hormone
DI	diabetes insipidus	SDS	standard deviation score
DKA	diabetic ketoacidosis	SED	spondylo-epiphyseal dysplasia
DNA	deoxyribonucleic acid	SGA	small for gestational age
DNS	diabetes nurse specialist	SHBG	sex hormone binding globulin
DSD	disorder of sex development	SIADH	syndrome of inappropriate antidiuretic hormone secretion
EPP	ectopic posterior pituitary		
FASD	foetal alcohol spectrum disorder	SOD	septo-optic dysplasia
FBC	full blood count	SRY	sex determining region of the Y
FGFR3	fibroblast growth factor receptor-3	T3	triiodothyronine
FISH	fluorescent *in situ* hybridization	T4	thyroxine
FSH	follicle stimulating hormone	TBG	thyroid binding globulin
FT3	free triiodothyronine	TFT	thyroid function tests
FT4	free thyroxine	TRH	thyroid releasing hormone
GH	growth hormone	TSH	thyroid stimulating hormone
GHD	growth hormone deficiency	U and Es	urea and electrolytes
GHRH	growth hormone releasing hormone	WBC	white blood cells

1 Diabetes Mellitus

Definition

Diabetes is diagnosed in the presence of either a blood glucose concentration of >11.1 mmol/L (200 mg/dL) or a fasting glucose concentration of >7 mmol/L (126 mg/dL). A fasting blood glucose level of 5.6–6.9 mmol/L (100–125 mg/dL) is considered prediabetes, while a level < 5.6 mmol/L (<100 mg/dL) is normal. The diagnosis of diabetes, when symptoms are present, is usually straightforward and a glucose tolerance test is rarely needed. Glucose tolerance testing may be indicated following the identification of a borderline blood glucose concentration (e.g. in the sibling of a child with diabetes, or in children with disorders such as cystic fibrosis which predispose to diabetes and which, in the early stages, may be asymptomatic). The protocol for and interpretation of results from an oral glucose tolerance test is shown in Table 1.1.

Diabetes is a heterogeneous condition which may be classified on the basis of pathogenesis (Table 1.2). Most of this chapter focuses on type 1 diabetes, which is by far the most common form of diabetes in children. Other causes of diabetes are discussed on p. 30 and 35.

Incidence

The incidence of type 1 diabetes in children (0–18 years) is approximately 20/100,000 in the United Kingdom (prevalence 1 in 500), but varies from 0.6/100,000 in China to 42.9/100,000 in Finland. The reasons for these large variations are unclear, but may include genetic factors given the evidence of variations in the incidence of diabetes in different ethnic groups (e.g. in the USA, white people have a higher incidence than non-whites). There is a family history of type 1 diabetes in 10% of cases. The risk of

Practical Endocrinology and Diabetes in Children, Third Edition. Joseph E. Raine, Malcolm D.C. Donaldson, John W. Gregory, Guy Van Vliet.
© 2011 Blackwell Publishing Ltd. Published 2011 by Blackwell Publishing Ltd.

Table 1.1 Protocol for the oral glucose tolerance test.

Indications
Confirmation of the diagnosis of diabetes mellitus in uncertain cases and diagnosis of impaired glucose tolerance

Preparation
Perform in the morning after an overnight fast

Procedure
1. Pre test—plasma glucose sample
2. 0 minute—administer oral glucose 1.75 g/kg (up to a maximum of 75 g) diluted with water (consume over 5–10 minutes)
3. +2 hours—plasma glucose sample

Interpretation
1. Fasting plasma glucose $\geq$ 7.0 mmol/L (126 mg/dL) or 2 h concentration $\geq$ 11.1 mmol/L (200 mg/dL) are diagnostic of diabetes
2. 2 h plasma glucose concentration $\geq$ 7.8 mmol/L (140 mg/dL) and < 11.1 mmol/L (200 mg/dL) suggests impaired glucose tolerance
3. Fasting plasma glucose 6.1–6.9 mmol/L (110–125 mg/dL) suggests impaired fasting glycaemia

developing type 1 diabetes for an individual with an affected relative is outlined in Table 1.3. If a twin develops type 1 diabetes the lifetime risk to a non-affected monozygotic twin is approximately 60%, whereas that for a dizygotic twin is 8%. Environmental effects are probably important as the incidence rises in the winter months. The incidence of type 1 diabetes in children is set to rise over the next 10 years in Europe, especially in those under

Table 1.2 The American Diabetes Association Classification of Diabetes.

Type 1 Immune-mediated and idiopathic forms of β-cell dysfunction which lead to absolute insulin deficiency

Type 2 A disease of adult or occasionally adolescent onset ranging from predominantly insulin resistance with relative insulin deficiency to predominantly an insulin secretory defect with insulin resistance

Other specific types of diabetes
Includes a wide range of specific types of diabetes including the various genetic defects of β-cell function, genetic defects in insulin action and diseases of the exocrine pancreas (e.g. cystic fibrosis)

Gestational diabetes mellitus
Impaired glucose tolerance and impaired fasting glucose

Table 1.3 The risk of developing type 1 diabetes for an individual with an affected relative.

Relative with type 1 diabetes	Risk to individual (%)
Sibling	8
Mother	2–3
Father	5–6
Both parents	30

5 years of age. Currently, the peak incidence occurs in those aged 11–14 years.

Aetiology and pathogenesis

The precise cause of type 1 diabetes is unknown but there are a number of possible contributory factors.

Autoimmune
Several autoantibodies have been identified in newly diagnosed cases of type 1 diabetes and there is some evidence that this process starts as early as 6–12 months of age. These include islet cell antibodies (60–90% of new patients), glutamic acid decarboxylase antibodies (65–80%) and insulin antibodies (30–40%). Type 1 diabetes is also associated with other autoimmune disorders such as Hashimoto's and Graves' disease (3–5%), coeliac disease (2–5%) and Addison's disease (<1%). Some patients with type 1 diabetes have a negative autoantibody profile.

Genetic
Numerous susceptibility loci—genes that predispose to type 1 diabetes—have been found. The most important loci are located in the major histocompatibility complex (MHC) region on the short arm of chromosome 6, which contains genes that regulate the immune response. For example, the presence of DR3 and DR4 are associated with a high risk of developing diabetes. The homozygous absence of an aspartate residue at position 57 on the DQB chain leads to an approximate 100-fold increase in the risk of developing type 1 diabetes. Conversely, there are also protective alleles such as DRB1*1501 and DQB1*0602. Genetic factors play a greater part in the aetiology of type 1 diabetes in children diagnosed under the age of 5 years. The risk of a sibling developing diabetes is therefore higher in this group, being 12% by the age of 20 years.

Genetic and autoimmune markers have been used in research studies to try and predict the risk of siblings of patients with type 1 diabetes developing the disease.

Viral

Epidemics of viral infections and the autumn and winter months are associated with an increase in the incidence of diabetes. Several viruses (e.g. coxsackie B, enteroviruses, rubella virus, mumps virus and cytomegalovirus) have been implicated in the aetiology of type 1 diabetes. Possible mechanisms for their effect include molecular mimicry in which the immune response to the infection cross-reacts with islet antigens. Alternatively, viral infections, including those occurring antenatally, may have more direct effects on peri-insular or β-cells.

Nutritional

Breastfeeding seems to provide protection against the risk of developing type 1 diabetes. Whether this is a direct effect of breast milk or is related to the delayed introduction of cow's milk is unclear. Many new patients with type 1 diabetes have IgG antibodies to bovine serum albumin, a protein in cow's milk with similarities to the islet cell antigen. This protein may stimulate autoantibody production leading to islet cell destruction as a result of molecular mimicry.

Chemical toxins

Ingestion of the rodenticide vacor is associated with the development of type 1 diabetes.

Stress

Prior to the onset of type 1 diabetes, adults have been shown to experience more 'severe life events' than a control group. The cause for this effect is unclear but may relate to stress-induced impairment of resistance to infection in genetically susceptible individuals.

Biochemistry (Figure 1.1)

Insulin is an anabolic hormone with a key role in glucose metabolism and important effects on fat and protein metabolism. Following a meal, circulating concentrations of insulin rise, facilitating the entry of glucose into cells via glucose-specific transporters, particularly in the muscles and adipose tissue. Insulin stimulates glycogen synthesis in the liver and muscle, inhibits gluconeogenesis in the liver, and stimulates fat and protein synthesis. Conversely, during fasting, glucose concentrations and insulin secretion fall leading to absence of glucose uptake in muscle and adipose tissue, with stimulation of glycogenolysis in the liver and muscles and hepatic gluconeogenesis (from amino acids and ketones).

In subjects with type 1 diabetes, insulin deficiency results in hyperglycaemia which, when the renal threshold for glucose is exceeded, leads to an osmotic diuresis causing polyuria and secondary polydipsia. When fluid losses exceed intake, particularly when vomiting is also occurring, dehydration develops. Insulin deficiency also causes lipolysis with the production of excess free fatty acids and ketone bodies (3-hydroxybutyrate and acetoacetate) leading to ketonuria. The accumulation of ketoacids in the blood causes a metabolic acidosis which results in compensatory rapid, deep breathing (Kussmaul respiration). Acetone, formed from acetoacetate, is responsible for the sweet smell of the breath. Furthermore, there is an increase in stress hormone (glucagon, adrenaline, cortisol and growth hormone) production which, because of their effects on metabolism, leads to a further rise in blood glucose and other intermediary metabolite concentrations. Progressive dehydration, acidosis and hyperosmolality cause decreased consciousness and, if untreated, can lead to coma and death.

Clinical presentation

History

At diagnosis, the following symptoms may have been present from 1 week to 6 months:
- Polyuria (may cause nocturnal enuresis)
- Polydipsia
- Weight loss
- Anorexia or hyperphagia
- Lethargy
- Constipation
- Infection (especially candidal skin infections)
- Blurred vision
- Hypoglycaemia (rare, probably represents islet cell instability in the early stages of diabetes)

Although most school-aged children will report polyuria and polydipsia, these symptoms may be less obvious in the very young child who may be relatively asymptomatic (e.g. polyuria will be less obvious in an infant in nappies) in whom the other less characteristic symptoms may predominate.

Patients with diabetic ketoacidosis (DKA) may also have:
- vomiting;
- abdominal pain; and
- symptoms of systemic infection.

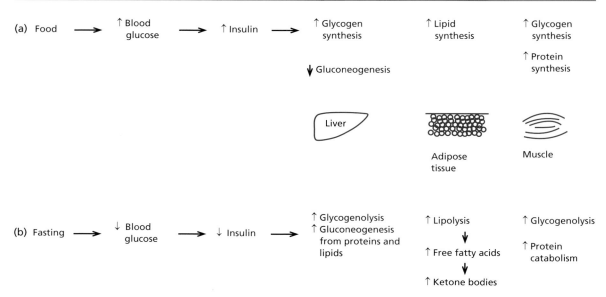

Fig. 1.1 Glucose homeostasis—a comparison of (a) fed state and (b) fasting state.

Examination

At diagnosis, most (approximately 75%) patients will not have DKA. These individuals may only have evidence of weight loss or, possibly, candidal skin infection. Patients with DKA may demonstrate the following:

- *Dehydration:*
  - 5%—dry mucous membranes, decreased skin turgor
  - 10%—sunken eyes, poor capillary return
  - >10%—hypovolaemia, tachycardia with thready pulse, hypotension
- Sweet smelling breath
- Kussmaul breathing (tachypnoea with hyperventilation)
- Depressed consciousness/coma
- Signs of sepsis (fever is not a feature of DKA and suggests sepsis)
- Ileus
- Signs of cerebral oedema (e.g. deteriorating level of consciousness)

Children less than 5 years old are more likely to present with DKA partly as a result of their clinical presentation not having been recognized by health professionals as being compatible with diabetes, leading to a delay in diagnosis and referral to hospital. Other factors that increase the risk of presenting with DKA include low socio-economic status, medication with high dose steroids and the absence of a first degree relative with type 1 diabetes.

Children diagnosed with diabetes should be referred to hospital on the same day.

Differential diagnosis

In the vast majority of cases the diagnosis of type 1 diabetes is obvious because of the presence of the classical symptoms of polyuria, polydipsia and weight loss, associated with a random blood glucose >11 mmol/L (200 mg/dL) and glycosuria with or without ketonuria. Diabetes should be considered in the differential diagnosis of any child presenting with impaired consciousness and/or acidosis.

Tachypnoea and hyperventilation in DKA may lead to the erroneous diagnosis of pneumonia. However, the lack of a cough or wheeze and the absence of abnormal findings on auscultation and/or a normal chest radiograph should raise the possibility of an alternative diagnosis such as diabetes. Abdominal pain and tenderness in DKA may suggest a surgical emergency such as appendicitis. However, appropriate fluid, insulin and electrolyte therapy will usually ameliorate the abdominal symptoms within hours. Diabetes should also be considered as a possible diagnosis in children with secondary nocturnal enuresis.

Acute illnesses, for example severe sepsis or a prolonged convulsion, may occasionally cause hyperglycaemia, glycosuria and ketonuria. However, these features are almost always transient and are rarely associated with previous polydipsia and polyuria. If in doubt, a fasting blood glucose or oral glucose tolerance test (Table 1.1) should be performed.

A family doctor who suspects or has made a definitive diagnosis of diabetes should refer the child promptly to a paediatrician. Children should be assessed on the day of referral or, if not unwell and in the absence of signs of DKA, the following day.

Investigations

At diagnosis, it is advisable to perform the following investigations:
• Plasma glucose concentration.
• Venous blood gas measurement (venous blood has a very similar pH and pCO_2 to arterial blood).
• Serum electrolytes, urea and creatinine concentrations (sodium and potassium measurements from the blood gas machine give provisional figures till the laboratory values are back).
• Full blood count (FBC) (leukocytosis, and a raised CRP, are common in DKA and do not necessarily mean that infection is present; an increased haematocrit will reflect the degree of extracellular fluid loss).
• A minority of children will have signs of sepsis and need appropriate investigations (e.g. blood culture, chest radiograph, urine microscopy and culture).
• Thyroid function tests (TFTs) and coeliac antibodies (to monitor these associated conditions).

At diagnosis, most patients have ketonuria but the presence of an abnormally low pH (i.e. venous pH<7.30) is suggestive of DKA.

Management of the child presenting without ketoacidosis

Hospitalization vs. outpatient (home) treatment

Hospital admission is necessary if intravenous (IV) therapy is required to correct dehydration, electrolyte imbalance and ketoacidosis, or if there are psychosocial difficulties. Children who are ≤ 5% dehydrated, not nauseas or vomiting, who are not particularly unwell and who have a pH ≥7.30 usually tolerate subcutaneous insulin and oral rehydration. Whether such a child with newly diagnosed diabetes can be treated at home will depend primarily on the availability of diabetes nurses who will need to visit at least daily in the first few days and maintain regular telephone contact, often outside normal working hours. The size of the geographical area that needs to be covered is also a factor. The advantages of home treatment include giving the family more confidence in dealing with diabetes at home, a more comforting environment, and less disruption and financial cost to the family. There is also some evidence that home treatment is cheaper, reduces subsequent readmissions and improves glycaemic control. The disadvantages include the risk of complications such as hypoglycaemia, which may occur before the family are sufficiently experienced to cope with it. To avoid this, home-managed children are often started on a dose of insulin of slightly less than 0.5 units/kg per 24 hours with the dose gradually being increased over the next few weeks according to the blood glucose concentrations. Some families prefer the security of being in hospital.

Many centres also offer the alternative of ambulatory care and provide diabetes education and training in a day care unit for several days following diagnosis.

Main topics for discussion following diagnosis

If several members of the 'diabetes team' are to be involved in educating the newly diagnosed child and his or her family, good communication between team members to ensure consistency in the information given is important. The following topics should be discussed with the child and family following diagnosis:
• Their pre-existing knowledge of diabetes.
• Our current knowledge of the cause of diabetes.
• The consequences of having diabetes and its lifelong implications.
• The concept of the 'diabetes team' of professionals who will be involved in their care.
• The role of insulin in type 1 diabetes management.
• Practical details of insulin injections.
• Practical details regarding when and how to monitor and interpret blood glucose concentrations.
• Appropriate dietetic advice (see section 'Diet').
• The effect of exercise on carbohydrate and insulin requirements.
• The causes and consequences of hypoglycaemia and how to treat it.
• When and how to measure blood or urinary ketone concentrations.
• Management of diabetes during intercurrent illness.
• The 'honeymoon period' of relatively reduced insulin requirements following diagnosis.
• Long-term microvascular complications.

- Who to contact in an emergency (including phone numbers).
- Details of outpatient follow-up.
- The importance of carrying identification (e.g. medical bracelets, etc.) indicating that the individual has diabetes.
- Additional sources of information about diabetes.
- Availability of support groups.
- Sources and entitlement to financial aid.
- Future developments.

Diet

In view of the important effects of diet on glycaemic control and other longer term adverse effects of diabetes, a newly diagnosed patient and their family should be referred to a dietitian who specializes in childhood diabetes within days of diagnosis. Several education sessions with the dietitian, preferably as part of the family's visit to the diabetes outpatient clinic, are usually required in the first weeks following diagnosis.

Principles of diet

Children should be encouraged to eat regular meals containing complex carbohydrates (e.g. potatoes and cereals), to reduce their intake of refined sugars, fats and salt, and to increase their dietary fibre content. The advice should be tailored to the patient's lifestyle and, where possible, should avoid drastic changes. No particular food should be considered forbidden as this may lead to disturbed attitudes to food. Furthermore, to deprive children of some foods such as sweets, which their friends consume regularly, may be psychologically damaging. Foods with high sugar content can be taken before exercise, incorporated into a main meal or used as a source of energy during illness when children have a poor appetite.

Dietary compliance may be improved if the whole family can make similar dietary modifications and the concept of a 'healthy' diet should be encouraged. Families should also be educated about the dietary treatment of the child experiencing hypoglycaemia or intercurrent illness and dietary management during parties and holidays.

Timing of meals and snacks

Children receiving twice daily injections of combined rapid- and intermediate-acting insulin require three main meals at regular intervals and usually also need a bedtime snack as a precaution against nocturnal hypoglycaemia. Occasionally, extra snacks are required if there are significant delays with meal times or if the child has only eaten a small proportion of a main meal. Preschool-aged children may have unpredictable eating habits and may require frequent, small meals.

Those on a basal bolus regimen with a long-acting insulin analogue such as glargine or detemir should not require a bedtime snack though one may wish to give this snack for the first few weeks following the commencement of that regimen. Children on a basal bolus regimen or continuous subcutaneous insulin infusion (CSII) need to have the ability to adjust the dose of their bolus rapidly-acting insulin in line with their carbohydrate intake.

Dietary composition

Caloric intake does not need to be calculated or altered unless the child is over- or underweight. It is recommended that approximately 35% of dietary energy intake should be derived from fat (mainly mono- and polyunsaturated fats), 15% from protein and 50% from carbohydrate.

There are several approaches to the dietetic management of diabetes:

1 Children can be encouraged to choose a certain number of carbohydrate-containing foods ('portions') from a list of such foods, at each meal and snack.

2 Food intake is based on the principles of a normal healthy diet.

3 In the past, families were taught about the carbohydrate exchange system in which 10 g of carbohydrate was equivalent to one exchange and meals were calculated on the basis of the number of 'exchanges' required. Because of uncertainties about the precise carbohydrate content of food and its physiological effects, dietary education on the basis of the carbohydrate exchange system was to a large extent abandoned in the 1990s. However, recently there has been renewed interest and emphasis in a quantitative rather than a qualitative approach to diet in diabetes management. In fact, so-called carbohydrate counting has now become standard for all patients on basal bolus and CSII regimens. A dietary regimen called Dose Adjustment For Normal Eating (DAFNE) has been introduced in many centres for the management of adults with diabetes. Modified schemes for children are also used in many hospitals. Computerized nutritional weighing scales can facilitate this process. The food is weighed, the nature of the food inputted and the carbohydrate content of the food is calculated by the computer. Various books are also available with information on the carbohydrate content of different foods. Detailed education is given on the carbohydrate content of food and the dose of rapidly-acting insulin required for a set amount of carbohydrate.

Most prepubertal children are started on 0.5 units of rapidly-acting insulin for every 10 g and most pubertal children on 1 unit of rapidly-acting insulin per 10 g of carbohydrate. However, these ratios can change and pubertal children in particular may need much higher doses of rapidly-acting insulin, sometimes up to 3 units per 10 g of carbohydrate. In children on insulin pump therapy, the '500 rule' is usually used to calculate the amount of carbohydrate (in grams) for every 1 unit of rapidly-acting insulin. This is worked out by dividing 500 by the total daily dose (TDD) of insulin and this provides the number of grams of carbohydrate covered by 1 unit of rapidly-acting insulin. For example, if the TDD of insulin is 25 units, then we get 500/25 = 20. Therefore, 20 g of carbohydrate will be covered by 1 unit of rapidly-acting insulin. This is equivalent to saying that 0.5 unit of rapidly-acting insulin should be given for every 10 g of carbohydrate.

A more liberal diet is permissible with this approach with multiple insulin boluses being given in line with the carbohydrate intake. It is common for pubertal children, who often have a large appetite, to have a snack on return from school and a bolus of rapidly-acting insulin can be given with this frequently large snack. Good control has been achieved with these regimens, which is partly due to improved dietary management and the additional education involved when commencing these regimens. An improved quality of life has also been associated with these regimens.

There is a risk of unwanted weight gain with basal bolus and CSII regimens and the diet should be closely supervised in these patients. Weight gain can be due to glucose calories no longer being lost in the urine as glycaemic control improves. These regimens can also be associated with an increased frequency of hypoglycaemia which may lead to more food being eaten to counteract it. There may also be excessive eating of desserts and sweets, as confidence in carbohydrate counting grows. Weight gain can also occur if the fat content of food is not considered or if patients eat more high-calorie foods and larger portions.

When carbohydrate counting, one should also be aware of the glycaemic index (GI) of food. Low-GI foods will lead to a slow and gradual absorption of carbohydrates whereas high-GI foods will lead to fast carbohydrate absorption and a rise in blood glucose. The amount of fat, protein and fibre in food will influence the GI and carbohydrate absorption. For example, the greater the amount of fat, the slower the absorption.

The numerous commercially available 'diabetic foods' are not generally recommended for children with diabetes as such foods tend to be expensive and have no particular advantages over a healthy diet based on normal foods.

Some diabetic foods also contain the sweetener sorbitol that may lead to diarrhoea. Diabetic foods may also have a high calorie and fat content. Non-alcoholic drinks containing sugar should be replaced with those containing artificial sweeteners.

Insulin therapy

A number of different insulin regimens are available. It is important to be flexible when choosing an insulin regimen and to bear in mind the families' needs and wishes. The initial insulin regimen may require changing if glycaemic control is poor or if there are practical difficulties. Following diagnosis, most children will require approximately 0.5 units of insulin per kilogram body weight daily although this may decrease substantially during the first few months of therapy (occasionally to the point where patients may be transiently, completely weaned off insulin) during the so-called 'honeymoon period'. This period, which represents partial recovery of the existing β-cell mass, may last from a few months up to 2 years. Parents should be warned that insulin requirements will increase significantly at the end of the 'honeymoon period'.

For most children, a basal bolus regimen is most appropriate. Basal bolus regimens comprise injections of rapidly-acting insulin prior to each main meal with an injection of a long-acting insulin analogue prior to bedtime. The latter provides a basal 'peakless' level of insulin for up to 24 hours (Table 1.9). There is also some evidence that nocturnal hypoglycaemia is less common with the long-acting insulin analogues as compared to isophane. Normally, approximately 40% of the TDD of insulin is given at bedtime as a long-acting insulin analogue (glargine is usually given at bedtime but as it lasts for 24 hours it can be given at any time of day and in some children is given at breakfast time, detemir is usually given at bedtime but can be given at breakfast time or occasionally is required both at bedtime and breakfast time). The remaining insulin is given as rapidly-acting insulin and is split between the pre-breakfast, lunch and evening meal injections. Carbohydrate counting and correction doses determine the precise amount of insulin given with each meal. The correction dose is calculated by dividing 100 by the TDD. One unit of rapidly acting insulin will decrease the glucose level by approximately 100/TDD. The correction dose is usually used to normalise an abnormally raised glucose level, typically to 6–8 mmol/L.

Basal bolus regimens allow flexibility with regard to the timing and size of meals, and are popular with teenagers as they lead to greater independence. In those children who are on a ratio of 1 unit or less of rapidly-acting insulin to every 10 g of carbohydrate, a carbohydrate snack of up to

15 g can be ingested without a bolus. However, in those on an insulin to carbohydrate ratio of >1 unit: 10 g, an insulin bolus may be required with carbohydrate snacks of <15 g. In children reluctant to administer a pre-lunch injection at school or in whom there are difficulties with a full basal bolus regimen, an intermediate solution is to give mixed insulin before breakfast, rapidly-acting insulin prior to the evening meal and intermediate-acting insulin (isophane) prior to bedtime.

Possible alternative regimens in children under 4 years of age include a CSII, once daily glargine/detemir or isophane before breakfast, once daily glargine/detemir or isophane before breakfast with rapidly-acting insulin prior to the evening meal, twice daily isophane and twice daily mixed insulin with approximately 70% of the TDD being given at breakfast time.

In older children the use of twice daily injections, using a mixture of rapidly-acting and intermediate-acting insulin most commonly in a ratio of 25–30%:70–75% with approximately 70% of the TDD being given at breakfast time is also a possible alternative which can provide good control, especially in the first year of treatment during the 'honeymoon period'. CSIIs are a further alternative.

Although hypoglycaemic episodes are unusual in newly diagnosed patients, care should be taken to avoid these in children treated at home until the family have had the appropriate training. Children initially treated in hospital are less active than at home and most will experience a fall in their blood glucose following discharge.

It has been suggested that aggressive insulin therapy to achieve early onset of normoglycaemia may help maintain residual β-cell function and lead to a prolonged 'honeymoon period'. However, there is insufficient evidence to prove this and the possible benefits of tight glycaemic control may be outweighed by the risks of hypoglycaemia.

Psychological support

The diagnosis of diabetes is invariably a shock to the child and family. Psychological or psychiatric problems may arise, particularly at diagnosis or during adolescence (see p. 28). Psychological support can be provided by a psychologist or psychiatrist as well as by diabetes nurses, other parents, and local and national support groups.

Requirements on discharge from hospital

The family doctor should be informed of the child's diagnosis and discharge from hospital, and the school or nursery should be visited by the diabetes nurse and ideally also by the dietitian to ensure that suitable information and arrangements are in place. The equipment that a child will need on discharge is shown in Table 1.4.

Table 1.4 Equipment required on discharge.

Lancets or other finger-pricking devices

Blood glucose testing strips

Blood glucose meter

Oral glucose gel

Glucagon kit

Blood or urinary ketone testing sticks

Sharps bin

Literature on diabetes and how to obtain medical bracelets/necklaces

Pen-delivery system, disposable pre-filled pens or syringes with needles for insulin injections

Insulin cartridges for pen-delivery system or insulin vials

Rapid-acting insulin

Alcohol swabs

Needle clipper

Management of the child presenting with ketoacidosis

Approximately 25% of new patients with type 1 diabetes will present with DKA (in type 2 diabetes, DKA is a presenting feature in <10% of patients). In children with established diabetes, the risk of DKA is increased in those with poor metabolic control and previous episodes of DKA, adolescent girls, children with psychiatric disorders including eating disorders and those with psychosocial difficulties. Inappropriate interruption of insulin pump therapy may also lead to DKA. 75% of DKA episodes are associated with insulin omission or treatment error. The majority of the remainder are due to inadequate insulin treatment during an intercurrent illness.

The diagnosis can be made on clinical and biochemical grounds. The biochemical criteria for the diagnosis of DKA include hyperglycaemia (glucose>11 mmol/L (200 mg/dL)) with a venous pH<7.30 and/or bicarbonate < 15 mmol/L (15 mEq/L). The blood glucose concentration is usually elevated but in 8% of cases may be <15 mmol/L (270 mg/dL). Blood ketone levels are generally > 3.0 mmol/L but some well children who do not fulfill the DKA criteria may have ketone levels >6.0 mmol/L. There is also ketonuria. DKA can be further classified by its severity – mild (venous pH<7.30 and/or bicarbonate<15 mmol/L (15 mEq/L)), moderate (pH<7.2 and/or bicarbonate<10 mmol/L) and severe (pH<7.1 and/or bicarbonate <5 mmol/L).

The mortality rate from DKA is approximately 0.2%. Death is usually caused by cerebral oedema but may also be caused by hypokalaemia-induced dysrhythmias, sepsis and aspiration pneumonia.

Resuscitation

DKA is a medical emergency and resuscitation should follow the 'ABC' scheme. The protocol which follows for the treatment of DKA is largely based on that published by the European Society of Paediatric Endocrinology and the Lawson Wilkins Paediatric Endocrine Society (Dunger, D.B. *et al.* 2004) and by the British Society of Paediatric Endocrinology and Diabetes (BSPED) (Edge, J.A. 2009).

- *Airway:* If the child is comatose, an airway should be inserted and if the conscious level is depressed or the child is vomiting, a nasogastric tube should be passed, aspirated and left on free drainage.
- *Breathing:* If there is evidence of hypoxia, give 100% oxygen and consider the need for intubation and ventilation. However, airway and breathing problems are rare.
- *Circulation:* An IV cannula should be sited and blood samples (including a venous blood gas) taken for investigations (see p. 5). In cases of circulatory impairment (suggested by the presence of poor capillary refill and tachycardia), give 10 mL/kg body weight of 0.9% saline intravenously as quickly as possible. This can be repeated with further boluses (subsequent boluses can usually be given more slowly) to a maximum total of 30 mL/kg until the circulation is restored.

If at presentation the child is too ill to weigh, for the purposes of calculating fluid requirements, weight can be estimated from a recent clinic weight or from a centile chart.

Antibiotics should be given if sepsis is thought likely after appropriate samples for culture have been taken.

Initial monitoring

The child should ideally be nursed in either a high dependency or intensive care unit. In hospitals without a high dependency unit, high dependency care can still be given by providing a high level of nursing care, often on a 1:1 basis. If the child is under 2 years of age, has a pH <7.1, is severely dehydrated with shock, has a depressed level of consciousness with a risk of aspiration from vomiting or if staffing levels are poor then the case should be discussed with a paediatric intensive care unit (PICU) consultant as the child may require intensive care.

The following should be documented:

- Hourly BP and basic observations.
- Weight should be measured twice a day.
- A strict fluid balance chart should be kept which should include measurement of urine volumes and fluid losses from vomiting and diarrhoea.
- Hourly blood glucose measurements should be performed. Ideally, an additional cannula should be inserted for blood sampling to prevent recurrent, painful finger pricks.
- Venous or capillary blood ketone testing 1–2 hourly, which measures the main ketone – β-hydroxybutyrate – should be performed to quantify the suppression of ketogenesis (urine testing for ketones is an inferior test which measures acetone which is not the main ketone produced).
- Blood gases, electrolyte and urea concentrations.
- A cardiac monitor should be used to monitor abnormal serum potassium concentrations (hypokalaemia is suggested by flat T waves and dysrhythmias, whereas hyperkalaemia is indicated by the presence of tall, peaked T waves with dysrhythmias).
- All patients with DKA should have at least hourly neurological observations and if comatose the Glasgow Coma Score should be recorded. The development of a headache or change in behaviour should be reported immediately to medical staff as this may be the first sign of cerebral oedema.
- If the patient is comatose or there is difficulty monitoring fluid losses, a urinary catheter should be inserted.

Fluid therapy

Calculation of fluid requirements

Once the circulating fluid volume has been restored, ongoing fluid requirements can be calculated as follows:

$$\text{fluid requirement} = (\text{fluid maintenance} + \text{fluid deficit})$$
$$- \text{fluid used for resuscitation}$$

The fluid deficit should be replaced over 48 hours and can be calculated from:

$$\text{fluid deficit (L)} = \%\text{dehydration} \times \text{body weight (kg)}$$

The extent of dehydration is usually 3–8%. Grades are mild 3%, moderate 5%, severe 8%, and shock. Most children are classed as 5 or 8% dehydrated. Dehydration is often overestimated and, for the purposes of calculating fluid requirements, the fluid deficit used should not exceed

Table 1.5 Maintenance fluid requirements in DKA.

Weight (kg)	Maintenance fluid requirements (mL/kg/24h)
0–12.9	80
13–19.9	65
20–34.9	55
35–59.9	45
> 60	35

N.B.: Neonatal DKA requires special consideration and larger volumes of fluid than those quoted may be required, usually 100–150 mL/kg/24 h.

8% of body weight. The fluid used during initial resuscitation to restore the circulation should be taken into account when calculating fluid requirements and deducted from the total. Maintenance fluid requirements can be estimated from Table 1.5.

The hourly infusion rate is calculated using the following formula:

$$\text{hourly rate} = \frac{48 \text{ hour maintenance} + \text{deficit} - \text{resuscitation fluid already given}}{48}$$

Significant ongoing fluid losses, such as vomiting or excess diuresis, should also be replaced. An example of calculations to estimate fluid requirements for a child with DKA is shown in Table 1.6. It is always important to double-check these calculations. The BSPED DKA guideline has a link to both a fluid calculator and an observations and results flow chart.

Table 1.6 Example of fluid volume calculation.

An 8-year-old boy weighing 27 kg who is 8% dehydrated and who required 10 mL/kg 0.9% saline during resuscitation will need:
Daily maintenance = 27 kg × 55 mL = 1485 mL
Deficit = 27 kg × 8% = 2160 mL
Resuscitation fluid = 270 mL
Total requirements over 48 hours = (2 × 1485) + 2160 − 270 = 4860 mL
Hourly rate = 4860/48 = 101 mL/h

Ongoing fluid prescription

At presentation in DKA, the serum sodium concentration is usually low. This is mainly caused by a deficit in body sodium. Hypernatraemia may be present if water loss has been severe and has exceeded sodium losses. The following solutions should be available from the pharmacy: 500 mL bag of 0.9% saline/5% dextrose containing 20 mmol KCl and 500 mL bag of 0.45% saline/5% dextrose containing 20 mmol KCl. Following resuscitation, 0.9% saline with 20 mmol KCl in 500 mL should be used. This sodium concentration should be used for at least the first 12 hours of rehydration. After 12 hours, if the plasma sodium level is stable or increasing the bag can be changed to 500 mL of 0.45% saline/5% dextrose/20 mmol KCl. However, if the plasma sodium is falling continue with 0.9% saline/20 mmol KCl in 500 mL. Glucose may also be required in the bags depending on the blood glucose level. Some authorities believe that corrected sodium levels give an indication of the risk of cerebral oedema. The corrected sodium can be calculated from the formula: corrected Na = Na + 0.4 (glucose − 5.5 mmol/L). A rougher, quicker estimate is to add 0.3 mmol/L of sodium for every 1 mmol of glucose above 5.5 mmol/L. Corrected sodium levels should rise with therapy. Once the plasma glucose concentration has fallen to 14 mmol/L (250 mg/dL) glucose should be added to the fluid.

In the early stages of DKA, patients often experience marked thirst and request oral fluids. In severe dehydration with impaired consciousness, no fluids should be allowed by mouth. A nasogastric tube may be necessary in the case of gastric paresis, vomiting or impaired consciousness to decrease the risk of aspiration pneumonia. Oral fluids should only be allowed following a significant clinical improvement with no vomiting. If a substantial clinical improvement has occurred prior to the 48 hours of rehydration, oral intake can proceed and the IV infusions reduced to take account of the oral intake.

Potassium administration

Potassium is mainly an intracellular ion and at presentation in DKA there is invariably a large depletion of total body potassium even though initial serum potassium concentrations may be normal or even high. Early addition of potassium to the fluid regimen (40 mmol/L) is essential even if the serum concentration is normal as insulin will drive glucose and potassium into the cells producing a rapid fall in serum potassium concentrations and increased potassium requirements.

Following resuscitation potassium should be added to the IV fluids as soon as urine output has been established. In the rare cases where there is doubt about the urine output, the patient should be catheterized. Early potassium therapy should be avoided if anuria is present as a result of acute tubular necrosis. The serum potassium concentration should be maintained between 4 and 5 mmol/L. Very occasionally, more than 40 mmol/L may be required.

Phosphate

Depletion of intracellular phosphate also occurs. The fall in plasma phosphate levels is exacerbated by insulin therapy as phosphate re-enters the cells. Phosphate depletion may last for several days after the DKA has resolved. Prospective studies have failed to show any significant benefit from phosphate replacement, and phosphate administration may lead to hypocalcaemia.

Insulin therapy

Rehydration alone will lead to a fall in plasma glucose and ketone concentrations. There is some evidence that cerebral oedema is more likely if insulin is started early. Insulin therapy should therefore only be started at least 1 hour after the start of fluid therapy. Insulin helps reverse the underlying metabolic abnormalities by further reductions in the glucose concentration and by prevention of ketone body formation.

The insulin infusion should be prepared by adding 50 units (0.5 mL) of soluble insulin (e.g. actrapid) to 49.5 mL of 0.9% saline in a 50 mL syringe pump to produce an insulin concentration of 1 unit/mL. This may be connected to the fluid infusion through a Y-connector and prescribed as follows:

- The insulin solution should run at 0.1 mL/kg/h.
- When the blood glucose has fallen to 14 mmol/L (250 mg/dL), alter the fluid to one containing 5% dextrose.
- The insulin infusion should not be stopped before the acidosis has corrected as insulin is required to switch off ketone production. Nor should it be stopped whilst glucose is being infused. If the blood glucose falls to <4 mmol/L (72 mg/dL), a bolus of 2 mL/kg of 10% dextrose should be given and the dextrose concentration in the fluid increased. Insulin can temporarily be reduced for 1 hour.

- If needed, a solution of 10% glucose with 0.45% saline can be made up by adding 50 mL 50% glucose to a 500 mL bag of 0.45% saline/5% glucose with 20 mmol KCl.
- When the pH is >7.30, the blood glucose concentration ≤ 14 mmol/L (250 mg/dL), and a glucose infusion has been started, the insulin infusion rate can be reduced, but not to less than 0.05 units/kg/h.

In children who are already on long-acting insulin (especially glargine (lantus)), this can be continued at the usual dose and time throughout DKA treatment, in addition to the IV insulin infusion, in order to shorten the length of stay after recovery from DKA. In children on CSII pump therapy, the pump should be stopped when starting DKA therapy.

Acidosis and bicarbonate therapy

Adequate hydration and insulin therapy will reverse even a severe acidosis. Appropriate hydration will also reverse any lactic acidosis, which may account for 25% of the acidaemia, due to poor tissue perfusion and renal function. Continuing acidosis usually reflects inadequate fluid resuscitation or insulin therapy. The use of bicarbonate therapy is very rarely required. Bicarbonate should only be considered to improve cardiac contractility in patients who are severely acidotic (arterial pH<6.9) with circulatory failure despite adequate fluid replacement. **Bicarbonate should never be given without prior discussion with a senior doctor.**

Anticoagulant prophylaxis

There is a significant risk of femoral vein thrombosis in young and very sick children with DKA who have femoral lines inserted. Therefore, anticoagulation with 100 units/kg per day as a single dose of fragmin should be considered in these children. Children who are significantly hyperosmolar may also require anticoagulant therapy.

Subsequent management

Although plasma glucose concentrations may fall to near normal levels within 4–6 hours of treatment of DKA, the metabolic acidosis may take 24 hours or longer to resolve. Subsequent management should include the following:
- Blood gases and electrolyte and urea concentrations should be re-evaluated 2 hours after the start of treatment and 4 hourly thereafter, or more frequently if there are clinical concerns, until the child has recovered.
- The rate and composition of the IV fluid prescription should be reviewed regularly and adjusted according to the electrolyte results and fluid balance.

- If there is continuing massive polyuria, the rate of infusion of IV fluids may need to be increased. If there are large gastric aspirates, these will need replacing with 0.45% saline with KCl.
- Once the blood gases and electrolyte concentrations normalize, the frequency of blood sampling can be decreased and discontinued once the child is tolerating oral fluids and food.
- The frequency of bedside capillary blood glucose measurements may be reduced to 2 hourly if plasma glucose concentrations are relatively stable while the child is receiving IV dextrose.
- If the acidosis or hyperglycaemia do not improve after 4–6 hours, the patient should be reassessed by a senior doctor. Insufficient insulin and insulin errors, inadequate rehydration, sepsis, a hyperchloraemic acidosis, or salicylate or other prescription or recreational drugs may be the cause. More insulin, further 0.9% saline or antibiotics may be required.
- Use bedside blood (or urine) ketone testing to confirm that ketone levels are falling. If they are not falling check the infusion lines, the calculation and dose of insulin and consider giving more insulin.
- IV fluids should be continued until the child is drinking well and able to tolerate food. Once the blood ketone levels are below 1.0 mmol/L, subcutaneous insulin can be started (urinary ketones may take longer to clear).
- When the patient is started on a conventional subcutaneous insulin regimen (see above for regimen for new patients, established patients can return to their previous regimen), the insulin infusion should be discontinued 60 minutes (if using actrapid) or 10 minutes (if using Novorapid or Humalog) after the first subcutaneous injection to avoid rebound hyperglycaemia. In the case of patients on CSII therapy, this can be restarted when blood ketones are < 0.6 mmol/L.

Cerebral oedema

Cerebral oedema has a mortality rate of approximately 25%. Significant neurological morbidity is present in 10–26% of survivors. It occurs in approximately 0.3–1% of cases of DKA.

Aetiology

The aetiology of cerebral oedema is poorly understood and even with optimum management of DKA, cases still occur. It is more common in children under 5 years of age and in newly diagnosed cases. A fall in sodium concentration following treatment, a severe acidosis, the use of bicarbonate, marked hypocapnia and a high urea at presentation have all been implicated as risk factors. Much of the treatment is aimed at minimizing these possible contributory factors.

Clinical features

Cerebral oedema usually occurs 4–12 hours after the start of treatment and often follows an initial period of clinical and biochemical improvement. However, in some cases the patient's state of consciousness may decline from admission onwards, whereas in others cerebral oedema may occur after 48 hours. Typical symptoms and signs include:

- onset or worsening of headache (this is often present initially in DKA and should improve with treatment);
- confusion;
- irritability;
- reducing conscious level (patients are often drowsy at presentation but this should improve with treatment);
- pupillary abnormalities/cranial nerve palsies;
- hypertension and bradycardia;
- decerebrate or decorticate posturing; and
- oxygen desaturations and respiratory impairment.

More dramatic signs such as convulsions, papilloedema and respiratory arrest are late signs associated with a very poor prognosis.

Treatment

If cerebral oedema is suspected, senior staff should be informed immediately and the following measures should be taken urgently whilst arranging transfer to a PICU:
- Hypoglycaemia should be excluded.
- Give hypertonic (2.7%) saline (5 mL/kg over 5–10 minutes) or mannitol 0.5–1 g/kg (= 2.5–5 mL/kg 20% mannitol over 20 minutes). This should be given **as soon as possible** if warning signs such as a headache and pulse slowing occur.
- Fluids should be restricted to half maintenance with the deficit replaced over 72 rather than 48 hours.
- The child should be discussed with a PICU consultant and transferred to a PICU. Do not intubate and ventilate until an experienced doctor is available.
- Once the child is stable an urgent computed tomography scan should be performed to exclude other problems such as cerebral thrombosis, haemorrhage or infarction.
- A repeat dose of mannitol may be required after 2 hours if there is no initial response.

Other complications

- *Infections:* Antibiotics are not routinely given unless a significant bacterial infection is suspected.

- *Abdominal pain:* This is common and may be due to liver swelling, gastritis, bladder retention or ileus. However, surgical conditions such as appendicitis rarely occur and a surgical opinion may be required once DKA is stable. A raised amylase is common in DKA.
- Other problems are pneumothorax +/− pneumomediastinum, interstitial pulmonary oedema, unusual infections (e.g. tuberculosis) and hyperosmolar hyperglycaemic non-ketotic coma.

The diabetes clinic

General principles
Children with diabetes should be seen in a designated diabetic clinic supervised by a senior paediatrician trained in the care of diabetes. It has been recommended that, within a clinical service, there be a specialist nurse for every 70 children with diabetes. Where possible, the clinical service should provide care for a minimum of 40 patients with diabetes to allow the necessary accumulation of expertise. Age banding of the clinic may help bring families with similarly aged children together and facilitates group teaching of age-appropriate topics. The clinic should be held in a paediatric environment with facilities for auxology. Separate arrangements should be made for clinics for adolescents, which are described later in this chapter. Educational literature, DVDs and information about holidays for children with diabetes should be available.

The clinic visit
The following staff should ideally be available at each clinic:
- Paediatrician with expertise in diabetes.
- Diabetes nurse specialist (DNS) with paediatric training or expertise.
- Dietitian with paediatric experience.
- Psychologist.
- Social worker to provide financial and other advice to the family.

Any child with diabetes attending the diabetes clinic should undergo the following:
1 Documentation of general health and life events (e.g. changing school), recent hospital admissions, insulin regimen, details of hypoglycaemic episodes and school absences.
2 Review of practical aspects of blood glucose monitoring and insulin injections.
3 If necessary, provision of advice on adjustments to the insulin regimen in light of the results of blood glucose monitoring.

4 Measurement of height and weight.
5 Examination of injection sites.
6 Three-monthly measurement of glycosylated haemoglobin.
7 An annual review of all patients aged 11 years or older, who have had diabetes for ≥2 years, which should include:
- a physical examination for microvascular and other complications of diabetes (Table 1.7);
- TFTs;
- random cholesterol measurement;
- screening for microalbuminuria by measurement of the albumin:creatinine ratio in an early morning urine sample; and
- many centres perform retinal photography in addition to a clinical examination of the fundi (if the latter is abnormal then retinal photography is recommended to delineate the degree of retinopathy).

Details of the consultation (and non-attendance) should be documented using either paper records or computer software to enable future audit. Given the multidisciplinary nature of a diabetes clinic, it is often helpful to have a team meeting at the end of the clinic to share information about patients who have attended clinic.

Insulin treatment

Insulin delivery systems
Insulin has an effective shelf life of at least 2 years if kept in a refrigerator at 4°C and can be kept at room temperature for up to 1 month. However, if kept in tropical climates, car interiors or freezer compartments insulin may degrade more rapidly. Insulin is most commonly administered by a pen-delivery system, a pump or using syringes and needles. In general, vials of insulin are cheaper than insulin in pen cartridges, which in turn are cheaper than insulin-filled disposable pens. For children with needle phobia, spring-loaded automatic injection devices in which the needle is not visible, or transjector systems in which a jet of insulin is delivered at sufficiently high pressure that it penetrates the skin without the need for a needle may be helpful.

Insulin pens
Using a pen-delivery system, insulin may be administered using either a preloaded disposable device or cartridges fitted into a reusable pen device. Pen-delivery systems are generally preferred by children as they are quicker and easier to use than syringes and needles, and lead to greater independence.

Table 1.7 Points to note on clinical examination of patients with diabetes at annual review.

System	Points to note
Height	Growth failure
Weight	Poor or excessive weight gain
Puberty	Delayed puberty/menarche
Skin	Lipohypertrophy at injection sites Necrobiosis lipoidica
Mouth	Presence of caries or other signs of poor dental hygiene
Eyes	Presence of retinopathy/cataracts (through dilated pupils)
Feet	Signs of poor foot care (e.g. calluses from poorly-fitting shoes) verrucae
Hands	Finger-prick sites Limited joint mobility ('prayer sign')
Cardiovascular	Hypertension (if present, recheck at the end of the clinic visit)
Endocrine	Goitre or other signs of hypothyroidism or hyperthyroidism Increased pigmentation suggestive of Addison's disease
Neurological	Impaired vibration or pinprick sense Loss of ankle reflexes

Syringes and needles

Insulin for injection may be drawn up from a vial and injected using a syringe and needle system. A choice is available between using premixed insulin preparations or mixing separate supplies of rapid- and intermediate-acting insulins within the syringe by the patient. When mixing insulins the rapidly-acting clear insulin should be drawn up into the syringe prior to the intermediate-acting (isophane), cloudy insulin. Any preparation containing intermediate-acting insulin should be gently inverted several times prior to use. Although mixing of separate insulins allows, in theory, greater flexibility, there is little evidence that in routine clinical practice this leads to better glycaemic control than that which can be achieved using premixed insulins. Furthermore, mixing separate insulins is time-consuming and requires manual dexterity.

Injections

Depending on the maturity and confidence of the individual patient, children as young as 5 years can be taught to administer their own injections of insulin. However, the age at which children start to give their own injections is very variable. Peer pressure, such as that which may be experienced by a child attending a diabetic camp, where children may see their contemporaries, or even younger children, administering injections may help a child learn to self-inject.

Appropriate injection sites are demonstrated in Figure 1.2. The use of different injection sites and rotation of these sites should be encouraged to avoid the development of lipohypertrophy (Figure 1.3) which may be unsightly and lead to erratic absorption of insulin. If patients avoid injecting into these areas, lipohypertrophy will resolve, typically within 3 months.

Clinically significant variations in the amount of insulin absorbed from each injection can occur as a result of the factors listed in Table 1.8.

Injection technique

It is unnecessary to clean the skin prior to a subcutaneous insulin injection. It is recommended that patients be taught to give the injection at a 45° angle to the surface of the skin. When using the very short (e.g. 5 mm) needles the injection can be given vertically without pinching the skin unless the patient is very thin. In those who find injections painful, distraction techniques can be used or the skin can be rubbed with an ice cube prior to the injection. Pen needles can be used up to three times before

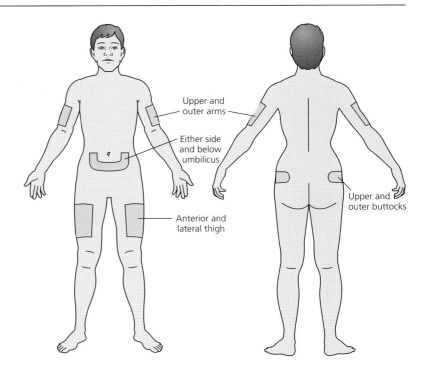

Upper and
outer arms

Either side
and below
umbilicus

Anterior and
lateral thigh

Upper and
outer buttocks

Fig. 1.2 Appropriate insulin injection
sites.

being changed. More frequent use will lead to blunting
and painful injections.

Insulin requirements
Suggested starting dosages of insulin are shown on
p. 7. In established patients, it is unusual for prepubertal children to require more than 0.8 units of insulin/kg
per day. In contrast, children in puberty may require up to
2 units/kg per day. Obese patients may be insulin resistant
and require relatively higher dosages.

Altering insulin dosage
In children under 10 years insulin dosage can be altered
by 1–2 units per day and in children over 10 years by 2–4
units per day, depending on the results of blood glucose

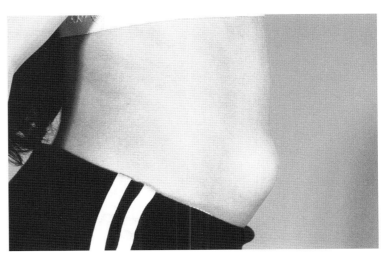

Fig. 1.3 Lipohypertrophy.

Table 1.8 Factors affecting insulin absorption.

Slower insulin absorption	Faster insulin absorption
Leg or arm injection sites	Abdominal injection site
Subcutaneous injection	Intramuscular injection
Lipohypertrophy	Exercise
Cold skin	Peripherally vasodilated
Obese subjects	Thin subjects

testing. Following any change in insulin dosage, blood glucose concentrations should be monitored carefully for 2–4 days to assess the effect.

Injecting small doses

In infants, the injection of doses of insulin as small as 1 unit can result in significant inaccuracies, with the dose actually delivered ranging from 0.89 to 1.23 units. In these circumstances, it is recommended that pen-delivery systems available from the manufacturers of insulin which allows injections of insulin in increments of 0.5 units are used.

Insulin preparations

In solution, human insulin forms hexamers (six-molecule units) which are slowly absorbed across endothelial barriers when insulin is injected subcutaneously. The rate of absorption is mainly determined by how quickly these hexamers dissociate into monomers (single molecules), which are rapidly absorbed at the injection site. Children with diabetes should be treated with human sequence or human insulin analogues. In the United Kingdom, this is usually available in a concentration of 100 units/mL (U100) although more dilute forms may be necessary for the treatment of infants receiving very small doses of insulin. Table 1.9 outlines the most common preparations of insulin available to treat children in the United Kingdom and their duration of action.

Most children are treated using basal bolus regimens or CSII. A minority are treated with twice daily injections of a premixed insulin. Several insulins are very similar in their duration of action. To simplify matters and to avoid confusion, it is therefore recommended that a 'diabetes team' limit the number of insulins they use.

Insulin analogues

Rapidly-acting insulin analogues incorporate amino acid substitutions which make them quickly dissociate into monomers and dimers following injection and therefore lead to rapid absorption. They can be given just prior to a meal or, in young children in whom there is concern about how much food they will actually eat or where there may be food refusal, within 15 minutes of starting a meal. Compared with short-acting insulin, they produce lower postprandial glucose excursions but higher preprandial glucose concentrations. They may, therefore, be helpful in children who become hypoglycaemic prior to lunch. They do not lead to a decrease in the overall incidence of hypoglycaemia but there is some evidence that they lead to a decrease in the incidence of severe hypoglycaemia. Compared with conventional insulin, these analogues are associated with a very small decrease in HbA1c of approximately 0.1%.

Rapidly-acting analogues are also available in a pre-mixed form with intermediate-acting insulin. They decrease postprandial glucose concentrations, but when compared to similar mixtures of conventional insulin have similar effects on the HbA1c and the incidence of hypoglycaemia.

Recently, two long-acting insulin analogues have been developed. They both lead to a consistent and prolonged release of insulin with no peaks. Insulin glargine has glycine instead of asparagine at position 21 on the A-chain and has two arginines added to the carboxyl terminal of the B-chain at positions 31 and 32. These changes result in a low solubility at neutral pH but total solubility at the pH of its injection solution (pH 4). Following injection, the pH of the insulin solution increases, leading to the formation of micro-precipitates, from which small amounts of glargine are gradually absorbed into the circulation. This leads to a prolonged duration of action (22–24 hours). It can be injected at any time but is usually given in the evening. There is some evidence that there is a decreased incidence of nocturnal hypoglycaemia when it is given at breakfast.

Insulin detemir has the terminal amino acid (B30) in the B-chain deleted and a 14-carbon fatty acid attached at position B29. This leads to a prolonged duration of action as a result of two mechanisms: albumin binding via a fatty acid side-chain retains insulin in the subcutaneous depot and strong self-association of insulin detemir hexamers at the injection site. The duration of action is partly dependant on the dose with lower doses lasting 12 hours and higher doses lasting up to 24 hours. It is administered once or occasionally twice daily. Glargine and detemir are licensed in the United Kingdom for patients aged 6 years and above, but have been used in younger children as well.

Insulin glargine and detemir have provided new opportunities to optimize glycaemic control. Both result in

Table 1.9 Insulin preparations commonly used to the treatment of children in the UK.

Preparation	Manufacturer	Formulations	Approximate time course of action		
			Onset	Peak	Duration
1) Rapidly acting insulin					
Humalog (insulin lispro)	Lilly	vial, cart, pen	15 mins	30–70 mins	2–5 h
Nororapid (insulin aspart)	Novo Nordisk	vial, cart, pen	15 mins	1–3 h	3–5 h
2) Short acting insulin (Soluble, neutral)					
Human Actrapid	Novo Nordisk	vial	30 mins	1–2 h	6–8 h
Humilin S	Lilly	vial, cart	30 mins	1–2 h	6–8 h
3) Intermediate acting insulin (isophane)					
Human Insulatard	Novo Nordisk	vial, cart, pen	2 h	4–6 h	8–12 h
Humilin I	Lilly	vial, cart, pen	2 h	4–6 h	8–12 h
4) Biphasic Insulins (mixed insulins)					
Human Mixtard 30 (30% actrapid /70% insulatard)	Novo Nordisk	vial, cart, pen	30 mins	2–6 h	8–12 h
Humilin M3 (30% Humilin S/70% Humilin I)	Lilly	vial, cart, pen	30 mins	2–6 h	8–12 h
Humalog Mix 25	Lilly	cart, pen	15 mins	1 h	8–12 h
Humalog Mix 50	Lilly	pen	Same time course as Mix25 but increased intensity of early action		
Novomix 30	Novo Nordisk	cart, pen	15 mins	1–4 h	8–12 h
5) Long acting Insulins					
Insulin glargine	Aventis Pharma	vial, cart, pen	2 h	Peakless	24 h
Insulin detemir	Novo Nordisk	cart, pen	2 h	Peakless	12–24 h

Vial: Stardard 10 ml bottle to use with Syringe. Cart: 3 ml Cartridges for reusable pen. Pen: disposable 3 ml pens
Aventis Pharma also produce Insuman rapid, Insuman basal and Insuman Comb 15, 25 and 50

glycaemic control that is at least comparable to that using isophane insulin. Some studies comparing basal bolus regimes with isophane or glargine have shown that the use of glargine leads to a small (0.1–0.5%) decrease in HbA1c, but other studies have shown no difference. There is some evidence that both glargine and detemir lead to a decrease in the incidence of hypoglycaemia including nocturnal hypoglycaemia. Weight gain with both these insulins may be less than that with isophane insulin.

Basal bolus regimen
This regimen is discussed on p. 7–8. When converting from twice daily insulin injections to a basal bolus regimen, the total number of units is often decreased by 10%

to reduce the risk of hypoglycaemia. Normally, approximately 40% of the TDD of insulin is given at bedtime as a long-acting insulin analogue with the remaining insulin being given prior to breakfast, lunch and the evening meal in the form of rapidly-acting insulin. When converting from a basal bolus regimen containing isophane to one with a long-acting insulin analogue, the same number of units of the analogue is usually given. In the case of glargine, and occasionally with detemir, the dose of rapidly-acting insulin prior to meals (the ratio of rapidly-acting insulin to carbohydrate when carbohydrate counting) may need to be lowered if there is good glycaemic control. If daytime blood glucose levels are generally high then the insulin to carbohydrate ratio can be left unaltered.

As with any significant change in insulin regimen blood glucose levels should be tested frequently to see what effect the change has had. It can take up to 2 weeks for the full effects of a change in regimen to become apparent.

Example of how to convert a patient from twice daily insulin to a basal bolus regimen

- Patient received 44 units of a 30:70 premixed insulin in the morning and 22 units of the same insulin in the evening.
- Decrease total daily dosage of insulin from 66 to 60 units.
- Initially, try 24 units (40%) of a long-acting insulin analogue prior to bedtime.
- Use rapidly-acting insulin and carbohydrate counting to determine the correct dose prior to each meal.
- Adjust doses of insulin in light of blood glucose test results (also use correction doses).

Once on this regimen, the bedtime dose should be slowly adjusted to achieve an average morning fasting glucose concentration of 6 mmol/L (110 mg/dL). Further adjustments can then be made to the preprandial doses. Typical pre-meal doses in adolescents vary from 4 units for a small breakfast to 20 units for a large meal.

Continuous subcutaneous insulin infusions (insulin pumps)

Insulin pumps are used in <5% of children in the United Kingdom and in about 25% of children in the USA. They can be used at all ages. The devices consist of a programmable pump (which may be as small as a match box) containing rapidly-acting insulin which is connected by an infusion line to a small plastic/metal cannula inserted subcutaneously usually in the abdomen (in toddlers and infants it is often inserted in the buttock) and fixed by tape. The cannula is usually left in place for 2–3 days. If the cannula is not changed regularly or if the same site is recurrently used, there is a risk of lipohypertrophy. Changes in the insulin infusion rate as small as 0.025 units/h can be made. Blood glucose should be tested at least four times a day including morning and late evening. A 24-hour profile including measurements before each meal, 2 hours following the meal, at midnight, at 2.00–3.00 a.m. +/− 5.00 a.m. should be carried out at least every other week to help enable any necessary changes to be made. The absence of a long-acting insulin depot means that if there is a problem with insulin delivery, blood glucose levels will rise quickly and ketosis can develop in 4–6 hours. CSII therapy is more expensive than current standard

therapy and in the United Kingdom costs £2500–3500 with consumables costing about £1800 per year.

The indications for CSIIs in the United Kingdom have recently been liberalized. Pumps are recommended as a treatment option for children aged 12 years and above with type 1 diabetes when multiple daily injections (MDI) insulin therapy results in disabling hypoglycaemia or fails to reduce the HbA1c level below 8.5%, and for children under 12 years of age whenever MDI therapy is impractical or inappropriate. It should only be continued if it reduces the HbA1c or the frequency of hypoglycaemic episodes. It is important that patients and their families are committed, competent and interested in using CSII treatment.

There is evidence that CSIIs reduce the HbA1c by 0.5–1% as well as decrease the incidence of hypoglycaemia. Most patients maintain the same weight following pump therapy. Some may gain weight if the HbA1c falls as they stop loosing glucose in their urine. The increased ease of administering boluses can also lead to overeating and weight gain. Others adopt a healthier dietary intake when they start pump therapy, eat smaller meals with smaller boluses and loose weight.

Before commencing CSII therapy, a lot of education about the pump is required and for the majority of patients further refining of carbohydrate counting skills. Patients should be allowed to choose the pump they prefer from the selection available. Pumps differ in size, weight, ease of use, features including dosage increments, cost and customer backup. Support and training are provided by the diabetes team with additional support from the company representative as necessary. Ideally, there should be a structured education programme over several days to teach families about CSII therapy. However, patients' and families' learning curves and working schedules vary and others spread the education over several half days over a period of 1–2 weeks. Daily contact is important over the first couple of weeks. Some units provide 24-hour diabetic support by their nursing/medical staff whilst others rely on a mixture of the 24-hour support provided by the pump manufacturer's company and out of hours by the support provided by the on-call medical staff and the resident ward nursing staff.

When commencing a patient on CSII therapy patients have the option of starting with a saline trial to get used to the pump and its controls for a few days or commencing directly on insulin. When changing a patient from their MDI regimen to CSII therapy the dose of glargine or detemir given the previous night is halved, or omitted if glargine or detemir is given in the morning. The normal dose of rapidly-acting insulin is given with breakfast and CSII therapy is usually commenced mid-morning. The TDD of insulin chosen is dependent on the patient's HbA1c, average blood glucose, weight and frequency of hypos. The difficulty is that it may be difficult to determine if the HbA1c is high because the patient is on insufficient insulin or whether that is due to their not taking their insulin. Most patients experience a significant decrease in their TDD of insulin when they convert to CSII therapy. For this reason, and to be cautious, the patient's TDD is often decreased by 25% at the start of pump therapy. Approximately 50% of the TDD is given as basal insulin. The remainder is administered as bolus doses. The same insulin to carbohydrate ratio may be maintained but often this ratio is lowered by about 20–25%; for example, the ratio may be changed from 1 unit of rapidly-acting insulin for every 10 g of carbohydrate (1:10) to a 1:12 ratio. The same correction dose (also known as 'insulin sensitivity factor') may be kept but again this is often reduced by about 20–25%; for example, the correction dose may be changed from 1 unit of rapidly-acting insulin to lower the blood glucose by 4 mmol/L (72 mg/dL) to 1 unit to lower the blood glucose by 5 mmol/L (90 mg/dL), the aim being to decrease the blood glucose to 7 mmol/L (125 mg/dL). These reductions are made to try and decrease the risk of hypoglycaemia following the commencement of pump therapy. When starting a newly diagnosed patient on CSII therapy (this is done in some centres, most often in children < 3 years), the TDD is often calculated as 0.5 units/kg per day with about 50% of the TDD being given as basal insulin (on occasion, a higher percentage of the TDD will be required as basal insulin). The '500 rule' (see page 7) is often used to calculate the insulin to carbohydrate ratio and the correction dose is worked out by dividing 100 by the TDD. There can be a lot of variability in glycaemic control following pump initiation and close monitoring is required in the initial stages.

A minority of patients use the pump at night only with multiple rapidly-acting insulin injections during the day and intermediate acting insulin (e.g. isophane) in the morning. This may be done in patients who are reluctant to wear the pump during the day, when there are difficulties with adult supervision during the day, if there are problems with night-time hypos, or if there are difficulties with high blood glucose levels in the early morning. A night-time pump may also be useful during a holiday when the patient may be exercising and swimming a lot during the day. In such cases, the morning intermediate insulin may not be necessary.

On occasion a patient may want to revert from CSII therapy to pen/syringe treatment; for example, if going on holiday. In such cases, the TDD should be increased by 10% with 30% of the TDD being administered as long-acting insulin. It may be best to make this change a few days before going on holiday to get used to this mode of treatment again.

Initially, we use the same basal rate for the whole day. However, different rates may be necessary for different parts of the day and temporary changes in the basal rate may be required when the patient is ill (usually an increase) or during exercise (a decrease). An increase in the basal rate may also be necessary in the days leading up to menses or if the patient is on a drug known to increase blood glucose levels, for example steroids. Young children often have their highest basal rate between 9.00 p.m. and 12.00 a.m. whereas adolescents who secrete a lot of GH overnight may require high basal rates in the early hours of the morning to counter the dawn phenomenon (see page 21). One way of altering the daytime basal rates is to divide the day into three with each time span containing a main meal. The blood glucose should be measured before the meal for several days to help evaluate the basal rate. If the blood glucose is <5 mmol/L (90 mg/dL), then the basal rate prior to the meal should be decreased by 0.05 units/h if the rate is <0.3 units/h, by 0.1 unit/h if the rate is 0.3 to 0.975 units/h and by 0.2 units/h if the rate is > 1 unit/h. Conversely, if the blood glucose is >10 mmol/L (180 mg/dL), then the basal rate prior to the meal should be increased by 0.05 units/h if the rate is <0.3 units/h, by 0.1 units/h if the basal rate is 0.3 to 0.975 units/h and by 0.2 units/h if the rate is >1 unit/h. A further way of adjusting the daytime basal rate is to miss breakfast and the accompanying bolus, and to measure the blood glucose hourly till lunchtime. If the blood glucose level rises then an increase in the basal dose is required and vice versa. This process can be repeated with the other meals. In children this period of fasting may be difficult to achieve but parents can try and give food containing virtually no carbohydrate (e.g. eggs or carrots).

Bolus doses are given at meal times, their size depending on the amount of carbohydrate ingested. Even a 10 g carbohydrate snack should be accompanied by a bolus (compare to basal bolus regime) page 7–8. Additional correction doses may be necessary at the same time if the blood glucose is high, or at other times when the blood glucose is raised; for example, during illness. There are different types of boluses. A standard bolus delivers the whole bolus immediately whereas a square or extended bolus administers it over a variable period of time, for example

2 hours. Dual or combination boluses can also be administered which deliver varied combinations of the above two boluses, for example 50% standard bolus and 50% square bolus. Square or dual boluses may be preferred for a meal rich in fat, for example a pizza; a meal with a low glycaemic index; or when food will be eaten over a protracted period of time, for example a party; or if it is uncertain how much food the child will eat.

CSIIs can help in calculations of the necessary bolus dose. Insulin pumps have a built-in calculator which can be pre-programmed with the relevant insulin to carbohydrate ratio, the insulin sensitivity factor and the blood glucose targets. If the glucose reading and the amount of carbohydrate to be eaten are entered, the pump can work out the bolus dose. This calculation will include any necessary correction dose and will also take into account any 'insulin on board' from the last bolus that was administered that may still be acting. Patients can input into the pump their favourite foods and their carbohydrate content to create a food list, thus further facilitating carbohydrate counting when the same food is eaten again.

There is some evidence that there is a slightly increased risk of DKA, especially in the first few weeks following the initiation of CSII therapy. However, a recent study showed a lower rate of DKA in CSII users. Patients and parents should be aware of the symptoms of insulin deficiency such as polyuria, polydipsia, nausea, vomiting, abdominal pain, tachypnoea and drowsiness. Blood ketone sticks are useful as they detect raised ketone levels several hours earlier than urine ketone sticks. If the blood glucose is >14 mmol/L (250 mg/dL) and blood ketones are ≥ 0.6 mmol/L (or urine ketones are moderate or large), this indicates an interruption in insulin delivery or an increased requirement for insulin, for example due to infection. 0.1 unit/kg of rapidly-acting insulin should be administered with a pen or syringe. The pump and infusion set should not be used as they may not be working properly. The blood glucose should be measured hourly. If it does not fall, the same insulin dose can be repeated every 2 hours. Blood ketones should also be measured 2 hourly to document if they are falling. If the situation is not improving then the insulin cartridge, infusion set and cannula/needle should be changed. The skin should also be examined for signs of erythema which would indicate infection, or moisture which would suggest an insulin leak. Large amounts of sugar-free fluids should be drunk. If the blood glucose is ≤ 11 mmol/L (200 mg/dL) and blood ketone levels are still elevated, then sugar containing fluids should be drunk and additional rapidly-acting insulin should be administered. One should **always** have

insulin to be administered with a pen or syringe in case of a problem with the pump.

Hypoglycaemia should be treated by administering 15 g of rapidly-acting carbohydrate; for example, 4–5 glucose tablets or 90 mL of a sugary drink or fruit juice (check the label). The glucose level should be checked after 15 minutes. If it is still <4 mmol/L, then the above procedure should be repeated. In contrast to MDI therapy, the rapidly-acting carbohydrate does not need to be followed up with a longer-acting source of carbohydrate as there is no long-acting insulin present. In the case of a major hypo with unconsciousness, the insulin pump should be stopped and appropriate action taken (see 'Hypoglycaemia' p. 26). The cause of the hypoglycaemia (basal rate too high, increased physical activity with an insufficient reduction in the basal rate, miscalculation of a meal bolus, or alcohol) should be determined and any necessary changes implemented.

During some exercises such as swimming or contact sports, the pump can be disconnected for 1 hour. Alternative approaches to exercise include having a snack prior to the exercise, or if one is exercising shortly after having had a meal with a premeal bolus, to decrease the meal bolus.

In other cases, and especially in the case of prolonged exercise such as a 4-hour tennis match, the best plan is to reduce the basal rate. This may need doing 1–2 hours prior to the exercise as it takes 1–2 hours before a decrease in the basal rate has an effect. This would be necessary especially if the hypos were occurring early in the course of the exercise. For instance, the basal rate may need decreasing by up to 50% 1–2 hours prior to the start of the exercise until 1–2 hours following the end of the exercise. Further decreases in the basal rate may be necessary and regular testing before, during and after exercise should help determine the appropriate basal rate. Exercise can also lead to hypoglycaemia up to 24 hours following the exercise. In the case of strenuous exercise carbohydrate will also need to be taken during the exercise and following the exercise. If the exercise has been in the afternoon or evening, the basal rate may need decreasing by 10–20% until the following morning. In children attending sports camps the basal rate should be decreased by about 20% on the first day of activities and then adjusted according to the blood glucose readings.

The approach to illness in children with a CSII is similar to that of high blood glucose readings with raised blood ketone levels. Fever and the stress of illness nearly always raise blood glucose levels. Meal boluses should be continued even if one is eating less. Correction doses should be given as appropriate. The basal rate should be increased by 10–20% if the blood glucose level remains high. The blood glucose should be checked every 2–4 hours and blood ketones should also be measured frequently. Further increases in the basal rate may be necessary. 0.1 unit/kg of rapidly-acting insulin should be administered if the blood glucose is > 14 mmol/L (250 mg/dL) with blood ketones ≥ 0.6 mmol/L. A further similar dose should be given every 2 hours until the blood glucose is < 10 mmol/L (180 mg/dL) and the ketone levels are falling. All extra insulin doses should be given with a pen or syringe if the blood glucose has risen suddenly in case the rise is due to a problem with the pump. Large amounts of glucose-free fluid should also be drunk to increase the excretion of ketones and to prevent dehydration. When the blood glucose is < 11 mmol/L (200 mg/dL), glucose containing drinks should be drunk. In the case of nausea, small amounts should be drunk frequently. If hypoglycaemia is a problem then sweet drinks should be drunk and the basal rate should be lowered.

Schools and nurseries should be told that a pupil in their class is about to start or has started on insulin pump therapy. Ideally the DNS, but if that is not possible the parent, should teach the patient's carers how to administer a bolus.

Problems with the CSII may be due to the pump itself (failure, flat batteries), the insulin reservoir/cartridge (empty or plunger stuck), the infusion set (blocked), the cannula (blocked or dislodged), or the insertion site (infected, lipohypertrophy). Furthermore, there may be leaks between the connections. The first sign of a malfunction may be a rise in the blood glucose that may precede the pump alarming. The pump safety features can be personalized to alert the user before the insulin cartridge or battery run too low. Various other alarms are also programmed into the pumps. These include occlusion alarms. If an alarm occurs in the middle of a bolus the pump will state how much of the bolus it has delivered. However, how much of the bolus the patient has received will depend on whether the occlusion was partial or total and how far down the infusion line it occurred. The alarm can also go off if no buttons have been pressed for a set length of time. It can also be programmed to limit the maximum basal and bolus rates to avoid overdosage. The pump can also be 'locked' to prevent the accidental pushing of buttons.

Clinic visits involve reviewing the blood glucose levels to identify if there are any patterns that would justify alterations in the basal or bolus rates, measurements of the HbA1c, discussions of any problems with the pump, dietetic issues, etc.

Some CSIIs have remote controls that enable the bolus dose to be given more easily and discretely. Some remote controls can also be used as glucose meters and to input data into the pump.

Recently, a new type of pump called a 'patch pump' has been developed, for example the OmniPod. Patch pumps comprise of a micro pump, an insulin reservoir (patch) and a cannula, and attach directly to the skin. Insulin is delivered through the very small integrated subcutaneous catheter. Patch pumps are free of tubing which makes them more discrete and allows greater freedom with activities. They are disposable or semi-disposable and many are lighter and smaller than conventional pumps. They are controlled by a remote control device that communicates wirelessly with the patch pump and which often doubles up as a glucose meter. They usually need to be reapplied every 3 days.

CSIIs can also be used with continuous glucose monitoring sensors that measure glucose levels in the interstitial fluid every few minutes. These sensors are usually used for a few days in a month rather then continuously. The data can be transferred to the pump using Bluetooth technology so that if the blood glucose is below a certain value, for example 4 mmol/L (72 mg/dL), the insulin pump alarms and stops. Some insulin pumps can also be set to alarm if the glucose level is falling rapidly. It is hoped that in the near future, the two will be combined to provide a reliable closed loop system, i.e. an artificial pancreas. There is evidence that such systems increase the number of readings in the target range and decrease hypoglycaemia. Various algorithms for such a device to cope with situations such as exercise (where absolute glucose values and trends are looked at) are currently being devised in this promising research avenue that could greatly improve the management of diabetes.

The use of CSIIs is increasing in the United Kingdom and in many other countries, especially as technology improves. The pump enables a flexible life style and eating patterns and is associated with a high degree of satisfaction in appropriately motivated patients.

Potential problems with insulin therapy

The dawn phenomenon

The dawn phenomenon describes the rise in insulin requirements and blood glucose concentrations in the latter part of the night, approximately 5.00–8.00 a.m. It occurs mainly in puberty and is thought to be caused by the insulin resistance produced by nocturnal GH secretion. This is a difficult problem to resolve in those using twice daily insulin regimens. Possible benefit may be obtained in such patients by dividing the evening injection so that rapid-acting insulin is given prior to the evening meal and intermediate-acting insulin prior to bedtime. Alternatively, in patients on a basal bolus regimen the pre-bedtime dose of intermediate-acting insulin or long-acting insulin analogue can be increased.

The Somogyi phenomenon

This is said to be the 'rebound' morning hyperglycaemia which may occur following nocturnal hypoglycaemia caused by the release of counter-regulatory hormones such as glucagon, adrenaline and cortisol. Whether this phenomenon exists is open to debate and it may be the consequence of the excessive ingestion of refined carbohydrates used to treat the episode of nocturnal hypoglycaemia.

Monitoring glycaemic control

Blood glucose testing

A number of studies have shown that greater frequency of blood glucose monitoring improves metabolic control. The following principles for home blood glucose monitoring are recommended:

• Children should be encouraged to perform their own finger-prick blood glucose testing at as young an age as they feel able to do so (sometimes as young as 5 years old).
• Finger pricks should be performed on the sides of the fingertips.
• Finger-pricking devices with variable depth settings can make testing less painful.
• Forearm blood glucose testing is an acceptable and accurate alternative to finger-prick testing.
• Electronic blood glucose meters with a memory, which may allow data to be downloaded onto a computer for discussion in clinic, are useful for recording results but need regular calibration.
• Date-expired blood glucose testing strips should be avoided as use of these may lead to inaccurate blood glucose estimations.
• The child should be encouraged to monitor blood glucose concentrations regularly, prior to each main meal and at bedtime. On rare occasions, it may be helpful to monitor values 2 hours after a main meal.
• More frequent blood glucose testing may be indicated if the child is unwell, partaking in unusual amounts of physical activity or feels hypoglycaemic.
• Devices that regularly monitor glucose readings, in some cases at intervals of <5 minutes have recently become available. The devices are inserted subcutaneously and measure interstitial fluid glucose, which with the best devices is within 15% of blood glucose. They can be left in place for 3–6 days and are usually used intermittently; for example, on an ad hoc basis or for a few days a month. These devices, that can be used with injections or CSII therapy, have been shown to detect hypoglycaemia more frequently than conventional monitoring, and may also have hypoglycaemia and hyperglycaemia alarms. Conventional blood glucose testing is still required to calibrate the device. The monitoring can be performed retrospectively, when there is no contemporaneous display of sensor readings or in real time. Real-time monitors will demonstrate trends in glucose levels. However, there is a lag of at least 15 minutes between blood and interstitial glucose levels which increases when the blood glucose is changing rapidly, for example during exercise. Absolute interstitial glucose values are, therefore, not always the same as blood glucose levels and the interstitial glucose value should be checked with a blood glucose value prior to any therapeutic action being taken. Data can be analysed in relation to insulin doses, carbohydrate intake and exercise. These devices are helpful in monitoring suspected nocturnal hypoglycaemia and/or early morning hyperglycaemia, suspected unrecognized hypoglycaemia (for example low HbA1c without reported hypoglycaemia), disabling hypoglycaemia especially in those with hypoglycaemia unawareness and to help with further optimization of MDI or CSII when the HbA1c cannot be lowered in spite of apparent optimal treatment. There is some evidence that such devices can help lower the HbA1c and decrease the incidence of severe hypoglycaemia.
• The child should aim for pre-meal blood glucose concentrations of approximately 4–8 mmol/L (72–145 mg/dL), pre-bedtime values of 7–10 mmol/L (125–180 mg/dL) and <10 mmol/L (180 mg/dL) 1–2 hours after meals.
• In children under 5 years of age acceptance of slightly higher blood glucose concentrations may be necessary to avoid hypoglycaemia which may be a consequence of variable feeding patterns.

Blood and urinary ketone testing

Blood ketone sticks measure β-hydoxybutyrate which is the main ketone produced in insulin deficiency states. Urine sticks measure acetoacetone which is a less important ketone. Blood ketones also provide a more up to date assessment of the body's ketone production and the patient's status in the same way as blood glucose does when compared to a urine glucose measurement. Ketone levels

Table 1.10 Interpreting glycosylated haemoglobin values.

DCCT-HbA1c (%)	IFCC-HbA1c (mmol/mol)	Comment
4.0–5.9	20–41	Within non-diabetic reference range, possibility of frequent hypoglycaemia
6.0–6.9	42–52	Ideal glycaemic control
7.0–7.5	53–59	Very good glycaemic control in the absence of complications
7.6–8.9	60–74	Associated with increased risk of microvascular complications. Advise to improve glycaemic control
9.0–10.9	75–96	Compliance likely to be a problem. Associated with high risk of microvascular complications
> 11.0	> 97	Poor compliance, probably associated with omission of insulin injections and unrestricted diet

should be measured during illness or when blood glucose concentrations are unusually high, particularly when associated with symptoms of polyuria, polydipsia, nausea or abdominal pain. The presence of hyperglycaemia and significantly raised blood (> 1.5 mmol/L) or urine (+++) ketone levels indicates that DKA may be present or that urgent increases in the dosage of insulin are required to avoid this happening.

Glycosylated haemoglobin measurement

HbA1c is formed by the adduction of glucose to adult haemoglobin and reflects average blood glucose values during the previous 2–3 months. It has been recommended that to assist audit, laboratories should report their results adjusted to give comparable values to the assays used in the Diabetes Control and Complications Trial (DCCT). The DCCT-aligned normal, non-diabetic range is 4–6%.

For clinics, bench-top machines for the measurement of blood HbA1c concentrations are now available and have the advantage of providing results for discussion with the patient while they are attending clinic. Such machines, however, require careful maintenance and quality control.

Haemoglobin variants may interfere with the HbA1c assays (DCCT and International Federation of Clinical Chemistry and Laboratory Medicine (IFCC)) and lead to misleading results. In such cases, the HbA1c can be used to look at trends, the patient's glycaemic control needs to be inspected more closely, and the serum fructosamine assay which provides a measure of glycaemia in the previous 2 weeks and which is less accurate than HbA1c values may be used if available.

The American Diabetes Association (ADA) have recommend aiming for a HbA1c of <8.5% in toddlers, <8% in children and <7.5% in teenagers. The clinical interpretation of HbA1c measurements is shown in Table 1.10. Recently, many laboratories have changed to the IFCC standardized values which are more accurate and are reported in mmol/mol of haemoglobin and as whole numbers. Currently, many laboratories supply HbA1c results both as a % (DCCT-aligned) and as mmol/mol (IFCC). It is planned to change in 2011 from DCCT-aligned values to the more specific IFCC standardized values. This will also make global comparisons of HbA1c easier. Depending on glycaemic control, HbA1c concentrations should be measured every 3–6 months.

Diabetes control and complications trial (DCCT)

This trial, published in 1993, is arguably the most important publication on diabetes in the last 17 years. A total of 1441 subjects with diabetes aged 13–39 years were randomized to either: (1) continue with their conventional treatment; or (2) receive intensive therapy with increased support from the 'diabetes team' and insulin administered either by a pump or by three or more injections daily. After a mean time interval of 6.5 years, compared with conventional therapy, intensive treatment resulted in a reduction in:

- mean HbA1c concentration of approximately 2%;
- the risk of retinopathy by 76%;
- the occurrence of microalbuminuria by 39%; and
- the occurrence of neuropathy by 60%.

The trial found that for every 10% reduction in HbA1c (e.g. 8 vs. 7.2%), there was a 44% reduction in the risk of microvascular complications.

The disadvantages of intensive treatment included a two-to-three-fold increase in severe hypoglycaemia and a mean weight gain of 4.6 kg when compared with conventional treatment. This study clearly demonstrated the reduction in risk of the microvascular complications of diabetes which can result from improved glycaemic control. Furthermore, for a given mean HbA1c there was a significantly lower incidence of complications in the intensively treated group suggesting that this form of therapy produces less glycaemic excursion, thereby lowering the risk of complications. The challenge for clinicians, however, is to discover how to apply an intensive therapeutic regimen in standard clinical practice in a manner that will be acceptable to most adolescents.

Effect of exercise on blood glucose control

Exercise is beneficial to children with diabetes as it results in:
- reduced blood glucose concentrations;
- increased insulin sensitivity;
- reduced serum lipid concentrations; and
- reduced risks of hypertension and heart disease.

Ideally, blood glucose monitoring should occur before and after exercise. Hypoglycaemia can be avoided by taking complex carbohydrate in the form of a snack before exercise and/or by decreasing the dose of insulin by approximately 10–20%. In school, the teacher should be aware that the child has diabetes and carbohydrate (e.g. glucose tablets or drinks) should be available for the treatment of hypoglycaemia. Exercise can also lead to delayed hypoglycaemia (e.g. during the night) and in such circumstances additional complex carbohydrate should be taken with the bedtime snack. Occasionally, short-duration exercise can cause hyperglycaemia because of the increased secretion of counter-regulatory hormones (e.g. adrenaline) which raise blood glucose.

Diabetes in preschool-aged children

There are a number of factors which are pertinent to the management of very young children with diabetes as shown in Table 1.11.

Table 1.11 Characteristics of preschool-aged children with diabetes.

Atypical symptoms at diagnosis

Increased insulin sensitivity

Practical difficulties administering insulin injections

Prolonged night-time fast

Frequent bottle feeds in infancy

Food refusal

Inability to communicate symptoms of impending hypoglycaemia

Frequent infective illnesses often associated with vomiting

Rapid growth and neurodevelopment

Complete dependency on others to supervise their diabetes

Diabetes in adolescence

Transition clinics

Transition refers to the period between childhood and adulthood. Adolescence is accompanied by many physical and psychosocial changes. There is also a gradual change from total dependence on one's parents for treatment to independent self-management. These changes can be difficult to negotiate for patients and parents, and there is often a deterioration in glycaemic control in adolescents. It has been increasingly recognized in recent years that transition clinics (sometimes also called adolescent, teenage or young person's clinics) are of benefit to adolescents with significant chronic conditions and their families.

Ideally, in these clinics patients should be seen jointly by the paediatric and adult physician with the paediatrician introducing the patient to the adult physician. In some clinics, joint consultations are only done initially whilst in others this pattern is maintained.

The venue of the clinic varies according to local circumstances. Usually, it takes place in the hospital adult clinic but it may also take place in the paediatric clinic or in a community clinic. The environment should be appropriate for teenagers with appropriate literature, computer games and so forth.

Young adults from 14–25 years are seen in these clinics with the age range of individual clinics being very variable. Some clinics focus on the 14–18 year age group whilst others will see mainly 18 to 25-year-old patients. When to transfer a patient to the transition clinic should depend primarily on the wishes of the young person and their family. The doctor's wishes (e.g. wanting to see a patient with type 2 diabetes with an adult physician) and local protocols will also influence this decision. Surveys have suggested that young people favour the age of approximately 18 for transfer to adult care. Discussion and planning will improve clinic attendance. The transfer may need to be planned well in advance to avoid overly long gaps between appointments.

Attendance rates can be very low and a telephone call and/or a text message 1–2 days prior to the appointment, in addition to the standard letter, can help improve attendance.

The patient may be seen with their parent(s), on their own or with a friend. Group sessions held at the same time as the clinic, for instance organized and facilitated by the DNS, where young people can exchange views about their diabetes and their ways of coping with it can be useful. As well as the doctor, DNS and dietitian, the presence of a psychologist or psychiatrist at these clinics can be very helpful. Attendance at 3–4 monthly intervals is advocated as frequent attendance is associated with better control. Though diabetic control often deteriorates in adolescence, one study demonstrated that the HbA1c improved on transfer to an adult clinic.

Paediatric clinics often permit laxer glycaemic control and focus more on particular areas such as school progress. It is important that paediatric and adult physicians get on well in transition clinics, and have agreed strategies and education programmes. Transition clinics may focus more on subjects such as exercise. Tighter glycaemic control is advocated aiming for preprandial blood glucose levels of 4–7 mmol/L (72–125 mg/dL) and levels of ≤ 9 mmol/L (160 mg/dL) postprandially, as control should be easier post puberty and with increasing maturity. A more intensive approach to insulin therapy is advocated and the use of insulin pumps is often discussed. In the United Kingdom, there is often no routine screening in adult clinics for thyroid disease or coeliac disease as these conditions are uncommon in adults. In contrast, there is a greater focus on screening and monitoring for microvascular and macrovascular complications which increase in incidence with age.

The clinics should also provide a forum for the education and discussion of subjects of particular relevance to teenagers such as contraception, alcohol and smoking.

It is also important for the patient to know which doctor, DNS and dietitian they should liase with and whether they would be admitted to a paediatric or adult ward should they require admission.

Insulin requirements

Insulin requirements increase in puberty partly because of the rapid increase in size and appetite, and partly because of increasing growth hormone secretion which leads to a degree of insulin resistance. This results in increased difficulty in maintaining good glycaemic control (including the dawn phenomenon) and, particularly for girls, an increased tendency to be overweight. Insulin requirements may be greater than 1.3 units/kg per day and on occasion may be as large as 2 units/kg per day. Inadequate insulin therapy may cause delayed puberty and impaired growth.

Insulin regimens

The results of the DCCT suggest that the basal bolus regimen or CSII should be used in children over 13 years. For some adolescents, giving an injection before lunch at school may not be practical. In such patients, a three-injection regimen – mixed insulin before breakfast, rapidly-acting insulin prior to the evening meal and intermediate-acting insulin (isophane) or the long-acting insulin analogue detemir before bedtime – may provide a useful compromise. Adolescents may be more concerned with short-term problems such as an increased risk of hypoglycaemia, which may lead to loss of a driving licence, than with decreasing the risk of longer term complications.

Psychological and psychiatric problems

Psychological problems are common during puberty. The presence of a psychologist or psychiatrist in clinic is particularly valuable in this age group. It is important to differentiate between the normal psychological changes of adolescence and a pathological response to a chronic disease. The latter may lead to depression and require skilled psychiatric care.

Many patients will not comply with the diet and some may even binge. A higher than average number of diabetic children, particularly girls, have eating disorders. Abnormal eating patterns may develop as a means of manipulating parents. Most eating disorders are mild and do not require formal intervention. However, occasionally a patient will develop anorexia nervosa or bulimia. These conditions can be very difficult to treat in a patient with diabetes and often necessitate a prolonged admission to an adolescent psychiatric unit. Some adolescents may smoke and others may start using recreational drugs. They should be strongly dissuaded from both.

Not infrequently, adolescents fail to comply with their insulin treatment, experimenting with omission and/or reduction of their insulin doses, sometimes in an effort to manipulate their weight. Poor compliance may also occur in their failure to monitor blood glucose concentrations. Results in the record book can be fabricated. Recordings which for many days have been documented in the same pen, a significant discrepancy between the results and the HbA1c value, apparently excessively large insulin requirements (>1.75 units/kg per day) and poor clinic attendance are suggestive of poor compliance. Negotiating appropriate solutions to these difficult problems may take considerable patience and skill, and psychological support may be particularly helpful. There is some evidence that motivational interviewing, a counselling approach to behaviour change, may improve well-being and glycaemic control in adolescents with diabetes.

The problems listed above can lead to an increased incidence of DKA and hypoglycaemia. Furthermore, puberty is the time when the early signs of microvascular complications, such as background diabetic retinopathy, may become evident.

Miscellaneous problems
There is an increased incidence of polycystic ovary syndrome and menstrual irregularities in girls with diabetes. The menstrual cycle may also affect blood glucose control with rising values in the 2–3 days prior to the start of the period. In those in whom this occurs regularly, insulin dosage can be increased during this time.

Hypoglycaemia

In children with diabetes, hypoglycaemia may be defined as a blood glucose concentration less than 4 mmol/L (72 mg/dL). However, children whose glycaemic control is poor may experience hypoglycaemic symptoms at concentrations above 4 mmol/L (72 mg/dL) if a rapid fall in blood glucose has occurred.

Causes of hypoglycaemia
Although in up to half of cases there may be no obvious cause, hypoglycaemia may be caused by:
• a missed or delayed snack or meal;
• exercise (may also cause delayed hypoglycaemia);
• alcohol;
• an overdose of insulin;

• impaired food absorption as a result of gastroenteritis or coeliac disease; or
• Addison's disease.

Symptoms and signs of hypoglycaemia
Symptoms of hypoglycaemia are unusual with blood glucose concentrations above 3 mmol/L (55 mg/dL) and a surprising number of children, particularly those with very good glycaemic control or those with recurrent blood glucose values below 4 mmol/L (72 mg/dL), will have no symptoms even with glucose values below 2 mmol/L (36 mg/dL) (so-called 'hypoglycaemia unawareness'). The inability to respond to the usual warning signs of hypoglycaemia can lead to severe hypoglycaemia.

Fortunately, most school-aged children are quickly able to recognize the symptoms of hypoglycaemia (see Table 2.1). In young children symptoms are less obvious and may result in more severe hypoglycaemia. Chronic mild hypoglycaemia may affect concentration, school performance and intellectual function. Early age of onset of diabetes is associated with mesial temporal sclerosis. Hypoglycaemic seizures may lead to deficits in perceptual, motor, memory and attention tasks, and may also have an effect on grey matter volume.

Nocturnal hypoglycaemia
Nocturnal hypoglycaemia is common. Blood glucose concentrations fall to their lowest levels between 3.00 a.m. and 4.00 a.m. Severe hypoglycaemia is more common at night. This may be because the patient is asleep and unaware of symptoms of impending hypoglycaemia or because of an impaired response from the counter-regulatory hormones. Nocturnal hypoglycaemia may be suggested by disturbed sleep, excessive sweating, morning headaches, difficulty waking from sleep or convulsions. Continuous glucose monitoring systems (e.g. GlucoWatch Biographer) may be helpful in monitoring nocturnal blood glucose concentrations in patients with suspected or confirmed nocturnal hypoglycaemia. Parents may be afraid that their child will die in the middle of the night from hypoglycaemia – the so-called 'dead in bed' syndrome. This syndrome, thought to be caused by hypoglycaemia, is extremely rare (no recorded cases under 7 years of age) and parents should be reassured that it is very unlikely because of the effect of the counter-regulatory hormones.

Treatment of hypoglycaemia
Good glycaemic control is likely to be associated with occasional hypoglycaemic episodes which, if mild, may be acceptable. Avoidance of recurrent blood glucose

concentrations below 4 mmol/L (72 mg/dL) may prevent the development of hypoglycaemia unawareness. Hypoglycaemia may be treated by:
• the ingestion of short-acting carbohydrate (e.g. glucose tablets or drinks or a snack-sized chocolate bar) followed by complex carbohydrate (bread, cereal or pasta) to prevent a recurrence;
• application of a glucose gel (e.g. glucogel) to the inside of the mouth and its massage into the buccal mucosa or gums in a child who refuses or is unable to take any food or drink;
• intramuscular glucagon (0.5 mg if body weight <25 kg, 1 mg if weight >25 kg) in unconscious or fitting patients who should be placed in the 'recovery position'. Side effects of glucagon include nausea, vomiting, diarrhoea and hypokalaemia. Glucagon can also be administered subcutaneously. There is some evidence to show that it is equally efficacious when administered this way; and
• in hospital with 2 mL/kg of 10% dextrose given intravenously.

A hypoglycaemic convulsion may be accompanied by a normal blood glucose concentration because of the effect of the counter-regulatory hormones. In patients with neurological signs and in those who remain in a coma following treatment, other disorders (e.g. epilepsy or meningitis) should be considered.

Nocturnal hypoglycaemia may be prevented by:
• decreasing the evening/bedtime insulin dose;
• increasing the evening snack;
• the use of rapid-acting human insulin analogues;
• the use of long-acting human insulin analogues;
• the use of CSII; and
• ensuring that young children on twice daily or basal bolus regimens going to bed at 07.00 p.m. have a blood glucose concentration >10 mmol/L (180 mg/dL) and older children going to bed at 10.00 p.m. a value >7 mmol/L (125 mg/dL). If the blood glucose concentration is below these levels, a snack, a larger than usual snack or, if a snack has already been eaten, a second snack should be consumed.

Recurrent DKA

Recurrent DKA is a particular problem in adolescents and may be fatal. It may be precipitated by:
• poor compliance with insulin therapy or diet (when responsible adults administer insulin a tenfold reduction in episodes of DKA has been reported);

• infection;
• stress;
• alcohol; or
• psychosocial problems.
The treatment of DKA is described earlier in this chapter (page 8).

Management of diabetes during intercurrent illness

Acute febrile illness often leads to a rise in blood glucose due to raised levels of stress hormones and gluconeogenesis which may progress to DKA. Conversely, diseases associated with diarrhoea and/or vomiting such as gastroenteritis may lead to a fall in blood glucose and hypoglycaemia. Families should have clear guidelines on the management of diabetes during intercurrent illness ('sick day rules').

The following are the important principles for the management of diabetes during intercurrent illnesses:
• Do not to stop insulin therapy.
• Monitor blood glucose concentrations frequently, at least prior to each meal and prior to bedtime. Sometimes much more frequent monitoring, for example hourly, is required.
• Eat carbohydrate regularly. If the child has a poor appetite this may take the form of regular small snacks and/or sugary drinks, rather than large meals.
• Drink plenty of water and/or reduced sugar fluids to counteract the potential dehydration that may be associated with glycosuria and a febrile illness.
• Test blood or urine regularly for ketones.
• Adjust the dosage of insulin, increasing as necessary to treat hyperglycaemia and ketosis. For example, in cases where the blood glucose is > 14–22 mmol/L (250–400 mg/dL) with blood ketones <0.6 mmol/L (or urine ketones negative or trace) give 0.05 units/kg of rapidly-acting insulin. If these glucose readings are accompanied by blood ketones ≥1.0 mmol/L (or urine ketones moderate or large) give 0.1 unit/kg. If the blood glucose is >22 mmol/L (>400 mg/dL) then 0.1 unit/kg of rapidly-acting insulin should be administered irrespective of the presence or absence of blood or urinary ketones. If the blood glucose and/or ketones do not decrease then the dose of rapidly-acting insulin can be repeated after 2 hours. This scheme is easiest to implement in children on a basal bolus regimen. In those on a twice daily mixed insulin regimen it will entail additional injections of rapid-acting insulin following the standard injections and

Table 1.12 Suggested insulin infusion rates during surgery (same sliding scale can be used in cases of diarrhoea and vomiting).

Blood glucose concentration in mmol/L (mg/dL)	Suggested insulin infusion rate (units/kg/h)
< 4 (72)	0.01 with 2 mL/kg bolus of 10% dextrose
4–6.9 (72–124)	0.02
7.0–11.0 (125–199)	0.04
11.1–17.0 (200–306)	0.06
17.1–22.0 (307–396)	0.08
> 22.0 (> 396)	0.10

Do not stop the insulin infusion if the blood glucose is < 4 mmol/L (72 mg/dL) as this will cause hyperglycaemia. Reduce the rate of the insulin infusion further. Continue with the glucose infusion and increase the rate if required.

during the day. Blood glucose should be measured frequently when additional insulin is required. The approach to intercurrent illness in children on CSII therapy is discussed on p. 20.
• If hypoglycaemia occurs, particularly in association with gastroenteritis and mild ketosis, ensure that the child takes regular, frequent amounts of carbohydrate snacks and/or sugary drinks. Oral rehydration solutions are sometimes necessary. Occasionally, glucogel or glucagon are required to treat hypoglycaemia and to help re-establish oral feeds. Vomiting may be treated with a single injection of an anti-emetic to try and improve carbohydrate intake. The insulin dosage may need to be reduced to two-thirds or a half of the regular dose.
• In cases of severe gastroenteritis and in those with severe or persistent vomiting, IV fluids may be necessary (e.g. 5% dextrose/0.45% saline with 10 mmol of potassium per 500 mL). In such cases, it is often best to also administer IV insulin. Insulin infusion rates such as those outlined in Table 1.12 may be used, initially with hourly blood glucose measurements.
• To treat the underlying illness, antibiotics may be required for some infections and antipyretics are also often required. Sugar-free medicines are preferable if available.
• If, despite these measures, the child has persistent vomiting and/or diarrhoea, significant hypoglycaemia, abdominal pain, drowsiness, tachypnoea, the blood glucose and/or ketone concentrations fail to respond to changes in insulin treatment, or the child is under 5 years,

or the parents remain concerned, then they should contact the diabetes nurse, doctor or hospital for further advice.

Management of diabetes when travelling

When travelling, the following principles are recommended for the management of the diabetes:
• At least twice as much insulin and equipment as would normally be required should be taken with one set of supplies taken as hand luggage. Supplies should include glucogel and glucagon.
• A letter for Customs stating the diagnosis and outlining the equipment required should be taken.
• Appropriate insurance must be arranged.
• In very hot climates, insulin should be kept refrigerated. In patients on CSII the insulin cartridge should be changed every 1–2 days.
• Snacks should be kept with the hand luggage in case the child does not like the food on the plane or the meals contain inadequate carbohydrate.
• With short flights or where the time zone between departure and arrival changes by less than 4 hours, no major changes to the insulin regimen are required.
• With long-haul flights crossing time zones, the most straight forward approach is to give 15–20% of the TDD of insulin as rapidly-acting insulin before main meals on the plane and to revert to the usual regime on arrival at the new destination.

When on holiday, especially those involving physical activities, children with diabetes often require less insulin than usual to avoid hypoglycaemia. At the start of the holiday, the child should be advised to monitor blood glucose concentrations regularly to help decide what changes in insulin treatment are required.

Psychological aspects of diabetes management

Ideally, a psychologist should meet with the family in clinic and be involved in the patient's care from the time of diagnosis. Additional support for the family can be gained by introducing them to other families with children with diabetes, local support groups or national diabetes associations. The child may benefit from meeting other children with diabetes by going on clinic 'away-day' trips, adventure weekends or holidays for children and families with diabetes. Whenever possible, positive encouragement should be given to the patient as constant negative criticism by the clinical staff and/or family is unlikely to encourage compliance.

Needle phobia occasionally occurs in younger children. This problem may be helped by the child watching the parents performing blood tests or giving injections to themselves or to a teddy bear or doll. Spring loaded and jet injectors can also help (see p. 13). Various blood-testing devices exist which allow the depth of penetration of the needle into the skin to be altered. Behaviour therapy under the supervision of a clinical psychologist can also help.

Psychological problems which are common in adolescence are described on p. 25. In addition to these, severe stress, obsessive behaviour in relation to monitoring and occasionally problems from overprotective parenting may be encountered.

Management of diabetes during surgery

There are many protocols for the perioperative management of children with diabetes. These need to be agreed by the diabetes, anaesthetic and surgical teams in the hospital. The main goals of the management of diabetes during surgery are to avoid hypoglycaemia, hyperglycaemia and DKA. Blood glucose control should be optimized in the weeks preceding elective surgery. Ideally, surgery should be performed in the morning with the patient first on the list whenever possible. In the case of an afternoon list, the patient should be first on the list if possible.

Evening prior to elective surgery
The day prior to elective surgery, blood glucose should be measured before each meal and before bedtime. Blood or urinary ketones should also be measured. In patients treated with glargine or detemir pre-bedtime, half the dose should be administered. Severe hyperglycaemia or ketosis will require overnight correction, using maintenance IV fluids and IV insulin. If ketosis persists, surgery may need to be delayed or postponed.

Morning operations
- No solid food from midnight.
- Clear fluids may be taken up to 4 hours pre-operatively.
- Omit morning insulin dose (in patients on CSII the normal basal rate can be continued till the IV fluids and insulin are commenced).
- Measure FBC, urea and electrolytes (U and Es), and blood or urinary ketones pre-operatively.
- Start IV fluids, 5% dextrose/0.45% saline with 20 mmol of KCl/litre, at a maintenance rate (for the first 10 kg body

weight – 100 mL/kg per day, for each kg between 10 and 20 kg – 50 mL/kg per day, and for each kg above 20 kg – 25 mL/kg per day) between 6.00 and 8.00 a.m.
- Simultaneously start an insulin infusion. Insulin should be administered as a continuous infusion, using a syringe pump (1 unit of short-acting insulin/mL) and the rate adjusted according to the sliding scale shown in Table 1.12 aiming for a blood glucose concentration of 6–12 mmol/L.
- Hourly blood glucose monitoring pre-operatively and half hourly monitoring perioperatively.
- Hourly blood glucose monitoring 4 hours postoperatively and subsequently 1–2 hourly depending on the blood glucose until the usual regime is restarted.
- Measure U and Es postoperatively and subsequently as indicated.
- Continue IV fluids and insulin until the patient tolerates oral fluids and snacks (this may not be until 24–48 hours after major surgery).
- Change to the usual subcutaneous insulin regimen before the first meal is taken. The insulin infusion can be stopped 10 minutes after administering subcutaneous insulin containing a rapidly-acting insulin analogue. Food can be given at the same time as the insulin injection. In the case of children on CSII, this should be started 15 minutes prior to stopping the IV insulin. A bolus dose using the CSII can then be given with the meal.
- Following minor operations it may be possible to discharge the patient after the evening meal if the child has fully recovered.

Afternoon operations
- Patient can have breakfast with the usual dose of rapidly-acting insulin. In patients on CSII, the normal bolus can be given with breakfast and the basal rate can be continued until the IV fluids and insulin are commenced.
- Can have clear fluids up to 4 hours pre-operatively.
- Measure FBC, U and Es, and blood or urinary ketones pre-operatively.
- Start IV fluids and an insulin infusion at midday (see 'Morning operations').
- Then follow protocol for morning operations.

Emergency surgery
- Remember that DKA may present with severe abdominal pain, which may be mistaken for a 'surgical abdomen'. Acute illness may also precipitate DKA.
- Keep patient nil by mouth.
- Obtain IV access.

• Check weight, FBC, U and Es, blood glucose, a venous gas and blood or urinary ketones pre-operatively.
• If ketoacidosis is present, follow the DKA protocol and delay surgery until the circulating volume has been restored and any electrolyte imbalances have been corrected.
• In the absence of ketoacidosis, start maintenance IV fluids and an insulin infusion as for elective surgery.

Minor procedures requiring fasting (e.g. endoscopy, grommets)

For short procedures (with or without sedation or anaesthesia) where a rapid recovery is anticipated, a simplified protocol can sometimes be followed by the diabetic/anaesthetic team. For instance, for an early morning procedure between 8.00 and 9.00 a.m. insulin and breakfast can be delayed and given immediately after completion.

Type 2 diabetes mellitus

Type 2 diabetes is most common over the age of 40 years but is becoming more frequent in adolescence. In the United Kingdom at present, approximately 1% of children under 16 years of age with diabetes have type 2 diabetes. In contrast, data from the USA shows that up to 33% of newly diagnosed patients with diabetes aged 10–19 years have type 2 diabetes. Prevalence rates in the USA suggest that 0.41% of teenagers have type 2 diabetes. More specifically, in obese children and adolescents in the USA, the prevalence of impaired glucose tolerance was 25% and of silent type 2 diabetes 0.4%, independent of ethnicity. Many of these patients had high risk factors for type 2 diabetes including a positive family history, a sedentary lifestyle predisposing to obesity, and African, Hispanic or Asian ancestry. Type 2 diabetes is also more common in females and in infants born small for gestational age who have remained short.

Type 2 diabetes is characterized by diminished pancreatic insulin secretion and insulin resistance. Islet cell and glutamic acid decarboxylase (GAD) antibodies are absent. Children with type 2 diabetes may be asymptomatic and therefore those at high risk (primarily children who are obese and have a family history of type 2 diabetes) should be screened. Most children with type 2 diabetes are overweight at diagnosis and present with absent or mild polyuria and polydipsia, little or no weight

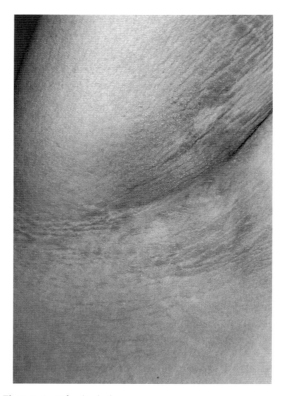

Fig. 1.4 Acanthosis nigricans.

loss, hyperglycaemia and glycosuria without ketonuria. However, up to one-third have ketonuria at diagnosis and 5–25% of patients who are subsequently classified as having type 2 diabetes have ketoacidosis at presentation. It can therefore be difficult, initially, to distinguish between type 1 and type 2 diabetes (especially in overweight adolescents). Acanthosis nigricans (see Figure 1.4), polycystic ovary syndrome, hypertension, fatty liver disease and lipid disorders may also be present.

As with type 1 diabetes, the aims of treatment are the normalization of blood glucose measurements and HbA1c, and to decrease the incidence of long-term microvascular complications. The mainstay of treatment of type 2 diabetes involves restriction of dietary carbohydrate, increased physical activity and weight reduction if obese. These measures may lead to good glycaemic control but most patients also require drug therapy at diagnosis or subsequently. The following medications can be considered:
• Biguanides (e.g. metformin), which in the presence of residual endogenous insulin secretion reduces insulin

resistance, thereby reducing β-cell demand and prolonging β-cell life.

- Sulphonylureas (e.g. gliclazide), which augment insulin secretion and therefore requires residual β-cell activity to be effective.
- Insulin therapy.

Metformin is the only biguanide therapy available. With metformin treatment, hypoglycaemia is very rare and less common than with the sulphonylureas. Oral treatment with metformin can be started with a dosage of 250 mg twice daily and increased, depending on the response, to 500 mg three times daily, or 1 g twice daily. The tablets should be taken with meals as they can cause nausea, abdominal discomfort and diarrhoea. If monotherapy with metformin is unsuccessful after 3–6 months, then a sulphonylurea or insulin can be added. Insulin is required at diagnosis in patients who present acutely with hyperglycaemia and significant ketosis or ketoacidosis. At a later stage insulin may be required if blood glucose control is poor with HbA1c >7% in spite of intensive oral medication and appropriate diet and exercise. About 10% of patients with type 2 diabetes eventually require insulin. In extremely obese diabetic adolescents with type 2 diabetes significant weight loss, an improvement in cardiovascular disease risk factors such as hypertension, and remission of type 2 diabetes may occur after bariatric surgery.

There is some evidence that in type 2 diabetes presenting in adolescents microvascular complications may be present at diagnosis and their rate of progression may be faster than in patients with type 1 diabetes. Patients should therefore be screened at diagnosis for microalbuminuria, have their blood pressure measured and have LFTs to screen for fatty liver disease. Retinal photography should be performed shortly after diagnosis and fasting lipids should be measured 1–3 months after diagnosis following metabolic stabilization. Patients may require treatment with anti-hypertensives or statins.

It is often useful to discuss treatment with an adult diabetologist as they have greater experience than paediatricians of this disorder.

Long-term complications of diabetes

Long-term complications may be microvascular (retinopathy, nephropathy, neuropathy) or macrovascular (ischaemic heart disease, peripheral vascular disease). Microvascular complications may develop in puberty or early adulthood whereas macrovascular complications affect older adults. Low socio-economic status is the single strongest predictor of poor diabetic outcome. The longer the duration of diabetes, the greater the risk of complications which increase significantly following puberty. The risk of complications may also be increased by genetic factors, poor glycaemic control and behaviour such as smoking. Diabetes is associated with a decreased lifespan of up to 15 years.

Nephropathy

The prevalence of microalbuminuria is approximately 25% and 50% after 10 and 20 years of diabetes, respectively. Diabetic renal disease may lead to chronic renal failure and necessitate dialysis or renal transplantation. Risk factors include poor glycaemic control, long-standing diabetes, smoking, and a family history of diabetic nephropathy and hypertension.

Nephropathy is preceded by the development of persistent microalbuminuria, which affects approximately 10% of children and adolescents. The urinary albumin:creatinine ratio (ACR) is used as a screening tool for this complication as timed urine collections can be difficult in children. It can be measured at any time but the most accurate measurements are those done on the first voided morning urine sample. In practice, we measure the ACR at whatever time we see the child and if it is raised (which may be due to orthostatic proteinuria) we repeat the measurement on the first voided morning urine. It should also be remembered that proteinuria may be secondary to other causes such as periods and urinary tract infections. In the United Kingdom, annual ACR measurements of the first voided urine and annual blood pressure measurements are recommended from 12 years of age onwards. In the case of raised values (which equates in many laboratories to values above 3.5 mg/mmol in females and above 2.5 mg/mmol in males and in the USA to values ≥ 30 μg/mg), the ACR should be repeated at least 3 monthly. The presence of persistent microalbuminuria may be defined as a raised ACR in two out of three early morning urines within a 3–6 month period. About 50% of patients with microalbuminuria revert to normoalbuminuria. The significance of this intermittent type of protein leak is unknown. A proportion will maintain normoalbuminuria whilst others will re-develop microalbuminuria and of those some will develop macroalbuminuria.

In patients with microalbuminuria, attempts should be made to improve glycaemic control, ideally lowering the HbA1c to < 6.5%, and this may lead to normoalbuminuria. Stopping smoking, exercise, a low-protein diet and blood pressure control should also be advocated. Patients with persistent microalbuminuria should have their blood pressure and their serum urea, electrolytes and creatinine concentrations measured and a renal ultrasound performed. This is required to help exclude other causes of microalbuminuria and to quantify the extent of any renal damage.

If the microalbuminuria persists treatment with an angiotensin-converting enzyme (ACE) inhibitor, for example lisinopril, should be considered, even in the absence of hypertension. There is good evidence in adults with type 1 diabetes and microalbuminuria that ACE inhibitors can lead to a reduction in the ACR and in some cases to reversion to normoalbuminuria, and these drugs are recommended for these patients. In the United Kingdom, there is no clear guidance on the use of ACE inhibitors in the paediatric population. It may have the same benefits as in adults. However, there is currently no evidence of any long-term benefit and ACE inhibitors can have side effects such as a cough and hyperkalaemia (serum electrolytes, urea and creatinine concentrations should be measured 5–7 days after starting treatment). Further research is necessary to evaluate their role and their current use in children under 16 years of age is controversial. It is advisable to discuss these cases with an adult diabetologist or a nephrologist.

Eye disease

The prevalence of retinopathy in adolescents varies from 18 to 47%. More than 90% of patients with type 1 diabetes will eventually develop some degree of retinopathy. Risk factors include poor glycaemic control, increased duration of diabetes, hypertension, hyperlipidaemia and smoking.

The earliest sign of diabetic eye disease is the development of background retinopathy, which consists of microaneurysms and haemorrhages with exudates which do not involve the macula (Figure 1.5). This stage is asymptomatic and does not damage vision. It may stabilize, regress with improved glycaemic control or progress if poor control continues.

Background diabetic retinopathy may, but rarely in childhood, progress to proliferative retinopathy. This can be successfully treated in its early stages with laser photocoagulation therapy. All patients with retinopathy should be referred to an ophthalmologist.

Cataracts may affect patients with diabetes but is very rare under the age of 20 years. In the United Kingdom, annual screening for diabetic retinopathy using digital retinal photography takes place from 12 years onwards.

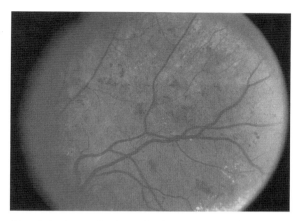

Fig. 1.5 Background retinopathy showing scattered 'dots and blots' (microaneurysms and haemorrhages) and exudates.

Neuropathy

The earliest symptoms include numbness and paraesthesia of the feet or hands with evidence of decreased vibration sense, loss of ankle jerk reflexes and a diminution in sensation to pinprick on clinical examination. However, clinically significant neuropathy in adolescence is very rare, although subclinical neuropathy demonstrated by abnormalities of motor nerve conduction velocity have been reported in 20–57% of children with diabetes.

Lipids

There is evidence that lipid levels are raised in children with type 1, and even more so in those with type 2 diabetes. However, in the United Kingdom routine screening of lipid levels in children and adolescents with type 1 diabetes is not recommended. Nevertheless, it is performed annually in some centres. If raised, the possibility of familial hyperlipidaemias should be considered. Treatment using dietary measures, life style changes or statins may need to be considered. Statin therapy is controversial in adolescents and there is no long-term outcome or safety data.

Mortality

Mortality in young adults with diabetes is increased primarily as a result of poor glycaemic control resulting in DKA or hypoglycaemia. Mortality in older individuals is raised mainly as a result of circulatory disorders, especially myocardial infarction. A reduction in life expectancy of up to 15 years has been reported. However, because of improvements in treatment, the prognosis in diabetes is constantly improving.

Miscellaneous practical matters

Driving

Patients with diabetes have a 1.23-fold increased relative risk of accidents compared with those without diabetes, which is the same order of risk as for those with epilepsy. If a teenager with diabetes wishes to drive, the following measures are required:

• The patient needs to inform the driving authorities (in the United Kingdom, the Driving and Vehicle Licensing Authority) who may request a medical form to be completed by the patient's physician. In the United Kingdom, assuming the patient has satisfactory health, is not affected by recurrent hypoglycaemia or hypoglycaemia unawareness and has visual acuity greater than 6/9, a licence for 3 years may be granted.

• Prior to driving, blood glucose concentrations should be checked, and a long journey should be broken by frequent rests and meals with blood glucose concentrations remeasured as required.

• If the patient feels hypoglycaemic, the car should be stopped, the engine turned off, the keys removed from the ignition and carbohydrate consumed.

• Stores of carbohydrate should always be kept in the car in case of unexpected delays.

School examinations

The stress of examinations can lead to impaired blood glucose control with adverse effects on academic performance. Glycaemic control should be optimized prior to examinations to try and ensure optimal performance.

Employment

Patients with diabetes should be aware that they are ineligible for certain careers. In the United Kingdom, these include the armed forces, being an airline pilot and driving heavy goods or public service vehicles.

Alcohol

Ingestion of alcohol may cause a number of problems including an increased risk of hypoglycaemia and DKA with symptoms that may make it difficult for the patient or others to distinguish between drunkenness and hypoglycaemia. The following guidelines are advised:

• The importance of avoiding drinking alcohol and driving should be stressed.

• Not to drink alcohol on an empty stomach.

• To eat while drinking or shortly afterwards.

• If drinking in the evening, to take a snack prior to bedtime.

• Not to substitute the carbohydrate content of alcohol for that contained in meals and snacks when estimating dietary carbohydrate requirements.

• To avoid beers with low sugar content as these tend to contain higher alcohol concentrations and may lead to hypoglycaemia.

• To limit consumption of low-alcohol beers with increased sugar content.

• To consume dry or medium wines in preference to sweet wines.

• To use sugar-free mixers when drinking spirits.

Drug abuse

Cigarettes and recreational drugs are widely available to adolescents and their use should be strongly discouraged. Little is known about the effects of recreational drugs on diabetes. Marijuana may stimulate the appetite and lead to binge eating with a rise in the blood glucose concentration. Drug addiction may lead to neglect of the management of diabetes with adverse effects on glycaemic control. As with alcohol, it may be difficult for a patient with diabetes and others to distinguish between the effect of drugs and hypoglycaemia.

Contraception and pregnancy

To avoid unwanted pregnancies, most teenagers with diabetes should be advised to choose between using a condom or the combined oral contraceptive pill. Using a condom has the advantage of protection against sexually transmitted diseases. Adolescents with good glycaemic control and without microvascular complications can safely use a low-dose combined oral contraceptive pill containing ≤35 μg ethinyloestradiol. Prior to prescribing the pill, hypertension and a family history of deep vein thrombosis should be excluded. Caution should also be exercised in patients with epilepsy and liver dysfunction.

Patients with microvascular disease or risk factors for coronary artery disease can safely use the progesterone-only 'mini-pill', which is marginally less effective than the combined oral contraceptive. Further advice should be sought from a gynaecology or family planning clinic.

Poor glycaemic control in pregnancy may increase the risk of congenital abnormalities and stillbirth. There is also an increased risk of macrosomia, preterm birth and neonatal hyperinsulinism with hypoglycaemia. To reduce the risk of adverse effects of maternal diabetes on the foetus, pre-pregnancy clinics have been developed to provide advice to women with diabetes in advance of conception.

Topics discussed at these clinics include the optimization of control, diet, cessation of smoking and alcohol, possible changes in other medications (e.g. angiotensin converting enzyme inhibitors), folate therapy and assessment of retinal, renal and thyroid status. Should a teenager with diabetes become pregnant, their medical supervision should be shared with an adult physician and an obstetrician with experience in managing pregnant women with diabetes.

Endocrine and other disorders associated with diabetes

Thyroid disease

This is the most common autoimmune endocrinopathy associated with diabetes. The possibility of occult thyroid disease should be considered at diagnosis and when a patient is assessed at the annual review. Thyroid microsomal antibody titres are abnormally elevated in 7–24% of children with diabetes, although their predictive value for the development of clinically significant thyroid disease is poor. Hypothyroidism affects approximately 3.9% of children with diabetes. It may be asymptomatic and significant changes in glycaemic control are not usually observed, although hypothyroidism may on occasion lead to a decrease in insulin requirements and to hypoglycaemia.

Hyperthyroidism affects 1% of children with diabetes and may also be relatively asymptomatic. However, hyperthyroidism may also be associated with increased insulin requirements. Further details of the investigation and treatment of thyroid disease can be found in Chapter 6.

Addison's disease

Addison's disease is a potentially life-threatening autoimmune disorder which affects 0.03% of individuals with diabetes. It commonly presents with evidence of recurrent hypoglycaemia and unexpectedly falling insulin requirements. Other classical symptoms include fatigue, hyperpigmentation of the skin and mucous membranes, weight loss, abdominal pain or presentation with an adrenal crisis during an intercurrent illness.

The diagnosis of Addison's disease should be confirmed by the presence of adrenal autoantibodies and inappropriately low circulating serum cortisol concentrations. Further details of other relevant investigations and of treatment with glucocorticoids and mineralocorticoids can be found in Chapter 8.

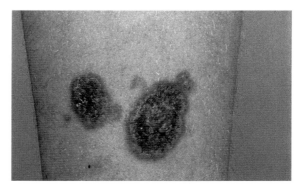

Fig. 1.6 Necrobiosis lipoidica diabeticorum on the shin.

Coeliac disease

Coeliac disease affects 3–5% of the diabetic population and may be present prior to the onset of diabetes. It is usually asymptomatic although it may present with diarrhoea, abdominal distension, anaemia or poor weight gain and linear growth. Malabsorption may lead to a fall in insulin requirements and to a predisposition to hypoglycaemia. The possibility of coeliac disease can be further investigated by the measurement of coeliac antibodies (the antitransglutaminase and antiendomysium antibodies are the most specific) and the diagnosis can be confirmed by the demonstration of the classical histological findings on a jejunal biopsy.

Treatment of coeliac disease requires a gluten-free diet. The combination of the dietary implications of a gluten-free diet and the appropriate diet for a child with diabetes can pose particular difficulties for the family and specialist dietetic advice is needed as compliance may be poor.

Necrobiosis lipoidica diabeticorum

Necrobiosis lipoidica diabeticorum affects 0.3% of people with diabetes. In childhood, it is most likely to occur in teenagers but is more common in adults. The aetiology is unknown. The lesions consist of slowly growing round or irregular non-scaling plaques with atrophic yellow centres, surface telangiectasia and livid, sometimes raised, erythematous borders (Figure 1.6,). They usually occur on the shins but may also affect the feet, arms, hands or face. The development of necrobiosis lipoidica diabeticorum is not influenced by glycaemic control. Complications include infection and ulceration of the lesions.

Approximately 20% of lesions resolve spontaneously. Treatment is difficult and consists mainly of a cosmetic approach using camouflage skin creams. Limited success has been achieved from the use of topical and systemic steroids and in extreme cases skin grafts may be necessary.

Unusual causes of diabetes in childhood

Maturity onset diabetes of the young (MODY)

MODY is a rare form of autosomal dominant diabetes mellitus developing before the age of 25 years which affects 1–2% of people with diabetes. Patients have a strong family history of diabetes in two or more consecutive generations. It results from β-cell dysfunction with the severity of the dysfunction depending on the underlying gene mutation. To date, nine mutations have been shown to cause MODY and these account for > 80% of patients.

MODY2 is caused by a mutation of the glucokinase gene on chromosome 7p. This leads to mild hyperglycaemia that develops in childhood and rarely requires specific treatment or results in complications.

MODY1 is caused by a mutation of the hepatic nuclear factor 4 alpha gene on chromosome 20q and MODY3 by a mutation of the hepatic nuclear factor 1 alpha gene on chromosome 12q. These forms of MODY lead to diabetes in adolescence which, unlike MODY2, requires treatment with sulphonylureas or occasionally insulin and may lead to microvascular complications. The identification of the gene mutation in a child with MODY confirms whether or not treatment is necessary, predicts the risk of future complications and allows specific genetic counselling.

Neonatal diabetes mellitus

Transient neonatal diabetes is rare with an incidence of 1 in 400,000 births. Most genetic mutations causing these cases are spontaneous but some of these patients have been shown to have paternal uniparental isodisomy of chromosome 6. Transient neonatal diabetes is thought to be caused by a delay in the maturation of the β-cells leading to hypoinsulinaemia. Intrauterine growth retardation (IUGR) is usually present. Permanent neonatal diabetes is even rarer and may be associated with neurological abnormalities. A proportion of these patients have activating mutations in the *KCNJ11* gene, which encodes the ATP-sensitive potassium channel subunit Kir6.2 in the pancreatic β-cell. Others may have insulin gene mutations.

The condition presents in the first few days or weeks of life with polydipsia, polyuria, marked weight loss, severe dehydration and vomiting. Hyperglycaemia and glycosuria are present but ketonaemia (or ketonuria) is unusual.

Initial treatment consists of rehydration and a continuous IV infusion of insulin. Thereafter, once daily subcutaneous injections of long-acting insulin can be introduced, though some patients are best managed by subcutaneous insulin pump therapy. Treatment in transient neonatal diabetes may be needed for a few days to 18 months (median 3 months). However, some of these patients may develop type 2 diabetes in later life.

Diabetes following pancreatectomy for persistent hyperinsulinaemic hypoglycaemia of infancy

Severe persistent hyperinsulinaemic hypoglycaemia of infancy may require treatment with a 95% pancreatectomy in early life (see Chapter 2). A proportion of these patients will progress to develop diabetes several months or years following surgery. It is usually relatively easy to achieve satisfactory glycaemic control in these patients, possibly because of residual pancreatic insulin secretion and reduced glucagon secretion.

Diabetes secondary to cystic fibrosis

Diabetes can develop in 5–10% of adolescents and young adults with cystic fibrosis and is thought to be caused by islet cell damage from chronic pancreatic inflammation. As with diabetes following pancreatic resection, glucagon secretion is reduced and DKA is rare, although these patients are at greater risk of hypoglycaemia than those with type 1 diabetes.

The diagnosis may be made on clinical grounds, by measuring the fasting glucose or the HbA1c. The most sensitive test is the oral glucose tolerance test.

Treatment consists of insulin therapy although the dosage of insulin required varies widely. These patients require close liaison between the paediatric diabetes and cystic fibrosis teams. The dietary management of these children may be rather different from that of type 1 diabetes because of difficulties with malabsorption and a frequently poor nutritional state. The adequacy of management of the diabetic aspects of these cases includes monitoring of both glycaemic control and weight gain.

Miscellaneous disorders

Diabetes is also associated with a number of other disorders such as Down's syndrome, Turner's syndrome, Klinefelter's syndrome, Prader–Willi syndrome, DIDMOAD syndrome, asparaginase and steroid treatment, thalassaemia and the autoimmune polyendocrine syndromes.

Audit

Auditing practice against agreed regional, national or international standards is an essential part of running a diabetes service. A register of all patients is essential to allow audit to take place. Increasingly, these registers are computer based. Several aspects of diabetes care can be audited including:
- HbA1c concentrations;
- evidence of normal growth, weight gain and puberty;
- the adequacy of management of newly diagnosed patients, DKA, hypoglycaemia or diabetes during surgery;
- the completeness of the annual review process;
- the incidence of complications;
- patient education; and
- the patients' satisfaction with the service.

Information gained from audit can be used to promote service developments.

Future developments

- Prophylactic therapy or earlier diagnosis through genetic and immunological screening of high-risk children.
- Immunotherapy to help prolong the life of insulin producing islet cells.
- Non-invasive methods of glucose monitoring.
- Improved versions of an artificial pancreas.
- Administration of insulin by alternative routes (e.g. oral, nasal, inhalation and transdermal).
- Glucagon-like peptide analogues which have glucose lowering effects and are used in type 2 diabetes may have a role in type 1 diabetes.
- Improvements in the management and outcome of pancreatic and islet cell transplantation.
- The development of stem cell therapy to generate a potentially limitless source of genetically modified, artificially cultured pancreatic β-cells suitable for transplantation.

Controversial points

- Should the initial insulin infusion rate for DKA be 0.05 or 0.1 units/kg per hour in young children?
- Why does cerebral oedema occur?
- Should mannitol or hypertonic saline be used in the treatment of cerebral oedema?

- Should a new patient with diabetes, but without DKA, be treated in hospital or at home?
- From what age and at what stage is an annual review necessary?
- What should the annual review comprise of?
- What are the indications for starting or changing a patient to an insulin pump?
- How much of a risk factor for future complications is poor glycaemic control before puberty?
- How can the implications of the results of the DCCT study be applied in routine clinical practice?
- In adolescents what is the role of ACE inhibitors in diabetic nephropathy and statins in those with hyperlipidaemia?
- What is the role of psychological support and motivational interviewing in helping children and adolescents to improve their glycaemic control and well-being?

Potential pitfalls

- Failure to realize that the blood glucose readings in a patient's book are fictitious (may all be written in the same pen, may not be in keeping with the HbA1c result).
- Recommending insulin doses in excess of 1.5 units/kg per day to help lower a high HbA1c when the most likely explanation is poor compliance and omission of injections.
- Failure to diagnose psychological/psychiatric problems, especially in adolescents, which may also be having an impact on glycaemic control.
- Errors in fluid calculations during therapy of DKA.
- Stopping the insulin infusion during therapy for DKA when hypoglycaemia occurs.
- Inappropriately advising the omission of insulin because the child is ill and not eating, thus increasing the risk of DKA.
- Omitting to perform annual reviews.
- Failure to identify the early signs of retinopathy when using direct ophthalmoscopy.
- Loosing track of patients, frequently adolescents, who often repeatedly fail to attend clinic (more likely to occur if no patient register is kept).
- Failure to consider Addison's disease as a possible cause for decreasing insulin requirements when the patient is beyond the 'honeymoon period'.
- Failure to distinguish between type 1 and type 2 diabetes resulting in inappropriate therapy.
- Failure to diagnose MODY in a patient with only mild abnormalities of glucose homeostasis and a relevant family history.

Significant guidelines/consensus statements

British Society of Paediatric Endocrinology and Diabetes (BSPED) Recommended DKA guidelines (2009). Website: www.bsped.org.uk/ professional/guidelines
  As well as the DKA guidelines, there is also a DKA calculator and a DKA flowchart. The guidelines include modifications made in light of the European Society of Paediatric Endocrinology/Lawson Wilkins Pediatric Endocrine Society consensus statement on diabetes mellitus (*Archives of Disease in Childhood* (2004) **89**, 188–194) and the guidelines produced by the International Society for Pediatric and Adolescent Diabetes (*Pediatric Diabetes* (2007) **8**, 28–43).
International Society for Pediatric and Adolescent Diabetes (ISPAD) Clinical practice consensus guidelines (2009). Website: www.ispad.org Contains up to date consensus guidelines on many aspects of paediatric diabetes.
Type 1 Diabetes: Diagnosis and Management of Type 1 Diabetes in Children, Young People and Adults (2004 with update in 2009). Guideline issued by the British National Institute of Clinical Excellence. Website: www.nice.org.uk/nicemedia/pdf/ CG015NICEguidelineUpdate.pdf
Lawson Wilkins Pediatric Endocrine Society. Continuous subcutaneous insulin infusion in very young children with type 1 diabetes (2006). Website: www.lwpes.org/policystatements/policyStatements.cfm

Useful information for patients and parents

Diabetes UK Website: www.diabetes.org.uk
American Diabetes Association (ADA) Website: www.diabetes.org
Juvenile Diabetes Research Foundation International Website: www.jdrf.org
Children with Diabetes Website: www.childrenwithdiabetes.com
These sites contain educational material, information on research, news and online support. Diabetes UK and the ADA have special sections for children and adolescents.
European Society for Paediatric Endocrinology Website: www.eurospe.org/patient. Information booklet on type 2 diabetes and obesity (available in English, French, Italian, Spanish and Turkish).

Case histories

Case 1.1
A 14-year-old girl had recurrent severe hypoglycaemia with two episodes leading to a convulsion and hospital admission. She was diagnosed with type 1 diabetes at 9 years of age and was treated with twice daily injections of premixed insulin with a ratio of short- to intermediate-acting insulin of 30:70, 30 units before breakfast and 18 units before the evening meal (0.9 units/kg per day). There had not been any recent changes in her diet or levels of physical activity.

Questions
1 What investigations would you consider doing?
2 If the results of these investigations proved normal, what further explanation could account for her recurrent hypoglycaemia?

Answers
1 Measurement of HbA1c concentration to assess overall glycaemic control, TFTs to exclude hypothyroidism and anti-endomysial antibody titres to exclude coeliac disease. Measurement of adrenal autoantibody titres and a Synacthen stimulation test may also be required to rule out Addison's disease.
2 Self-administration of high doses of insulin. This adolescent girl was not coping with her diabetes and the recurrent hypoglycaemic episodes were 'a cry for help'. The episodes stopped following a referral and advice from the child psychiatry service.

Case 1.2
A 15-year-old boy who had had type 1 diabetes for 5 years and who was a frequent non-attendee at clinic presented with short stature and delayed puberty. He was receiving premixed insulin with a ratio of short- to intermediate-acting insulin of 30:70, 24 units in the morning and 12 units in the evening (0.7 units/kg per day). His height had fallen from the 25th to the 2nd centile since diagnosis and his weight was on the 2nd centile. His testes were 4 mL in volume with Tanner stage 2 pubic hair. His HbA1c concentration was 11.4%.

Questions

1 How would you investigate this patient?
2 How would you manage this patient?

Answers

1 Detailed dietary assessment and measurement of TFT and anti-endomysial antibodies.
2 The patient appears to have delay in the onset of puberty which is likely to have contributed to his poor growth velocity in recent years. The dietary assessment revealed a poor calorie intake and the results of his tests for hypothyroidism and coeliac disease were normal. There had been little change in his diet or insulin dosage since diagnosis. Poor glycaemic control because of an inadequate dosage of insulin and an inadequate dietary intake is the most likely cause for his delayed puberty and short stature. Therefore, he should be advised to increase his dietary intake and significantly increase his daily dosage of insulin in an effort to improve glycaemic control. If this proves successful, this is likely to stimulate further progression of puberty and the pubertal growth spurt.

Case 1.3

A 15-year-old boy presented with a 6-week history of polyuria and polydipsia. His father had developed type 2 diabetes at the age of 35 years, which was controlled by diet. His paternal grandfather had developed type 2 diabetes at 48 years of age, controlled by diet and gliclazide. On examination his body mass index was 22.4 kg/m^2 and he was well and not dehydrated. His blood glucose was 19 mmol/L. He had glycosuria but no ketonuria.

Questions

1 What is the likely diagnosis?
2 How would you investigate this boy?
3 Why is it important to establish a precise diagnosis?

Answers

1 The most likely diagnosis is MODY. As hyperglycaemia in MODY may be mild and asymptomatic, the age of diagnosis can be considerably later than the age of onset which is the likely explanation for the late age of diagnosis in the father and grandfather.

2 By screening of genes, mutations of which are known to cause MODY. This patient was demonstrated to have a mutation of the glucokinase gene (MODY2).
3 The patient can be reassured that he is most unlikely to experience complications from his MODY, and he and his family can be counselled about the autosomal dominant inheritance of MODY.

Case 1.4

A 3-year-old girl presents for the first time with type 1 diabetes in DKA. She is dehydrated and acidotic with a pH of 7.08. She is resuscitated in accordance with the local DKA protocol and improves. However, 11 hours after admission she becomes restless and irritable, and more difficult to communicate with. She has one vomit. The nurse looking after her notes that her pulse has dropped from 120/min to 88/min.

Questions

1 What is the likeliest reason for this change in her condition?
2 What immediate investigation should be done?
3 What should be the management?

Answers

1 The likeliest explanation is that she has developed the complication of cerebral oedema. This can be present at diagnosis but more usually presents 4–12 hours after treatment has commenced. A headache (which in this girl may have been the cause of her irritability) and a decrease in the pulse rate of > 20/min (which cannot be explained by sleep or an improvement in the intravascular volume) are important early features.
2 A blood glucose should be done to rule out hypoglycaemia as the cause of her behaviour. At a later stage, a CT scan will be required to rule out other intracerebral complications such as a thrombosis or a haemorrhage.
3 A senior paediatrician and anaesthetist should be called urgently. Hypertonic (2.7%) saline or mannitol should be given as soon as possible. The patient should be nursed in a 20° head-up position to help venous drainage. Fluids should be restricted to half maintenance and the deficit replaced over 72 rather than 48 hours. The child

should be discussed with a paediatric intensive care consultant and transferred there as soon as is safely possible. She is likely to require intubation and ventilation to help maintain her $PaCO_2$ at 4.0–4.5 kPa.

Case 1.5

A 14-year-old Asian girl presents with a 6-week history of polyuria, polydipsia and weight loss. Her grandfather had developed diabetes when he was in his 50s and takes tablets. On examination, she appears overweight and her BMI is calculated as 29 kg/m² which is between the 98 and 99.6 percentiles on the BMI chart. She has some pink stretch marks and acanthosis nigricans. Her blood glucose is 26 mmol/L (468 mg/dL). She is not acidotic but has 3+ of glucose and moderate ketones in her urine.

Questions

1 What is the likely diagnosis?
2 What investigations would help clarify the precise diagnosis?
3 What treatment should be commenced?

Answers

1 The likeliest diagnosis is type 2 diabetes mellitus. She belongs to a high-risk ethnic group, has a family history, acanthosis and her BMI centile places her in the obese category. Pink stretch marks can occur in anyone who is obese. The ketonuria is unusual but does occur in a third of cases. In some cases, especially in one such as this where the patient has had weight loss and ketonuria, it can be difficult to distinguish between type 1 and type 2 diabetes.
2 Measuring islet cell and GAD antibodies would help (we don't usually measure insulin antibodies which are the least common). These would be negative in type 2 diabetes. Measuring C-peptide, which reflects the amount of natural insulin that the patient is producing, would also be useful. This would be normal or increased in type 2 diabetes but low in type 1 diabetes.
3 Though this patient is likely to have type 2 diabetes there is a possibility that it may be type 1. Some patients fall into a grey area between type 1 and type 2 diabetes. The results of the investigations listed in Answer 2 are likely to take several weeks.

In view of this, the high blood glucose and the ketosis, it would be advisable to start this patient on a basal bolus regimen. Dietary treatment and a good exercise regime are also very important. When the ketosis has resolved and the blood glucose has come down metformin should be gradually introduced with the aim of increasing the dose of metformin, decreasing the insulin dosages and eventually hopefully treating the patient with metformin alone.

When to involve a specialist centre

- Neonatal diabetes mellitus.
- Diabetes associated with hyperthyroidism or Addison's disease.
- Diabetes associated with cystic fibrosis or following pancreatic resection.
- If proliferative retinopathy or deteriorating renal function is present.

Further reading

American Diabetes Association (2000) Type 2 diabetes in children and adolescents. *Pediatrics* **105**, 671–680.

Amin, R., Widmer, B., Prevost, A. T. *et al.* (2008) Risk of microalbuminuria and progression to microalbuminuria in a cohort with childhood onset type 1 diabetes: prospective observational study. *British Medical Journal* **336**, 697–701.

Carel, J-C & Levy-Marchal, C. (2008) Renal complications of childhood type 1 diabetes mellitus. *British Medical Journal* **336**, 677–678.

Deary, I.J. & Frier, B.M. (1996) Severe hypoglycaemia and cognitive impairment in diabetes. *British Medical Journal* **313**, 767–768.

Diabetes Control and Complications Trial Research Group (1993) The effect of intensive treatment of diabetes on the development and progression of long-term complications in insulin dependent diabetes mellitus. *New England Journal of Medicine* **329**, 977–986.

Dunger, D.B., Loredana Marcovecchio, M & Chiarelli, F. (2008) Complications of type 1 diabetes mellitus in adolescents. *British Medical Journal* **337**, a770.

Edge, J.A., Ford-Adams, M.E. & Dunger, D.B. (1999) Causes of death in children with insulin dependent diabetes 1990–96. *Archives of Disease in Childhood* **81**, 318–323.

Hanas, R. (2010) *Type 1 Diabetes in Children, Adolescents and Young Adults*, 4th edn. Class publishing, London.

Lowes, L. & Gregory, J.W. (2004) Management of newly diagnosed diabetes: home or hospital? *Archives of Disease in Childhood* **89**, 934–937.

Shield, J.P.H. (1997) Relevance of the diabetes control and complications trial to paediatric practice. *Current Paediatrics* **7**, 85–87.

Torrance, T., Franklyn, V. & Greene, S. (2003) Insulin pumps. *Archives of Disease in Childhood* **88**, 949–953.

Update on Insulin Analogues (2004) Drug and Therapeutics Bulletin **42** (10), 77–80.

2 Hypoglycaemia

Physiology

Blood glucose is the main fuel for brain function and the brain is the main consumer of blood glucose. Important differences exist between children and adults in the mechanisms which maintain blood glucose concentrations within a relatively narrow normal range, and which protect the infant and child from the adverse consequences that may occur when blood glucose concentrations fall to below 2.6 mmol/L [46.8 mg/dL]. The infant and small children have relatively limited glycogen stores with larger brain:body ratios than adults and are therefore at greater risk of hypoglycaemia during prolonged starvation. However, in younger children, increased production of ketone bodies provides an alternative fuel source for cerebral metabolism when glucose supplies are restricted.

In response to feeding, blood glucose concentrations increase, stimulating insulin and suppressing glucagon secretion with the result that blood glucose concentrations are usually maintained below 9 mmol/L [162 mg/dL]. During prolonged fasting, blood glucose concentrations fall. To prevent hypoglycaemia, a counter-regulatory endocrine response occurs. The main counter-regulatory hormones are glucagon, adrenaline, noradrenaline, cortisol and growth hormone (GH). The endocrine responses to the fed and fasted states are summarized in Figure 2.1.

During progressively severe hypoglycaemia, a hierarchy of physiological responses occur with adrenaline-induced autonomic symptoms developing at higher blood glucose concentrations than symptoms resulting from neuroglycopaenia (Table 2.1). These symptoms are relatively non-specific and are particularly difficult to identify in the premature neonate and the newborn who is small for gestational age, and who is at greatest risk of developing hypoglycaemia.

Definition

There is considerable debate about the definition of hypoglycaemia. Blood glucose concentrations are influenced by the circumstances in which the sample is being taken (i.e. length of time since last meal) and to a lesser extent by the source of blood (e.g. arterial, capillary or venous) and whether measurements are to be made on whole blood, serum or plasma samples.

Hypoglycaemia can be defined in any of the following ways:
• Statistically (from the blood glucose responses of large samples of subjects).
• By the presence of physiological counter-regulatory hormone responses.
• By the presence of acute symptoms.
• In relation to evidence that a particular blood glucose concentration was associated with longer term neurodevelopmental sequelae.

When investigations into the cause of hypoglycaemia are being considered, blood glucose concentrations less than 2.6 mmol/L [46.8 mg/dL] should be taken as

Practical Endocrinology and Diabetes in Children, Third Edition. Joseph E. Raine, Malcolm D.C. Donaldson, John W. Gregory, Guy Van Vliet.
© 2011 Blackwell Publishing Ltd. Published 2011 by Blackwell Publishing Ltd.

(a) Fed state

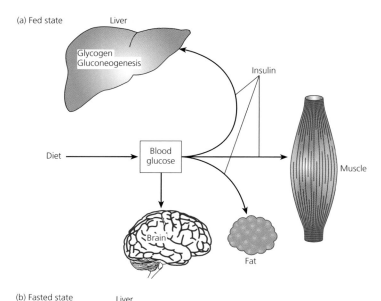

(b) Fasted state

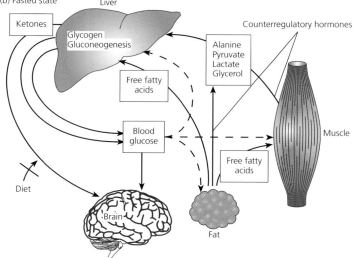

Fig. 2.1 The control of blood glucose in the fed state and the fasted state.

evidence of hypoglycaemia although it should not be assumed that such values are necessarily dangerous or that investigations are inevitably required (e.g. an asymptomatic term infant may utilize ketones for cerebral metabolism).

Aetiology

Hypoglycaemia occurs when blood glucose utilization exceeds supply and most commonly presents during prolonged fasting or at times of intercurrent illness, particularly when associated with anorexia or vomiting. Hypoglycaemia may also result when blood glucose production is limited by an impaired counter-regulatory response resulting from hormone insufficiency or an inborn error of metabolism or when excess blood glucose utilization occurs (e.g. hyperinsulinism). The main causes of hypoglycaemia are listed in Table 2.2.

Table 2.1 Symptoms of hypoglycaemia.

Neonate	Older infant or child
Autonomic	
Pallor	Anxiety
Sweating	Palpitations
Tachypnoea	Tremor
Neuroglycopaenic	
Jitteriness	Hunger and abdominal pain
Apnoea	Nausea and vomiting
Hypotonia	Pins and needles
Feeding problems	Headache
Irritability	Weakness
Abnormal cry	Dizziness
Convulsions	Blurred vision
Coma	Irritability
	Mental confusion
	Unusual behaviour
	Fainting
	Convulsions
	Coma

Table 2.2 Causes of hypoglycaemia.

Reduced glucose availability	Increased glucose consumption
Intrauterine growth retardation	Hyperinsulinism
Prematurity	Transient neonatal hyperinsulinism
Hypopituitarism	Infant of a diabetic mother
Adrenal insufficiency	Persistent hyperinsulinaemic hypoglycaemia of infancy
Growth hormone deficiency	
Hypothyroidism	Insulinoma
Glucagon deficiency	Rhesus haemolytic disease
Accelerated starvation (ketotic hypoglycaemia)	Beckwith–Wiedemann syndrome
Inborn errors of metabolism	Perinatal asphyxia
	Malaria
Drugs (alcohol, aspirin, β-blocker)	
Liver dysfunction	
Congenital heart disease	

Preliminary examination and investigation

History and examination

When hypoglycaemia occurs in the neonate, the following details should be obtained:

• Pregnancy (duration, maternal symptoms suggestive of diabetes).

• Mode of delivery (breech delivery is said to occur more often in infants with hypopituitarism).

• Birth weight (may be increased in the infant whose mother has experienced gestational diabetes or may be consistent with intrauterine growth retardation(IUGR)).

• Relationship between hypoglycaemia and feeding (evidence of hypoglycaemia related to excessive calorie intake is strongly suggestive of hyperinsulinism).

In the older child, clarify the following details:

• The maximum length of time that fasting has been tolerated without symptoms suggestive of hypoglycaemia.

• Any symptoms suggestive of hypopituitarism (e.g. prolonged jaundice in the neonatal period).

• Consider the possibility of accidental ingestion or factitious symptoms following administration to the child of oral hypoglycaemic agents or insulin.

• A careful family history, as parental consanguinity or unexplained infant death may be suggestive of an inborn error of metabolism.

• Hypoglycaemic or other symptoms, such as vomiting, diarrhoea, jaundice, hepatomegaly or failure to thrive following consumption of lactose or fructose and sucrose-containing foods, suggests galactosaemia or disorders of fructose metabolism, respectively.

Most individuals presenting with hypoglycaemia will have no abnormalities on clinical examination. Therefore, careful examination is required to identify abnormalities which may be associated with hypoglycaemia. Table 2.3 lists the most common signs and associated disorders.

Investigations

Although hypoglycaemia is a clinical emergency requiring prompt therapy, wherever possible, a blood sample for investigations should be drawn **prior to the administration of glucose**. Urine should be collected at the earliest opportunity and stored together with blood samples at $-20°$C or below. The processing of these samples should be discussed with the local biochemistry department to ensure proper storage of samples. Such samples may produce clear biochemical evidence of the cause of the

Table 2.3 Clinical signs on examination.

Clinical sign	Possible diagnosis
Optic atrophy	Septo-optic dysplasia
Cranial midline defects	Growth hormone deficiency
Short stature or decreased height velocity	
Microgenitalia	
Increased skin or buccal pigmentation	Addison's disease
Hypotension	
Underweight or malnutrition	Accelerated starvation
Tall stature or increased height velocity	Hyperinsulinism
Excess weight	
Abnormal ear lobe creases (Fig. 2.2)	Beckwith–Wiedemann syndrome
Macroglossia	
Umbilical hernia	
Hemihypertrophy	
Hepatosplenomegaly	Glycogen storage disorder

Table 2.4 Investigation of hypoglycaemia at time of presentation.

Sample	Investigation
Blood sample	Glucose
	Urea and electrolytes
	Bicarbonate or pH
	Liver function tests
	Ammonia
	Insulin and C peptide
	Cortisol and ACTH
	Growth hormone
	Free fatty acids and β-hydroxy butyrate
	Lactate
	Alanine
Administer glucose	
Next urine sample	Ketones
	Reducing sugars
	Dicarboxylic acids
	Glycine conjugates
	Carnitine derivatives
	Toxicology screen

Abbreviation: ACTH, adrenocorticotrophic hormone.

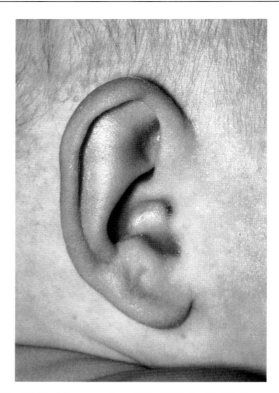

Fig. 2.2 Ear lobe creases in a child with Beckwith–Wiedemann syndrome.

hypoglycaemic episode, thus avoiding having to subject the child to further potentially hazardous investigations.

A protocol for the preliminary investigation of hypoglycaemia is shown in Table 2.4. If the blood and urine samples taken at the time of the initial episode of hypoglycaemia do not demonstrate the cause of the hypoglycaemia, then, depending on the level of clinical concern, additional investigations may need to be considered. These may include the measurement of intermediary metabolites before and after meals and the investigations listed in Table 2.4 following a prolonged fast. In addition to these, a blood sample may need to be taken for the measurement of pyruvate, glycerol, glucagon, lipids, urate, and free and acylcarnitine. It is most important to remember that any investigation, such as a prolonged fast which may render a child hypoglycaemic, is potentially dangerous. Such tests should therefore be discussed in advance with a specialist centre. The length of the fast will be determined by the age of the child (Table 2.5). Children undergoing these investigations should be closely supervised by staff who are experienced in dealing with hypoglycaemia. Therefore, the timing of the latter

Table 2.5 Length of fasts for children undergoing investigation of possible hypoglycaemia.

Age	Duration (hours)
<6 months	8
6–8 months	12
8–12 months	16
1–2 years	18
2–4 years	20
4–7 years	20
>7 years	24

stages of the fast when susceptible children are most likely to become hypoglycaemic should be planned to coincide with periods of the day when plenty of staff are available to monitor the patient and assist in any resuscitation which may be required. Intravenous (IV) glucose and hydrocortisone should be available at the bedside. All symptoms should be carefully documented, sample times clearly recorded, and on no account should a patient be left unsupervised until the test has been completed and the patient treated with glucose and/or food such that they are no longer at risk of hypoglycaemia. Should hypoglycaemia occur during investigations, the treatment is described below (see section 'Treatment').

Investigations frequently fail to identify a cause of hypoglycaemia which may occur in the context of a normal endocrine counter-regulatory response, associated with appropriately raised free fatty acids and ketone bodies. Plasma lactate and pyruvate concentrations may be normal but alanine low, suggesting a reduced supply of gluconeogenic precursors. This disorder of unknown aetiology is known as 'accelerated starvation' or 'ketotic hypoglycaemia'. It is more common in boys than girls, is often associated with a previous history of IUGR or a thin physique and usually resolves spontaneously by puberty. Accelerated starvation should only be diagnosed once other endocrine and metabolic causes of hypoglycaemia have been excluded.

Treatment

Acute treatment at initial presentation

Once the initial blood samples have been taken, the patient should be given IV dextrose (see box 'Emergency management of acute hypoglycaemia'). The response to treatment should be monitored and the infusion rate altered as nec-

essary to maintain blood glucose concentrations in excess of 4 mmol/L [72 mg/dL]. The use of intermittent boluses of glucose in concentrations in excess of 25% should be avoided because of the risk of cerebral oedema.

If the patient remains unconscious despite normalization of the blood glucose concentrations, then hydrocortisone should be administered intravenously in case of undiagnosed adrenal insufficiency. If the patient does not respond to hydrocortisone, then the possibility of an intracranial disorder or an inborn error of metabolism should be considered.

In the newborn, small-for-gestational-age baby with hypoglycaemia who is asymptomatic and tolerating feeds, increasing feed volume and frequency and, if necessary, the use of high-calorie milk formulae or the addition of calorie supplements to feeds may be all that is necessary to prevent further episodes of hypoglycaemia. If this fails, then IV dextrose should be added, starting at the rate described above.

Emergency management of acute hypoglycaemia

1 Take initial diagnostic blood sample.
2 Give 0.2–0.4 g glucose/kg body weight (2–4 mL/kg of 10% dextrose) intravenously over 4–6 minutes.
3 Start an infusion of IV 10% dextrose at an initial rate of 10 mg/kg body weight/min (6 mL/kg/h) and adjust according to longer term blood glucose response.
4 If patient remains unconscious give 25–100 mg (depending on size) hydrocortisone intravenously.
5 Collect next urine sample for diagnostic investigations.

Hyperinsulinism

Medical

There are several causes of hyperinsulinism which are listed in Table 2.2 and which should be considered when glucose requirements to avoid hypoglycaemia exceed 10 mg/kg body weight/min. Persistent hyperinsulinaemic hypoglycaemia is the commonest cause of persistent and recurrent hypoglycaemia in childhood and is heterogeneous in its clinical manifestations. Mutations of seven different genes (including those which encode the sulphonylurea receptor (*ABCC8*) and the associated potassium inward rectifying channel (*KCNJ11*)) have been described which lead to dysregulated insulin secretion from the β-cells of the pancreas.

Infants with hyperinsulinism should not be allowed to fast for significant lengths of time. In the presence of significant hyperinsulinism, enteral feeds may not prevent further episodes of hypoglycaemia and, in these circumstances, additional IV glucose should be given.

Glucose infusion rates may need to be increased up to 25 mg/kg body weight/min and increased concentrations of glucose will need to be administered through a central venous line. Most cases of hyperinsulinism presenting in the neonatal period will resolve spontaneously but, when the requirement for increased glucose infusion rates persists, the following specific treatments for hyperinsulinism should be considered:
• Diazoxide 5–25 mg/kg per day (subdivided 8–12 hourly) and chlorothiazide 20 mg/kg per day (subdivided 12 hourly); or
• Somatostatin analogue (Sandostatin) 6–40 mg/kg per day by subcutaneous injection (subdivided 4 hourly).

Side effects of long-term diazoxide therapy include hypertrichosis of the lanugo type, fluid retention and tachyphylaxis.

Surgical

In patients who do not respond to medical therapy, the only alternative is a partial pancreatectomy. Historically, histological and biochemical approaches have been used to differentiate focal (sporadic cases) from diffuse forms (inherited in an autosomal recessive or dominant manner) but recent advances in fluorine-18 L-3,4-dihydroxyphenylalanine ([^{18}F]DOPA) positron emission tomography (PET) scanning are now allowing non-invasive differentiation between these two forms. Where focal disease is demonstrated, a limited surgical resection in specialist centres of the affected area in the pancreas is usually curative. This surgery is associated with few side effects and is the treatment of choice in medically unresponsive patients. Unfortunately, in the presence of diffuse disease, a 95% subtotal pancreatectomy is required and may be associated with a risk of postoperative insulin-dependent diabetes mellitus, pancreatic exocrine insufficiency or recurrence of the disease. Where possible, therefore, surgery should be avoided in diffuse disease. If hypoglycaemia recurs postoperatively, then medical therapy should be restarted. If this is unsuccessful, further pancreatic tissue should be removed which may necessitate a total pancreatectomy.

Diabetes

See Chapter 1.

Hypopituitarism and adrenal insufficiency

Hypopituitarism in infancy may be associated with a recurrent predisposition to hypoglycaemia resulting from adrenal or growth hormone insufficiency. Hypoglycaemia should be prevented by the avoidance of prolonged periods of fasting and replacement of glucocorticoids (hydrocortisone 10–15 mg/m^2 per day) and GH (0.17 mg/kg per week) as necessary. At times of intercurrent illness, the dosage of oral hydrocortisone may need to be increased two- to three-fold, or the equivalent dosage of hydrocortisone may have to be given parenterally if the patient is vomiting or has gastroenteritis.

Inborn errors of metabolism

A detailed review of the treatment of inborn errors of metabolism is beyond the scope of this book. The principles of therapy involve the prevention of a catabolic state in such children by the use of frequent high-carbohydrate-containing meals and the avoidance of prolonged periods of fasting. In common with children who suffer from accelerated starvation, the use of uncooked cornstarch (1–2 g/kg body weight) mixed with a drink or yoghurt at bedtime is useful in the prevention of nocturnal episodes of hypoglycaemia. For advice regarding the management of inborn errors of metabolism at times of intercurrent illness so as to avoid hypoglycaemia, the reader is referred to an excellent review by Dixon & Leonard (1992).

Guidelines for follow-up

Infants who have experienced significant hypoglycaemia demonstrate electro-encephalographic abnormalities which persist for several hours after correction of the hypoglycaemia. There is also evidence to suggest that premature infants exposed to recurrent blood glucose concentrations below 2.6 mmol/L [46.8 mg/dL] are at an increased risk of neurodevelopmental abnormalities. It would, therefore, seem appropriate to undertake careful neurodevelopmental surveillance during childhood of all individuals who have experienced severe hypoglycaemia in early life so that appropriate support can be provided where necessary. Individuals who have been demonstrated to be at risk of significant hypoglycaemia require continued follow-up so that their tolerance to fasting with treatment can be re-evaluated as they grow older. In general, the older the subject, the greater is their tolerance to fasting.

When to involve a specialist centre

The management of infants and children with severe and potentially life-threatening hypoglycaemia, such as that can occur with persistent hyperinsulinaemic hypoglycaemia of infancy, requires urgent referral to a specialist centre for rapid diagnosis and adequate treatment to ensure that the patient does not experience preventable but irreversible brain damage. Such patients require a multidisciplinary team approach involving:
• paediatricians with expertise in endocrinology and metabolism;
• access to laboratories with facilities for undertaking the relevant endocrine and metabolic assays; and
• paediatric surgical and intensive care expertise to ensure adequate venous access for the emergency administration of IV glucose which may require insertion of central lines, etc.

Cases which should be discussed with a specialist centre are outlined below.
• Persistent hyperinsulinaemic hypoglycaemia of infancy.
• Panhypopituitarism.
• Addison's disease and other causes of adrenal insufficiency.
• Recurrent hypoglycaemia of unknown aetiology.
• Those whose planned investigations may include a prolonged fast.
• Inborn errors of metabolism.

Patients who are identified as having hypoglycaemia secondary to an underlying endocrine abnormality should be followed up in clinics in which specialist paediatric endocrine expertise is available to ensure optimization of therapy and to prevent further episodes of hypoglycaemia.

Transition

Many causes of hypoglycaemia such as accelerated starvation or hyperinsulinism are transient and resolve in early childhood or as a consequence of surgical intervention. These individuals do not, therefore, require follow-up into adult life. By contrast, children with hypoglycaemia that is secondary to disorders with life-long implications such as hypopituitarism or adrenal insufficiency will need to be followed up in adult life by physicians with expertise in the management of endocrine disorders. These individuals should be transferred to the adult service in their

mid- to late teenage years depending on local policies, once puberty has been completed. Ideally, this process should occur through joint 'transition' clinics involving both paediatric and adult specialist medical and nursing staff, facilitating a process of diagnostic review, retesting of endocrine function where appropriate, and coordination and 'streamlining' of therapeutic management.

Future developments

• Clinical studies are required to clarify uncertainties, which relate to the definition of hypoglycaemia and the relationship between severity of hypoglycaemia in the neonatal period and it's inter-relationship with other complications of prematurity which may affect neurological morbidity.
• New techniques, such as magnetic resonance spectroscopy, will allow sophisticated *in vivo* neurological studies to take place to assess further the acute adverse effect of hypoglycaemia and to evaluate mechanisms which may protect against these pathophysiological consequences.
• Identification of mutations in novel genes causing persistent hyperinsulinaemic hypoglycaemia in patients with no abnormalities in any of the known causative genes may give insights into as yet unknown pathophysiological pathways.
• Persistent hyperinsulinaemic hypoglycaemia in some patients is known to be a consequence of a mutation of a gene encoding the sulphonylurea receptor which is a regulatory subunit of the pancreatic β-cell ATP-sensitive K^+ channel. This defect leads to closure of this channel which results in membrane depolarization, uncontrolled calcium influx, and subsequent stimulation of insulin secretion. Knowledge of the pathophysiological basis of this disorder has led to interest in possible novel therapeutic approaches, including calcium-channel blockers such as nifedipine.

Controversial points

• How should hypoglycaemia be defined — symptomatically, physiologically or biochemically?
• Should clinically significant hypoglycaemia be defined by different blood glucose concentrations at different ages?
• Should hypoglycaemia be as aggressively managed in the neonate as in the older child?
• How extensively should a child with hypoglycaemia be investigated when initial tests fail to provide a diagnosis?

- What is the pathophysiological basis of 'accelerated starvation'?
- Why do some cases of persistent hyperinsulinaemic hypoglycaemia of infancy resolve spontaneously whereas others do not?

Potential pitfalls

- Failure to obtain blood samples for relevant investigations before treating a child to reverse hypoglycaemia.
- Failure to treat hypoglycaemia aggressively enough (e.g. with IV dextrose if necessary) to prevent further unnecessary episodes.
- Failure to refer infants with severe early-onset hypoglycaemia which is proving difficult to manage early enough to a specialist centre where adequate venous access can be secured surgically to prevent further unnecessary episodes of hypoglycaemia and results of investigations can be obtained relatively quickly.

- When subjecting children to a planned fast for further investigations into the cause of hypoglycaemia, inadequate skilled supervision, failure to extend the fast long enough to achieve hypoglycaemia, obtaining blood samples for measurement of hormones and intermediary metabolites before hypoglycaemia has occurred or failure to note time of blood sample on either the biochemistry request form or blood sample container.
- In children known to be at risk of hypoglycaemia, failure to make appropriate arrangements (e.g. planned use of IV dextrose and monitoring of blood glucose concentrations) to avoid hypoglycaemia while subjecting them to elective procedures requiring fasting.
- Failure to recognize the diagnostic significance of an excess glucose demand to avoid hypoglycaemia (implies hyperinsulinism) and the ineffective use of glucocorticoid treatment in these circumstances to prevent further episodes of hypoglycaemia.

Case histories

Case 2.1
A 2-day-old boy presented with sleepiness, jitteriness and hypoglycaemic convulsions. He required 20 mg glucose/kg body weight/min to avoid further episodes of hypoglycaemia. When IV glucose was temporarily discontinued, the following results were obtained from a blood sample drawn at the time of hypoglycaemia:

Glucose 1.8 mmol/L [32 mg/dL]
Cortisol 141 nmol/L [5.1 μg/dL]
GH 9.9 ng/mL
Insulin 72.4 mU/L
C-peptide 4.0 pmol/mL (fasting reference range 0.14–1.39)
Non-esterified fatty acids 0.13 mmol/L (fasting reference range 0.1–0.6)
3-β-hydroxybutyrate 0.45 mmol/L (fasting reference range 0.03–0.3)

Questions
1 What do the above results demonstrate?
2 Are further investigations indicated?
3 Is additional therapy indicated and, if so, what?

Answers
1 Hyperinsulinaemic hypoglycaemia with an inadequate cortisol response. With a blood glucose of

1.8 mmol/L [32 mg/dL], serum concentrations of cortisol should be >550 nmol/L [>20 mg/dL], growth hormone >20 mU/L [>7 ng/mL] and insulin should be undetectable.
2 A poor cortisol response in hyperinsulinaemic hypoglycaemia is not uncommon and does not usually indicate adrenal insufficiency in this circumstance. Nevertheless, a short Synacthen test may be necessary to ensure that there is no associated adrenal disorder.
3 Given that glucose requirements are markedly elevated, this infant should be given a trial of diazoxide and, possibly, chlorothiazide treatment. If this is unsuccessful, Sandostatin (octreotide) should be tried before subtotal pancreatectomy is considered.

Case 2.2
A 9-year-old boy presented to a hospital casualty department with a 2-month history of recurrent abdominal pain, vomiting and increasing lethargy. On examination, he appeared ill, dehydrated and hypotensive. An initial blood sample demonstrated the following:

Sodium 112 mmol/L
Potassium 7.9 mmol/L
Urea 28.4 mmol/L [30 g/dL]
Glucose 2.6 mmol/L [47 mg/dL]
Cortisol 290 nmol/L [11 mg/dL]

Questions

1 What additional investigations are necessary to confirm the diagnosis?
2 What emergency treatment is required?
3 What further clinical sign may help to establish the diagnosis?

Answers

1 Measurement of serum concentrations of adrenocorticotrophic hormone (ACTH), 17-hydroxyprogesterone, adrenal autoantibodies, and urinary steroid metabolite analysis should distinguish primary from secondary adrenal failure and the various causes of congenital adrenal hyperplasia from Addison's disease.
2 Ensure an airway and adequate respiratory support as required. Parenteral hydrocortisone (approximately 60 mg/m^2 per day, subdivided 6–8 hourly), IV glucose 200 mg/kg body weight given over 4–6 minutes and a bolus of 10–20 mL/kg body weight of IV saline (0.9%) should be given to restore the circulation. Thereafter, an infusion of 0.9% saline with dextrose (5–10% as required) should be continued. When able to take medication orally, fludrocortisone should be started.
3 Increased skin pigmentation, especially of the palmar creases, genitalia, nipples and areas exposed to sunlight, is a consequence of increased melanin production in primary adrenal failure.

Case 2.3

An 18-month-old boy presented to a hospital casualty department one morning with hypoglycaemia (confirmed laboratory plasma glucose of 1.7 mmol/l [31 mg/dL]) having refused his bottle of milk the night before and then having awoken vomiting. Most evenings when well, he consumes two rusks and a bottle of milk before bed. On examination, he had a depressed conscious level, his height and weight were just below the 0.4th centile but there were no other abnormal findings. An initial blood sample demonstrated the following:

Sodium 134 mmol/L
Potassium 3.5 mmol/L
Urea 5.8 mmol/L [6 g/dL]
Cortisol 1154 nmol/L [41.7 µg/dL]
GH 8.1 ng/mL
Insulin and C-peptide undetectable

Questions

1 What additional investigations are necessary?
2 What emergency treatment is required?
3 If no biochemical abnormalities of counter-regulation can be identified, what prognosis can the parents be offered?

Answers

1 An inborn error of metabolism should be excluded by measurement of blood pH, liver function tests, ammonia, free fatty acids, β-hydroxybutyrate, lactate, amino acids, and urinary amino and organic acids.
2 Ensure an airway and adequate respiratory support as required. IV glucose 200 mg/kg body weight should be given over 4–6 minutes and an infusion of 10% dextrose should be started at a rate of 6 mL/kg body weight per hour.
3 If no other biochemical abnormalities are identified, the likely diagnosis is 'accelerated starvation'. The use of high calorie bedtime feeds or addition of cornstarch to a bedtime drink is likely to prevent further episodes. This predisposition to hypoglycaemia of unknown origin is likely to resolve by school-age or shortly thereafter.

Case 2.4

A 5-year-old boy was admitted for an elective 20 hour fast 48 hours after discontinuation of anti-insulin therapy. He had been diagnosed with persistent hyperinsulinaemic hypoglycaemia aged 1 year following investigations into a 6-month history of convulsions. He had been clinically stable for 4 years on modest doses of diazoxide and chlorothiazide with no evidence suggestive of recurrent hypoglycaemia. He was asymptomatic during the fast with plasma glucose of 3.8 mmol/L after 15 hours and a blood sample at the end of the fast which demonstrated the following:

Glucose 3.4 mmol/L [61 mg/dL]
Insulin <3 mU/L
3-β-hydroxybutyrate 0.41 mmol/L (fasting reference range 0.03–0.3)
Non-esterified fatty acid 0.87 mmol/L (fasting reference range 0.1–0.6)

Questions

1 What does this result demonstrate?
2 What advice regarding management would you give?

Answers

1 The result demonstrates a persisting predisposition to hypoglycaemia though the absence of detectable insulin along with rising non-esterified fatty acid and ketone concentrations suggest that this is not due to persisting hyperinsulinism.

2 The results suggest that further treatment with diazoxide and chlorothiazide is no longer indicated. Whilst he will probably tolerate overnight fasting without difficulty, his parents should be advised to monitor blood glucose concentrations at times of illness, particularly if he is 'off his food' as he may be at increased risk of hypoglycaemia in such circumstances. In fact, 4 years after this test he remained well. Mutational screening of the sulphonylurea receptor, potassium inward rectifying channel, glutamate dehydrogenase and glucokinase genes failed to show any disease-causing mutations.

Significant guidelines

UK Baby Friendly Initiative (2008) Guidance on the development of policies and guidelines for the prevention and management of hypoglycaemia of the Newborn. Unicef.

Useful information for patients and parents

www.bsped.org.uk/patients/serono/index.htm and http://www.eurospe.org/patient/English/index.html are links providing downloadable booklets endorsed by the British Society for Paediatric Endocrinology and Diabetes (BSPED) and European Society for Paediatric Endocrinology which provide information for children and their families about the management of hypoglycaemia associated with endocrine disorders.

Further reading

Deshpande, S. & Ward Platt, M. (2005) The investigation and management of neonatal hypoglycaemia.–hidden weblink *Seminars in Fetal and Neonatal Medicine* **10**, 351–361.

Dixon, M.A. & Leonard, J.V. (1992) Intercurrent illness in inborn errors of intermediary metabolism. *Archives of Disease in Childhood* **67**, 1387–1391.

Gregory, J.W. & Aynsley-Green, A. (eds) (1993) *Ballière's Clinical Endocrinology and Metabolism: Hypoglycaemia*. Ballière Tindall, London.

Kapoor, R.R., Flanagan, S.E., James, C., Shield, J., Ellard, S. & Hussain, K. (2009) Hyperinsulinaemic hypoglycaemia. *Archives of Disease in Childhood* **94**, 450–457.

Matyka, K., Ford-Adams, M. & Dunger, D.B. (2002) Hypoglycaemia and counterregulation during childhood. *Hormone Research* **57**(Suppl 1), 85–90.

Mitrakou, A., Ryan, C., Veneman, T. *et al.* (1991) Hierarchy of glycemic thresholds for counter-regulatory hormone secretion, symptoms and cerebral dysfunction. *American Journal of Physiology (Endocrinology and Metabolism)* **260**, E67–E74.

Morris, A.A.M., Thekekara, A., Wilks, Z., Clayton, P.T., Leonard, J.V. & Aynsley-Green, A. (1996) Evaluation of fasts for investigating hypoglycaemia or suspected metabolic disease. *Archives of Disease in Childhood* **75**, 115–119.

3   Short Stature

Introduction

The term 'auxology' (Greek root, 'auxien' — to increase) is used to describe the study of human growth using repeated measurements of the same individual over successive time periods. It was Professor James Tanner in the 1970s who established auxology as a scientific discipline and introduced its routine use as an essential part of clinical growth assessment.

Definitions of short stature, failure to thrive and growth failure

Short stature can be defined both in terms of auxology and perception. In auxological terms, **short stature** refers to **height** which is less than two standard deviations below the mean for the population concerned; this corresponds to height below the 2nd or 3rd centile, depending on what growth charts are used. In terms of perception, short stature can be defined as small size sufficient to cause physical, psychological or social concerns in the child and family. Short stature should be distinguished from **failure to thrive** or weight faltering, a term usually applied to infants and pre-school children which denotes failure to gain **weight** at an appropriate rate; and **growth failure** –

failure to maintain a **height velocity** which is appropriate for both age and maturity.

In most patients, short stature is a variation of normal physiology rather than a pathological process. However, in order for the paediatrician to make a correct diagnosis, a logical process of assessment, based on clinical and laboratory procedures, is required.

Physiology of growth

Normal linear growth
Human linear growth can be divided into the three phases – infancy, childhood and puberty as described by Karlberg (see Figure 3.1). These are not distinct entities, for the process of growth is a continuum. However, during these periods of development distinct features of growth can be recognized, corresponding with subtly different regulatory mechanisms.

Infantile phase
This can be regarded as a continuation of the foetal growth curve, beginning at conception. The infantile curve is rapid but decelerating, with approximately 25 cm of growth in the first 12 months of life, and 12.5 cm during the second year. The major regulating influence on growth in infancy is nutritional status. Impairment of the infantile growth curve is seen both as a consequence, and continuation, of intrauterine growth retardation (IUGR).

Practical Endocrinology and Diabetes in Children, Third Edition. Joseph E. Raine, Malcolm D.C. Donaldson, John W. Gregory, Guy Van Vliet.
© 2011 Blackwell Publishing Ltd. Published 2011 by Blackwell Publishing Ltd.

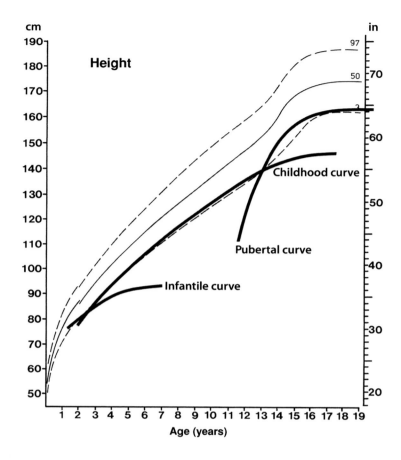

Fig. 3.1 The infancy, childhood and pubertal (ICP) concept of Karlberg showing the three growth curves. (After Karlberg 1989.)

Childhood

The childhood growth pattern starts from approximately 6 months of age and predominates from the age of 3 years. During this interval, nutrition becomes less important and hormonal influences, particularly the effects of the growth hormone (GH)–insulin-like growth factor axis and thyroid hormones – become the principal regulating mechanisms for linear growth. Impairment of the childhood growth curve may be seen as a consequence of GH or thyroxine (T4) deficiency.

Puberty

During puberty, the pattern of human growth changes dramatically, but differs in important ways between females and males (Figure 3.2). The adolescent growth spurt is caused by increasing levels of androgen and oestrogen production in males and females, respectively, as a result of hypothalamic–pituitary–gonadal activation, which results in a significant increase in GH secretion.

In females, the adolescent growth spurt starts approximately 2 years earlier than in males. Its onset coincides with the start of clinical puberty, namely breast development. The fastest point of the adolescent growth spurt, i.e. peak height velocity (PHV), occurs on average at approximately 12 years of age and the onset of menstruation (menarche) follows PHV by a variable interval, being close in early developers and more distant in late developers. Consequently, menarche occurs when height velocity is falling and is followed by approximately 2 years of gradually diminishing growth. A further difference between females and males is the amplitude of PHV which, in females, reaches approximately 8 cm per year compared with 10 cm per year in males.

In males, the adolescent growth spurt begins when puberty is already well established and coincides with a testicular volume of 10–12 mL. PHV is reached at an average age of approximately 14 years (15 mL testicular volume). The average difference in adult height between

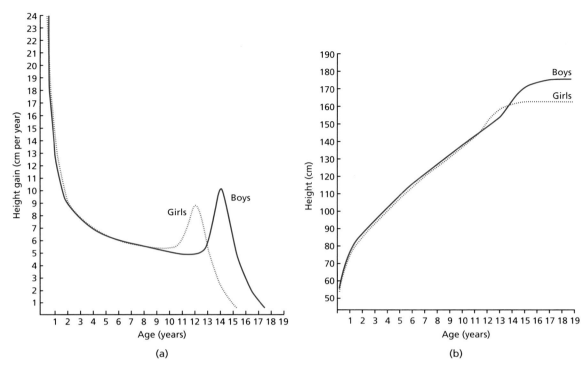

Fig. 3.2 (a) Height velocity and (b) typical individual height curves in girls and boys throughout childhood and adolescence. (From Tanner 1986.)

males and females is 12.5–14 cm, (roughly 5 inches) according to UK standards, being accounted for by two additional years of prepubertal growth, a greater amplitude of the adolescent growth spurt, and a larger prepubertal height in males.

Absence of the pubertal curve, with prolongation of the childhood curve, will be seen in delayed puberty. Failure of the pubertal growth spurt despite normal pubertal development is seen in GH (and T4) deficiency.

Endocrine control of growth

GH secretion

GH is the major endocrine regulator of linear growth. GH is a single-chain polypeptide consisting of 191 amino acids which circulates in the blood bound to one or more GH binding proteins (GHBP). The predominant form (75%) of GH exists as a 22 kDa protein with 5–10% of pituitary GH release represented by a smaller 20 kDa form which lacks amino acids in positions 32–46. GH is secreted by somatotroph cells of the anterior pituitary gland under the dual regulation of two hypothalamic peptides: GH-releasing hormone (GHRH) which is stimulatory, and somatostatin which is inhibitory to GH synthesis and release. These two peptides are, in turn, influenced by central neurotransmitters. GH is secreted in an episodic or pulsatile manner, reflecting the interaction of GHRH and somatostatin. Secretion of GH, mostly via its hypothalamic control, is influenced by a wide variety of environmental, genetic and physiological factors including nutrition, sleep, exercise and stress.

GH–insulin-like growth factor axis
(Figure 3.3)
The insulin-like growth factors (IGF-I, IGF-II) are related peptides, which are thought to mediate many of the biological actions of GH. The IGFs were named as such because of their close structural relationship with pro-insulin and their weak insulin-like metabolic effects.

IGF-I is a single-chain polypeptide of 70 amino acids which is encoded from a complex gene on chromosome 12. IGF-I is the product of the binding of GH to its receptor in the liver and other target organs. The concentration

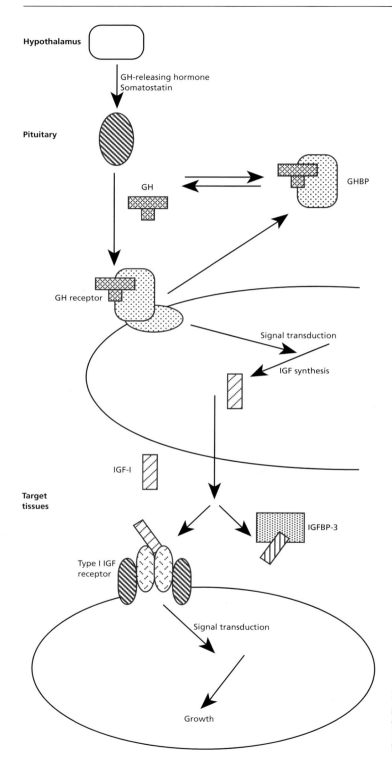

Hypothalamus

GH-releasing hormone
Somatostatin

Pituitary

GH

GHBP

GH receptor

Signal transduction

IGF synthesis

IGF-I

**Target
tissues**

IGFBP-3

Type I IGF
receptor

Signal transduction

Growth

Fig. 3.3 The growth hormone–insulin-like growth factor axis. GH = growth hormone, GHBP = growth hormone binding protein, IGF = insulin-like growth factor, IGFBP = IGF binding protein.

of IGF-I in the circulation is closely related to physiological secretion of GH, although this relationship may be disturbed in a number of pathological states. IGF-I interacts specifically with a number of soluble proteins called IGF-binding proteins (IGFBPs). The principal carrier protein for IGF-I is IGFBP-3, the systemic levels of which depend on GH status. When IGFBP-3 has an IGF molecule bound to it, it can then associate with a further GH-dependent glycoprotein, known as 'acid-labile subunit' (ALS), to form a ternary complex.

Consequently, unlike insulin, most IGF-I circulates in an inactive or bound form. The IGFBPs extend the half-life of the IGF peptides, transport them to target cells and modulate their interaction with their respective receptors. IGF-I binds to the type 1 IGF receptor in target tissues, such as the growth plate at the ends of long bones. Therefore, the GH–IGF axis is, according to our current knowledge, the predominant endocrine axis relating to growth and its integrity directly influences linear growth during infancy, childhood and puberty.

Clinical assessment of growth (see Appendix 2 for Growth Charts)

Techniques of measurement

Accurate measurement is essential for growth assessment and is therefore an important clinical skill. Errors may be the result of unreliable equipment, and due to measurement error. Ideally, a **single** trained measurer — or, at the most two – should measure children in a single clinic. Standardizing measurement techniques will minimise inaccuracies in measurement. The following techniques enable reliable data to be collected from the most commonly used measurements.

Weight

Ideally, babies and infants up to the age of 2 years should be weighed nude, using specialised digital baby/toddler scales. Nappies should always be removed. If the infant is especially fractious and will not lie or sit still enough for a reading to be taken it is acceptable to weigh the parent and child together and then the parent separately and calculate the child's weight by subtraction. For children over 2 years weight should be taken with the subject wearing the minimum of clothing on standing or sitting scales. In 2003, weighing scales used for monitoring, diagnostic and medical treatment purposes became subject to European Union regulations. Scales used for weighing patients in hospitals and medical centres must have a Grade III level of accuracy and use metric units only.

Measurement of standing height

The cost of equipment for measuring height varies considerably. The stadiometer is recommended for use with children from the age of 2 years. The subject stands with heels (without shoes and socks), buttocks and shoulder blades against the backplate and the measurer ensures that the imaginary line from the centre of the external auditory meatus to the lower border of the eye socket (the Frankfurt plane) is horizontal. The measurer then applies pressure on the mastoid processes and the reading is taken at maximum extension without the heels losing contact with the baseboard.

Measurement of supine length in children from birth to 2 years of age

Neonates and toddlers are notoriously difficult to measure accurately. The supine table and neonatometer, both consisting of a flat surface with a fixed headboard and moving baseplate, are two devices developed to reduce error in measuring babies and children too young to stand up (Figure 3.4). Two people are necessary to obtain a reliable measurement. The assistant holds the child's head in firm contact with the headboard, so that the Frankfurt plane is vertical; with neonates it is also advisable to use the forefingers to pin the shoulders down. At the same time, the legs of the (by now almost always bawling!) child are straightened and when the measurer is satisfied that the head is still in contact with the headboard, the measurement can be taken.

Sitting height

Technically more difficult to measure than standing height, sitting height is required to derive subischial leg length and thus assess body proportion. A sitting height table is required and the subject sits on the table with the back of the knees resting on the edge, with the feet supported on a variable height step so that the upper surface of the thighs is horizontal. The subject is then asked to sit up straight. The headboard is placed on the subject's head, upward pressure is then applied to the mastoid process and the measurement is taken.

Skinfold measurement

Skinfold measurements, traditionally using triceps and subscapular sites, are not essential in routine clinical paediatric endocrine practice. They are of value in research

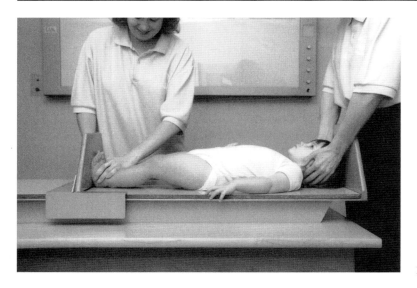

Fig. 3.4 Measurement of supine length.

studies of nutritional status and of therapy such as GH which influences subcutaneous fat.

Upper arm circumference

Upper arm circumference is also not used in routine clinical practice in the developed world. The site for measurement is mid-way between the acromion and the olecranon process.

Head circumference

Head circumference is an important measurement of normal growth and should be routine in children under the age of 2 years. The tape is slipped over the head and passed around the occipital prominence in order to measure maximal head circumference. Accurate positioning of the tape is vital to ensure reliability and the best of three measurements should be taken.

Reliability

Any competent measurer should be aware of their error of measurement. The error of measurement (Smeas) is calculated by using a small sample of subjects, i.e. at least 10. These individuals are measured twice and the difference between the two can be used to calculate the error:

$$\text{Smeas} = \sqrt{\text{S}d^2/2n}$$

where d is the difference between measurements and n is the number of subjects measured. With good technique, an error of ± 0.5 cm (2 SD) for height measurement by a single observer is achievable.

Other practical procedures for growth assessment

Decimal age

Expression of age as a decimal makes calculations, particularly height velocity, much simpler. The Table of Decimals of Year, which normally accompanies clinical growth charts, shows what decimal fraction of a year has elapsed by each day, for example 0.5 occurs near the beginning of July and 0.75 just after the end of September. So, on 2 July 1999 the year 1999 has passed 0.501 of the way to 2000 and that date can be expressed as 99.501.

To calculate the decimal age of a child seen at the clinic on 9 May 2009 and born on 26 August 1999, the decimal birthday (99.649) is subtracted from the decimal clinic appointment (109.351):

$$109.351 - 99.649 = 9.702$$

The decimal age is 9.702 years.

Calculation of height velocity

Height velocity should not be calculated from measurement intervals of less than 4 months. Intervals of 6 or 12 months are preferable. Height velocity is calculated by dividing the difference in height (cm) by the difference in interval (years). For example, a child born on 28 March 1992, measuring 132.6 cm on 3 February 2001 and 138.2 cm on 4 January 2002 will have decimal ages at the times of 8.854 and 9.772 so that the height velocity is:

$$\frac{138.2 - 132.6}{9.772 - 8.854} = \frac{5.6}{0.918} = 6.1 \text{cm/year}$$

An idea of height velocity can also be obtained by examining the growth curve constructed from a series of accurate measurements. If the height curve crosses the centile bands downwards, height velocity is abnormal and the child may require investigation.

Mid-parental height and target range

When a boy is seen in the clinic, the father's height centile should be indicated at the right-hand side of the growth chart. As the mother's height centile must be plotted on a male chart, this is done by adding 14 cm (or 12.5 cm in some centres). The mid-parental height (MPH) centile is the mid-point between these two centiles. The target range is calculated as the MPH ± 8.5 cm, representing two standard deviation confidence limits.

When a girl is seen in the clinic, 14.0 cm is subtracted from the father's height for the position of the father's height centile. The mother's true height is plotted. With normal parents and healthy children, the children's final heights will be normally distributed around the MPH, with only a 5% probability of falling outside the target range.

Pubertal staging

Staging of pubertal development using the criteria of Tanner and the Prader orchidometer in boys is **essential** in the clinical assessment of **all** patients irrespective of age. Details of the criteria for pubertal staging are given in Chapter 5.

Height and height velocity standard deviation score

Height for chronological age and bone age can be expressed as standard deviation scores (SDS) according to the following formula:

$$\text{Height SDS} = \frac{\text{child's height} - \text{mean height for age}}{\text{SD for height at that age}}$$

Height velocity SDS can be calculated according to the following formula:

$$\frac{\text{Child's height velocity} - \text{mean height velocity (for the mid age over which height velocity was measured)}}{\text{One SD for height velocity at that age}}$$

The SDS for height and height velocity at different ages can be obtained by consulting the original publications from which local growth standards have been derived. The advantage of using SDS to express height and height velocity values is that data on groups of children of both sexes and different ages can be pooled and compared statistically. Also, it is more informative to express extremely short or tall stature in SDS form than as < or << 0.4th centile, > or >> 99.6th centile, etc. When SDS values are calculated for patients in puberty, adjustments must be made for the pubertal stage of the child and the age at which PHV occurred.

Body mass index

The relationship between weight and height of an individual can be expressed by calculation of body mass index (BMI). BMI can be calculated using the formula:

$$\text{BMI} = \text{Body weight in kilograms}/(\text{height in metres})^2$$

This method has been criticized for assessment of obesity in children because the average values for BMI vary considerably with age. Normal standards for BMI in British children have recently been published (see Chapter 11 and Appendix 2).

Assessment of skeletal maturity

Skeletal age

Several methods have been developed to assess the skeletal maturity of growing children from an X-ray of the left wrist, commonly known as 'bone age'. The two most commonly used methods are the 'atlas method' (e.g. Greulich and Pyle) and the 'bone-specific scoring system' (e.g. Tanner–Whitehouse).

Greulich and Pyle method

In this method there is a published atlas of standard or typical X-rays of the left hand and wrist of normal girls and boys at specific ages throughout childhood and adolescence. The overall standard that most closely resembles the film in question is chosen and this becomes the bone age. Critics of this method claim that a single radiograph may yield bone ages that are several years apart when assessed by different observers. The standards, which are derived from North American children, are also relatively advanced (6–9 months) compared with European children. However, this method is the most widely used throughout the world, with relatively little specialized training being required.

Tanner–Whitehouse method

In this method criteria have been established for set stages in skeletal maturation. The most commonly used system is the TW2 method, which also incorporates a methodology for predicting adult height. The system is a bone-by-bone, stage-by-stage method and the assessor assigns a score to each bone according to written criteria. The composite score is the bone age. This system is generally considered by connoisseurs in the field as being superior to the atlas method as subjectivity is almost eliminated. However, specific training of the assessor is required and use of this method outside the United Kingdom is relatively limited. In 2001, this system of bone age assessment was updated to TW3 to take into account the secular trend towards more rapid physical maturation seen in many countries.

Growth charts

Growths charts are compiled using cross-sectional and/or longitudinal data. Cross-sectional charts are based on single measurements of a large number of individuals, covering the whole age range. Longitudinal charts are based on regular, serial measurements of a smaller number of individuals. Three main types of growth charts are currently available in the United Kingdom. The UK 90 charts published by the Child Growth Foundation in 1990 are cross-sectional and were compiled using contemporary UK data. They incorporate a novel nine-centile format with each centile 'band' being 2/3 SDS apart. The resultant growth curves are similar to the conventional 3rd –97th centiles, with additional curves −2.67 SD (0.4th centile) and +2.67 SD (99.6th centile) about the mean to give more useful cut-offs for stature screening. The Buckler–Tanner charts (1995) are a revised version of the former Tanner-Whitehouse charts and incorporate both cross-sectional (in the childhood curve) and longitudinal (in the pubertal curve) data, making them particularly useful for the interpretation of serial measurements. In 2010, UK–WHO growth charts for the age range birth to 4 years were introduced. These charts are based on the World Health Organisation (WHO) international child growth standards which describe the optimal growth of healthy breast-fed children from six countries. The UK-WHO charts, which were developed by The Royal College of Paediatrics and Child Health (RCPCH), combine UK90 and WHO data and incorporate both longitudinal and cross-sectional data.

Clinical assessment of short stature

Much of this is within the scope of all healthcare professionals who deal with children, including family practitioners, school nurses and health visitors. With meticulous

auxology, a thorough history and a focused examination it should always be possible to formulate a sensible diagnosis and management plan.

History
- **Presenting complaint**: Establish who is worried about what (e.g. parents but not child are concerned about small size).
- **History of presenting complaint** (three sections): Growth history (supplemented by previous measurements if available); general health including energy levels and activities; and degree of psychological upset.
- **Past medical history**: Birth weight, gestation and mode of delivery; history of atopy (an important factor in constitutional delay); relevant medical events (e.g. orchidopexy for cryptorchidism).
- **Family history**: Name, age and health of each family member; parental and sibling heights/height status; consanguinity; size during childhood and pubertal history in father and mother (including age at menarche in the latter).
- **Social and educational history:** Name and year of school; attendance, academic status, relationship with peers and authority figures; sport and leisure activities.
- **System review** (where appropriate).

Examination (with child standing initially)
- General appearance and nutrition
- Body proportions
- Dysmorphic features
- Systemic examination including heart and blood pressure measurements
- Fundi
- Pubertal status

Clinical diagnosis
The most likely diagnosis and differential diagnosis should be formulated **before** any investigations are contemplated.

Investigation of short stature

This is unnecessary in the majority of short children, for example those with normal genetic short stature and/or constitutional delay in growth and adolescence. Clinical features suggesting that investigation of short stature is indicated are given in Table 3.1. Investigation should always be seriously considered in a child whose height

Table 3.1 Clinical features suggesting that investigations for short stature are indicated.

Extreme short stature
Height centile below parental target range centiles
Subnormal/inappropriate height velocity
History suspicious of chronic disease
History of neonatal hypoglycaemia and prolonged jaundice
    (suggestive of hypopituitarism)
Dysmorphic features suggestive of underlying syndrome
    (e.g. Turner and Noonan syndromes)
Pubertal delay
Extreme parental concern

centile falls below the expected range, for example the target range centiles.

Laboratory investigations for short stature

Once the decision has been made to perform laboratory investigations on the child with short stature the doctor must proceed at this stage as a general paediatrician and not as a paediatric endocrinologist. If the approach is too specialized, disorders such as anaemia, malabsorption, renal disease, Crohn's disease or even Turner's syndrome can easily be missed. Baseline investigations for short stature are given in Table 3.2. Note that no investigations of GH status other than IGF-1 are included at this time.

The decision to investigate GH secretion in the patient is made only after the above investigations have been performed and have been documented to be normal. At the second and third consultations additional auxological information, particularly on height velocity, will be available. At this stage, further investigation of the child can be considered. Indications and procedures for investigation of possible GH insufficiency are covered in the section on the diagnosis of GH deficiency, which discusses this disorder in detail.

Differential diagnosis of short stature

The differential diagnosis of short stature is broad and involves a range of different mechanisms. The paediatrician needs, therefore, to take a broad view and to bear in mind that short stature can be the result of a combination of factors (composite short stature). For example, a child might be short due in part to IUGR but may also have short parents, poorly controlled asthma, and psychosocial difficulties. A suggested classification of the major aetiological categories is shown in Table 3.3. Several points should be noted. The classification shown separates idiopathic short stature from normal familial short stature, the former being given as a subset of endocrine causes. Also, there is some overlap between categories since some dysmorphic children are small-for-gestational age (e.g. foetal alcohol syndrome), while skeletal dysplasia is a component of other syndromes (e.g. Turner syndrome). Each category will be described briefly below.

Table 3.2 Baseline investigations for short stature.

Full blood count, ESR
Creatinine, urea, electrolytes
Calcium, phosphate, liver function tests
Ferritin, tissue transglutaminase (TTG) and endomysial
    antibodies (for coeliac disease)
Karyotype
T4, TSH
IGF-I, cortisol, prolactin
Skeletal survey if dysplasia suspected
X-ray of left wrist and hand for skeletal maturity ('bone age')

Table 3.3 Classification of short stature.

Normal short stature
• Genetic
• Constitutional delay
Short stature following smallness for gestational age (SGA)
Dysmorphic syndromes
• SGA a constant feature (e.g. Russell Silver and Foetal
    Alcohol Spectrum disorder)
• SGA not a constant feature (e.g. Turner and Noonan
    syndromes)
Skeletal dysplasias
Chronic disease (e.g. Crohn's disease, cystic fibrosis)
Psychosocial deprivation
Endocrine disorders
• GH insufficiency
• Thyroid deficiency
• Cortisol excess
• Idiopathic short stature

Causes of short stature

Normal short stature

Genetic short stature

This is the most common cause for referral of a child with short stature. Essentially, the child is perfectly healthy but has inherited short stature genes from one or both parents or, occasionally, a more distant relative. There is no endocrine abnormality and the bone age is usually not delayed, unless there is also a component of growth delay.

N.B.: Beware the diagnostic trap of assuming that familial short stature is always normal. If one of the parents is markedly short a dominant growth disorder, such as a skeletal dyplasia, neurofibromatosis or GH deficiency, should be considered (see below).

Constitutional growth delay

The diagnosis of constitutional growth delay is suggested when the child is healthy but looks younger than he/she actually is, has evidence of late maturation in terms of bone age and pubertal delay, and often the history that one parent or second degree relative (e.g. an uncle) was short during childhood with subsequent delay in puberty. Commonly, the child has a history of atopic asthma, often mild. The condition is more commonly seen in boys and in many cases there is a component of genetic short stature because it is the shorter children who tend to show slow maturation.

Frequently, the slow maturation starts in early childhood and the delay of physical development accumulates. Consequently, an 11-year-old boy could well have the physical maturity, bone age, height and appearance of an 8-year-old. Consistent with the delay in physical maturity, pubertal development is late as boys start their adolescent growth spurt only when they are well advanced in puberty with 10–12 mL testes. Constitutional growth delay can cause great anxiety to parents and also psychological disturbance in the patient due to the combination of slow growth and lack of meaningful virilization. Fortunately, effective treatment is available (see below). Typically, final adult height is within but in the lower half of the parental target range.

Short stature following smallness-for-gestational age (SGA)

The definition of SGA varies according to the paediatric discipline involved. The neonatologist defines SGA as birth weight less than the 9th or 10th centile, recognizing that this population is at risk of postnatal hypoglycaemia, and should be targeted for early feeding and capillary glucose monitoring. The endocrinologist defines SGA in auxological terms – birth weight below the 2nd or 3rd centile (i.e. more than 2 SD below the mean). Babies defined as SGA in endocrine terms will include many small normal babies but others will go on to demonstrate postnatal growth failure. The term IUGR, which implies actual intrauterine **growth failure** as opposed to **small birth size**, should, strictly speaking, be diagnosed only when serial ultrasound scans have shown impaired foetal growth. However, IUGR can often be inferred from the postnatal features and the degree of SGA.

SGA infants can be subdivided into those with symmetrical and asymmetrical growth restriction. **Symmetrical** foetal growth restriction consists of a reduction in weight, length and head circumference and is related to **early** growth failure. **Asymmetrical** SGA, with preservation of head growth, occurs because of **late** deprivation of nutrients usually related to placental insufficiency. Potential for postnatal catch-up growth is reduced in the foetus with symmetrical compared to asymmetrical growth failure. Follow-up studies on non-dysmorphic SGA infants indicate that all but 10–15% show catch-up growth by the age of approximately 5 years – it is these latter children who present to the growth clinic with short stature.

SGA can also be classified according to the cause – foetal, placental or maternal. The foetal defects can be of chromosomal origin, related to structural malformations or genetic syndromes (see section 'Dysmophic syndromes'), or to intrauterine infection. Impaired placental function can cause foetal malnutrition, hypoxaemia and acidaemia. Maternal causes include chronic illness such as renal disease and hypertension, smoking and alcohol.

In evaluating the short, previously SGA child the clinician must consider possible causes for the smallness at birth (such as foetal alcohol syndrome) whilst appreciating that other factors – familial height for example – may also be at play.

Dysmorphic syndromes

Dysmorphic syndromes can be defined as conditions arising from a specific event – chromosomal, genetic, environmental – during foetal life and resulting in a variable constellation of:
- unusual phenotype (especially face, hands, body proportions);
- growth problems – usually short but sometimes tall stature;
- developmental delay/learning disability;

- congenital anomalies (especially cardiac, renal and gastrointestinal); and
- gonadal problems.

The diagnosis of a dysmorphic syndrome is important not only in providing a diagnosis for the short stature but also in giving the child and family information about associated problems (e.g. ovarian failure in Turner syndrome) and the long-term prognosis, including the likely outcome in terms of final height.

The paediatrician seeing children with short stature needs to become experienced in recognizing clinical patterns suggestive of a dysmorphic process, and being aware of the heterogeneity of each syndrome. Professor James Tanner used to teach that identification of dysmorphic features is easier with the patient standing opposite the doctor who is sitting. Every patient in Professor Tanner's clinic was photographed, which also accentuated unusual features. The involvement of a clinical genetic colleague is invaluable, particularly in assessing the many patients with dysmorphism who do not fit into an obvious diagnostic category.

A detailed account of all the relatively common recognizable dysmorphic syndromes is clearly beyond the scope of this chapter, and is not necessary in the case of Down's syndrome, the commonest condition, in which the diagnosis will always have been made prior to referral to the growth clinic. Six syndromes which may present undiagnosed to the growth clinic will now be briefly described. Small size at birth is an integral feature of two disorders – Russell–Silver and Foetal Alcohol Spectrum Disorder – while birth weight typically falls within the normal population range in Turner, Noonan, Williams and Aarskog syndromes.

Russell-Silver syndrome

Birth weight is usually <2nd centile and almost invariably <9th, feeding difficulties are the rule, and nocturnal sweating (suggestive of hypoglycaemia) is common. On examination, affected individuals are short and thin, some showing asymmetry with hand, foot, arm or leg shorter on one side. Head is relatively large, often with expanded vault, and facies are characteristically triangular with down-sloping eyes. In our experience, intelligence is normal.

Foetal alcohol spectrum disorder (FASD)

In this condition birth weight is invariably reduced, and there is postnatal short stature associated with poor concentration, behaviour and learning difficulties. Facies are variable but may show smooth philtrum, short palpebral fissures, and malar hypoplasia. Head circumference is reduced. The history of maternal alcohol ingestion is often not available at initial presentation. Hence, SGA/IUGR children with developmental delay and poor concentration should be followed up so that FASD can be recognized.

Turner syndrome (see Table 3.4 and Figure 3.5)

This is defined as loss or abnormality of the second X chromosome in at least one major cell line in a phenotypic female and occurs in about 1 in 2500 liveborn girls. The principal features are outlined in Table 3.4 and include dysmorphic traits (see Figure 3.5), short stature (an almost constant sign) and ovarian dysgenesis (in about 90%). Associated problems include congenital heart disease including coarctation of the aorta and biscuspid aortic valve, renal anomalies which are rarely problematic, middle ear disease which can be very troublesome in over 50%,

Table 3.4 Principal features of Turner syndrome.

Features attributable to skeletal dysplasia
- Short stature (with disproportion affecting lower extremities)
- Short 4th/5th metacarpals
- Cubitus valgus
- High palate
- Micrognathia; dental overcrowding
- Broad chest

Ovarian dysgenesis

Chronic middle ear disease

Lymphoedema-related
- Hyperconvex nails +/– nail-fold oedema
- Neck webbing
- Lymphoedema hands/feet/limbs

CNS-related
- Sleeping difficulties and hyperactivity
- Specific learning difficulties: number work, visuo-spatial tasks
- Social vulnerability and isolation

Systemic malformations
- Cardiac abnormalities (aortic coarctation, biscuspid/stenotic aortic valve, aortic root dilatation/dissection)
- Renal abnormalities (horseshoe, duplex, elongated and posteriorly rotated kidneys)

Immune and inflammatory disease (e.g. Hashimoto's thyroiditis, coeliac, inflammatory bowel disease)

Miscellaneous – naevi, ptosis, epicanthic folds, oblique palpebral fissures, low set/rotated ears, low hairline

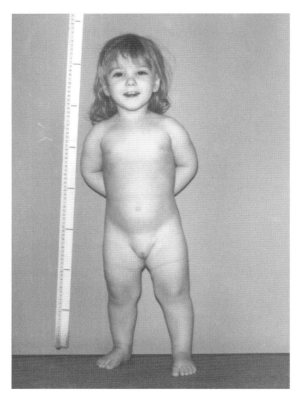

Fig. 3.5 Typical clinical features in a 3-year-old child with Turner's syndrome.

hypertension, specific learning difficulties particularly with mathematics, and a degree of social vulnerability.

Genetic aspects

Partial inactivation of the second X chromosome in all the body's cells from early foetal life goes some way to explaining the remarkably mild phenotype of Turner syndrome. However, about one-third of the genes on the short arm (Xp) are unsilenced including the *Short Stature Homeobox* (*SHOX*) gene. Loss of this and other genes results in skeletal dysplasia with short stature. Loss of genes controlling lymphogenesis, ovarian function and skin naevi result in lymphoedema, accelerated atresia of oocytes, and increased naevi (particularly on the face), respectively. The second chromosome may be completely lost (45,X), undergo duplication of the long arm (q) with concomitant loss of the short arm (p) to form an isochromosome (isoXq), undergo ring formation (rX), or deletion in the short or long arm (Xp− or Xq—). Complete 45,X monosomy accounts for 40–60% of the karyotypes on periph-

eral blood lymphocytes, while most of the remaining karyotypes show a mosaic pattern; for example, 45,X/46,XX, 45,X/46,X iXq, 45,X/46,XY, 45,X/46,XrX. There is little specific phenotype/genotype correlation for most karyotypes but phenotype is milder in the 45,X/46,XX and 45,X/47,XXX variants.

Growth

Ranke has divided growth in Turner syndrome into the following four phases:
1 IUGR (usually mild).
2 Subnormal growth during infancy and childhood.
3 Loss of 15 cm in height compared with normal girls between the ages of 3 and 12 years.
4 Absence of the pubertal growth spurt with prolongation of the total growth phase.

Final adult height in Turner syndrome from White European populations ranges from 142 to 147 cm. There is a positive correlation between final adult height and parental height. The assessment of skeletal maturity in Turner syndrome is particularly difficult because of structural abnormalities of the bones.

Diagnosis and follow-up

Because of the subtlety and variable incidence of many of these features, Turner syndrome cannot be diagnosed or excluded clinically. A karyotype analysis is therefore indicated in all girls presenting with short stature of unknown aetiology. Follow-up is required to pre-empt associated problems such as autoimmune thyroiditis, middle-ear disease, learning difficulties and hypertension and is best provided in designated Turner syndrome clinics, with good hand-over arrangements for specialist adult care.

Noonan syndrome (see Table 3.5 and Figure 3.6)

Noonan syndrome refers to a heterogeneous group of conditions resulting from various gene mutations, of which four have been identified – *PTPN11* (encoding SHP-2), *SOS1*, *KRAS* and *RAF-1*. Sporadic mutations are commonest, affected individuals then transmitting the condition in autosomal dominant fashion (see Figure 3.6). Its frequency in the general population is unknown but may be as common as 1 in 1000. Noonan's syndrome must be carefully considered in both boys and girls presenting with short stature. Its principal features are shown in Table 3.5. Growth is usually affected with height velocity being subnormal and puberty is typically delayed, with a blunted adolescent growth spurt. Ranke quotes final adult heights of approximately 162 cm in males and 152 cm in females.

Table 3.5 Principal features of Noonan syndrome.

Characteristic facies
- Hypertelorism
- Ptosis
- Low set, posteriorly rotated, prominent ears

Skeletal problems with:
- short stature
- scoliosis
- pectus excavatum
- cubitus valgus

Cardiac defects (usually pulmonary stenosis)
Cardiomyopathy
Gonadal problems (cryptorchidism in most males)
Delayed puberty
Lymphoedema (neck webbing)
Mild educational difficulties
Coagulation defect

Williams syndrome

This condition arises from a spontaneous deletion affecting 7q11.23 and may present with short stature in a child with developmental delay, increased fearfulness, hyperacusis and characteristic facies – button nose, full lips, and 'elfin' appearance. Associated problems include infantile hypercalcaemia, supravalvular aortic stenosis, pulmonary artery stenosis, hypertension, and scoliosis.

Aarskog syndrome

This condition results from a mutation in the *FGDY1* gene located on Xp11.21. The phenotype – hypertelorism, interdigital webbing, short broad hands, and shawl scrotum in males – is milder in affected females and more pronounced in their sons. Intelligence is normal and the degree of short stature usually insufficient to warrant intervention.

Skeletal dysplasias

This is a varied and complex group of disorders requiring input from colleagues in other disciplines including genetics, radiology and orthopaedics as well as endocrinology. Patients may present with severe short stature and obvious disproportion in which case the diagnosis of skeletal dysplasia is self-evident. In this situation, the family

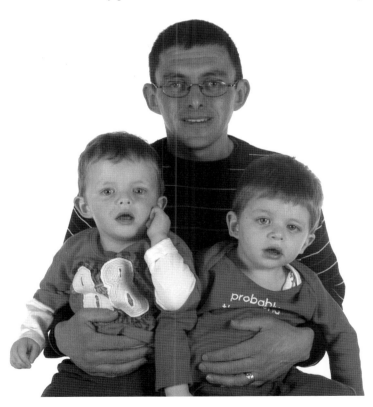

Fig. 3.6 Father and twin boys with Noonan's syndrome.

are wanting a specific diagnosis and an opinion on growth-promoting treatment options. Less severe cases may present with short stature of uncertain cause requiring a diagnosis, and shrewd assessment may be needed to detect mild disproportion. The limbs will be short in disorders principally affecting the long bones, for example achondroplasia, hypochondroplasia and metaphyseal dysplasia; the back will be short in disorders affecting the spine as well as the long bones, for example spondylo-epiphyseal dysplasia (SED). Table 3.6 gives the key features of three important disorders – achondroplasia, hypochondroplasia, and spondylo-epiphyseal dysplasia. The following points should be born in mind:

• Skeletal dysplasia may be only one component of a wider disorder, for example Turner syndrome, neurofibromatosis, and the mucopolysaccharidoses; careful evaluation of other systems including eyes, hearing, neurodevelopment and phenotype is therefore important.

• Many skeletal dysplasias are autosomal dominant in inheritance. The clinician should be wary of assuming normal familial short stature when one parent is particularly short.

• Sitting height must be measured, plotting both this and the derived leg length onto standard growth charts in both child and parent.

• Assessment should also include examination of the hands (looking for short, stubby fingers), the proportions of the upper and lower segments of the arms and legs, skull shape and circumference, and the spine for exaggerated lordosis.

• Typically bone age is advanced, and growth response to puberty blunted.

• Some children display a pattern of mild/no disproportion in the context of short stature with advanced bone age, normal skeletal survey, poor growth response to puberty, and lower adult than childhood height centile. It is possible that some of these cases (currently classified as idiopathic short stature (ISS)) will be found to represent mild forms of skeletal dysplasia which are undetectable with standard radiology.

Chronic paediatric diseases

It is well recognized that chronic illness may cause impairment of linear growth in childhood and adolescence (Figure 3.7). The child may already be diagnosed, and referred to evaluate the contribution of various components including the disease (e.g. chronic arthritis) and its treatment (e.g. systemic steroids) to the poor growth. By contrast, chronic disease may be an unsuspected

Table 3.6 Key features of achondroplasia, hypochondroplasia and spondylo-epiphyseal dysplasia

Achondroplasia
Activating mutation of *fibroblast growth factor receptor 3* (*FGFR3*) gene (located on 4p16.3) in 99% of cases
Usually *de novo* mutation; autosomal dominant transmission
Normal intelligence
Severe shortening of long bones
Relatively long trunk with lumbar lordosis
Large head with hypoplastic mid-face
Hypotonia and ligamentous laxity with associated limb pains
Narrow spinal canal with risk of symptoms from cord compression
Childhood height −5 to − 6 SDS
Adult height approximately 132 cm in males, 125 cm in females

Hypochondroplasia
Activating *FGFR3* mutation in 70% of cases
Autosomal dominant with variable severity
Normal head and face
Mild disproportion with short limbs
Short, broad hands and feet
Characteristic X-ray changes including narrowing of lumbar interpedicular distance
Blunted pubertal growth spurt
Approximate adult height 155 cm in males, 142 cm in females

Spondylo-epiphyseal dysplasia (SED)
Group of conditions including SED congenita due to mutations in the *COL2A1* gene encoding type II collagen (autosomal dominant); and SED tarda which can be X-linked (mutations in *SEDL gene)*, dominant or recessive
Shortening of trunk and limbs with disproportionately short back
Relatively normal-sized hands and feet
Atlanto–axial instability

Congenita
Associated with myopia and hearing loss
Pain, especially in hips and back
Thoracic kyphosis and barrel chest
Coxa vara with waddling gait

Tarda
Milder form with later presentation

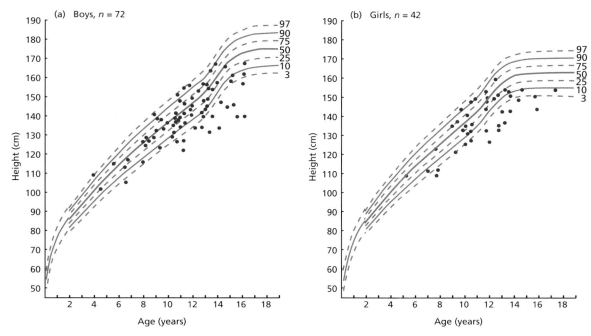

Fig. 3.7 Heights in (a) boys and (b) girls with Crohn's disease at referral to the Department of Paediatric Gastroenterology, St Bartholomew's Hospital, London.

cause of short stature. Gastrointestinal causes such as coeliac disease and inflammatory bowel disease can present in this way, while chronic renal disease is notoriously silent. The degree of growth failure varies considerably from a relatively mild effect, usually with constitutional delay, in asthma to potentially severe short stature in Crohn's disease and juvenile chronic arthritis. The mechanisms for poor growth and short stature in chronic disease are incompletely understood but include the following:

• Decreased calorie intake (cystic fibrosis, coeliac disease, Crohn's disease)
• Increased energy expenditure (e.g. cystic fibrosis, congenital heart disease)
• Pro-inflammatory cytokines (Crohn's disease, juvenile idiopathic arthritis (JIA))
• Hypoxia (cyanotic congenital heart disease)
• Metabolic disturbance (glycogen storage disease, renal failure)
• Partial GH resistance (Crohn's disease, renal failure)
• Prolonged steroid use (inhaled steroids in asthma, systemic steroids in chronic inflammatory disease)
• Delay in maturation and puberty

Psychosocial deprivation

There is an established relationship between socio-economic status and physical growth. However, it can be difficult to weigh up the contribution of the social environment to short stature and poor growth in the individual. This is because factors such as SGA, poor diet, respiratory illness related to parental smoking, and parental short stature may be contributory and of variable relation to the poor social circumstances.

It is also well recognized that particularly adverse family and social factors can delay a child's physical and emotional development. Skuse *et al.* (1996) have reported a striking variant of psychosocial growth failure known as 'hyperphagic short stature', which describes children who demonstrate abnormal behaviour with hyperphagia, polydipsia, growth failure, GH insufficiency and resistance to exogenous GH therapy. The GH insufficiency is reversible on moving the child to a favourable environment.

Psychosocial deprivation should always be considered when a child is referred with short stature, and the clinician must take a thorough family and social history. However, this diagnosis is seldom made exclusively in the consulting room. It is more likely that a child, who is found to be at risk, is noticed to be short and often underweight. The crucial role of the endocrinologist is to insist that the child be carefully measured and that height be documented. Sequential heights (and weights) may provide the only quantitative evidence of neglect and may thus be of enormous benefit to the child's future care.

Endocrine disorders

GH insufficiency and deficiency

Definition and cut-offs

These are controversial! **GH insufficiency** can be defined biochemically in terms of a peak GH level which is below an agreed cut-off level. Unfortunately, any cut-off level will be difficult to agree on, and arbitrary in nature since assays will vary between centres while the intra-patient variability of peak GH secretion is high. Severe GH insufficiency can be defined as a maximum stimulated GH concentration of <5 mU/L (μg/L), partial GH insufficiency as 5–15 mu/L (μg/L). It is important to recognize that low GH levels can be encountered in virtually any child with short stature and that low levels are not indicative of permanent impairment of the hypothalamo–pituitary (H–P) axis. It follows that GH status should be measured judiciously and carefully interpreted in the clinical context. A significant proportion of peripubertal children with short stature, slow height velocity, and low stimulated GH levels will show normal GH status on retesting once final height is achieved. In retrospect, many such children would have been displaying constitutional delay with hypothalamo–pituitary 'dormancy'.

The term **GH deficiency** (as opposed to insufficiency) can be used to refer to permanent impairment of the GHRH–GH axis, due to either congenital or acquired disease. According to this nomenclature, therefore, growth hormone deficiency is a subset of growth hormone insufficiency. We would recommend using the term 'GH deficiency' if actual impairment of GH secretion is either certain or very likely, and the term 'growth insufficiency' when GH levels are low but no definite H-P axis abnormality has been demonstrated.

While classic and severe growth hormone deficiency is clinically easy to diagnose (see Figure 3.8), milder forms are difficult to separate from normal variant short stature. The features of these two ends of the spectrum are shown in Table 3.7 and the causes of GH deficiency are shown in Table 3.8.

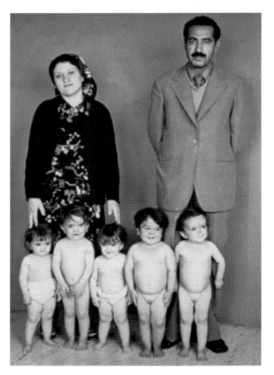

Fig. 3.8 Five children aged 2–7 years from two consanguineous families (two brothers married two first cousins who were sisters) with severe isolated GH deficiency. One parent from each family is shown in the picture. Note the excess subcutaneous fat, immature appearance and small genitalia in the affected boys. (Reproduced with kind permission of British Journal of Medical Genetics.)

Isolated GH insufficiency and deficiency

Idiopathic isolated GH insufficiency

In the majority (>80%) of cases, GH insufficiency is 'isolated', i.e. not associated with other anterior pituitary hormone deficiencies and may (see above) turn out to be a transient insufficiency rather than a permanent deficiency, falling into the 'mild' rather than 'severe' category described above. It is now known that the basic defect in most true isolated GH deficiency cases is in the synthesis or release of the hypothalamic peptide GHRH, but the precise pathogenesis is unknown. However, these patients respond to administration of exogenous GHRH by secreting GH, indicating that the somatotroph cells are functional and that the primary defect is in the hypothalamus. Magnetic resonance imaging (MRI) imaging and genetic studies are normal in this group of patients.

Table 3.7 Clinical features of severe and mild GH deficiency.

Severe GH insufficiency

    Presents before age 3 years (unless acquired)

    Obvious short stature

    Subnormal height velocity from birth, becoming more
       abnormal with age

    Hypoglycaemia

    Micropenis

    Possible associated anterior pituitary hormone
       deficiencies (TSH, ACTH, LH, FSH)

    Excess subcutaneous fat, increasing with age

    Mid-facial hypoplasia (only in extreme cases)

    Possible features of septo-optic dysplasia

    Delayed skeletal maturation

    Maximum stimulated GH concentration <5 mU/L

Mild GH insufficiency

    Unlikely to present before school entry

    Less severe short stature

    Subnormal height velocity documented by careful
       auxology over minimum interval of 12 months

    Isolated GH insufficiency

    Normal subcutaneous fat

    Delayed skeletal maturation

    Delayed puberty

Abbreviations: ACTH, adrenocorticotrophic hormone; FSH, follicle-stimulating hormone; GH, growth hormone; LH, luteinizing hormone; TSH, thyroid-stimulating hormone.

Table 3.8 Principal causes of GH insufficiency.

Transient GH insufficiency: Conditions in which GH levels may be < 15–20 mU/L on initial stimulation testing but normal on retesting

- Constitutional delay in growth and adolescence
- Short stature following smallness for gestational age
- Hypothyroidism
- Psychosocial deprivation

Permanent GH deficiency: Conditions in which GH levels are <15–20 mU/L due to impairment of hypothalamo–pituitary axis

Congenital

Inherited causes

- GHRH mutations
- GH-1 mutations (autosomal recessive, autosomal dominant, X-linked)
- *Pit-1, Prop-1* mutations

Structural defects

- Septo-optic dysplasia
- Agenesis of corpus callosum
- Holoprosencephaly
- Hypopituitarism with single central incisor

Hypothalamic disorders

- Prader–Willi syndrome

Acquired

Tumours adjacent to hypothalamo–pituitary axis

- Craniopharyngioma
- Suprasellar germinoma
- Optic glioma

Head injury

Surgery to the H–P axis

Cranial radiotherapy (e.g. for medulloblastoma)

Granulomatous disease

- Langerhans cell histiocytosis
- Sarcoidosis

True isolated GH deficiency related to genetic and structural MRI abnormalities

1 *GH deficiency of genetic origin:* These disorders are very rare in the general population, occurring in the context of consanguinity and closed communities. Severe GH deficiency is the rule. Disorders result from the following:

- GHRH receptor gene mutations.
- Deletions of the *GH-1* gene resulting in four variants of hereditary hGH deficiency:
    - type IA (recessive, absent GH, antibodies to hGH therapy);
    - type IB (recessive, low GH, response to hGH therapy);
    - type II (dominant, low GH, response to hGH therapy); and
    - type III (X-linked, low GH, response to GH therapy).

2 GH deficiency with MRI abnormality: The following three MRI abnormalities have been well documented in relation to either isolated GH deficiency or multiple pituitary deficiency (Figure 3.9):

- Small anterior pituitary
- Interrupted pituitary stalk
- Ectopic posterior pituitary (EPP)

Of these three features, EPP is the most strongly predictive of GH deficiency.

Multiple anterior pituitary hormone deficiencies

Idiopathic multiple anterior pituitary hormone deficiency

Multiple anterior pituitary hormone deficiency may present in the newborn period or early infancy with:

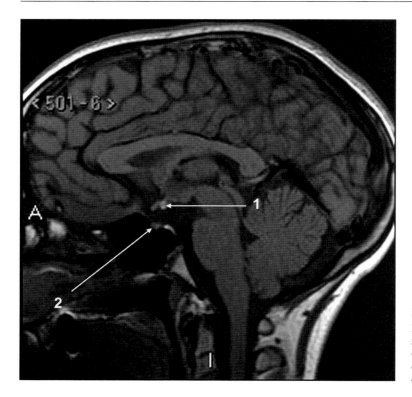

Fig. 3.9 MRI scan showing small anterior pituitary (1) and ectopic posterior pituitary gland (2) in a 15-year-old girl with GH deficiency and partial gonadotrophin deficiency. Her brother has isolated GH deficiency.

• hypoglycaemia, as a result of a combination of GH deficiency and adrenocorticotrophic hormone (ACTH) deficiency, leading to hypocortisolaemia;

• cholestatic jaundice related to low cortisol; and

• micropenis—caused mainly by prenatal testosterone deficiency secondary to luteinizing hormone (LH) deficiency and compounded by prenatal GH deficiency.

Hypothyroidism of pituitary origin is likely to be present, becoming manifest later, but usually without intellectual impairment. Subsequent imaging may show small anterior pituitary/interrupted stalk/EPP.

The treatment of congenital hypopituitarism is a neonatal emergency. It is crucial to give hydrocortisone to prevent persisting hypoglycaemia. If this is not effective, GH therapy must be added. T4 replacement will also be indicated. GH reserve should not be tested, as GH stimulation tests can induce serious and life-threatening hypoglycaemia. Low serum IGF-I and IGFBP-3 levels may be suggestive of GH deficiency.

Genetic causes of multiple anterior pituitary hormone deficiency

Gene mutations affecting the pituitary transcription factors Pit-1 (causing GH, thyroid-stimulating hormone (TSH), and prolactin deficiency) and Prop-1 (deficiency of GH, ACTH, TSH, LH, follicle-stimulating hormone (FSH)) are now well documented in families with hereditary multiple pituitary hormone deficiencies. Very rarely, genetic defects are found in structural central nervous system (CNS) defects (see below).

Congenital structural CNS defects

Congenital CNS defects occurring in the mid-line may cause GH insufficiency, usually with multiple pituitary hormone deficiencies. However, these lesions cause considerable endocrine heterogeneity.

The most frequent is the syndrome of septo-optic dysplasia consisting of two or three components of the triad:

• optic nerve hypoplasia (usually bilateral but may be asymmetrical);

- absent septum pellucidum; and
- hypothalamic hypopituitarism.

GH deficiency may be isolated, and evolve during childhood. ACTH and TSH deficiencies are common, vasopressin deficiency affects 20%. Interestingly, LH and FSH are often intact but may be partially or severely deficient in some patients. Presentation is usually in early infancy with either visual abnormality (roving nystagmus and failure of fixation), or hypopituitarism (hypoglycaemia, jaundice, poor feeding). Learning disability is a very variable associated feature, some patients being of completely normal intelligence, others severely affected. Defects in the *HESX-1* gene have been described in a very few cases, mainly familial in nature.

Other congenital defects which can cause GH insufficiency are agenesis of the corpus callosum, holoprosencephaly and arachnoid cysts. These conditions can be diagnosed by MRI scan, although the risks of general anaesthetic in the hypopituitary infant must be carefully considered.

Acquired causes of multiple anterior pituitary deficiency

CNS tumours

Craniopharyngioma

Although rare, this is the most common tumour in the hypothalamo–pituitary region to cause pituitary deficiency in childhood. The tumour arises in the region of the hypothalamo–pituitary axis and, although histologically benign, is locally invasive, involving adjacent structures including the hypothalamus, thus affecting pituitary function, and the optic nerves and chiasm. The three modes of presentation are:

- Raised intracranial pressure
- Visual disturbance because of the proximity of the optic chiasm
- Hypopituitarism with short stature, growth failure, diabetes insipidus

The management of craniopharyngioma is complex and controversial. Studies by Stanhope at Great Ormond Street Hospital, London, have emphasized the devastating endocrine and psychoneurological morbidity of radical surgery with removal of hypothalamic tissue. Complete macroscopic removal is now attempted only if damage to adjacent structures can be avoided. Otherwise the tumour is decompressed and debulked as safely as possible, following which radiotherapy is given.

Germinoma

This may present with diabetes insipidus alone for many years before the tumour itself and other pituitary deficiencies become manifest. Consequently, so-called 'idiopathic' diabetes insipidus must always be viewed with suspicion and investigated with regular CNS imaging. Bifocal germinoma with suprasellar and pineal lesions may occur. Pituitary stalk thickening may be the first radiological abnormality. Elevation of serum +/− cerebrospinal fluid human chorionic gonadotrophin (hCG) and α-fetoprotein (AFP) levels can be used as a tumour marker. Treatment is with chemotherapy and craniospinal radiotherapy.

Optic nerve glioma

Optic nerve glioma, which occurs more commonly in patients with neurofibromatosis, may also be associated with pituitary deficiency and, paradoxically, precocious puberty. Targeted radiotherapy is indicated if vision is threatened but most cases are managed conservatively, giving endocrine therapy as required.

Histiocytosis

The infiltrative lesion of histiocytosis typically involves the hypothalamus and causes diabetes insipidus. In a proportion of cases, this will be associated with GH deficiency.

Cranial irradiation

This topic is dealt with in Chapter 12. Children who have received CNS irradiation, whether for prophylaxis for leukaemia, for tumours distant from or adjacent to the hypothalamo–pituitary region or during total body irradiation are at risk for the development of GH deficiency, and thus constitute an important group for endocrine monitoring and follow-up.

Diagnosis of GH insufficiency and deficiency

As indicated earlier, most children with GH insufficiency do not come into this category of 'severe' GH deficiency (see Table 3.7). A combination of both auxological and biochemical criteria are required to make this diagnosis. GH therapy should not be prescribed without documentation of biochemical GH insufficiency.

Auxology

- Short stature
- Height inappropriately low for parental target range centiles
- Subnormal height velocity (<25th centile for age)

Biochemical diagnosis

Physiological tests

GH profile. GH secretion is pulsatile, with peaks occurring approximately every 3 hours. A pattern of GH secretion, demonstrating physiological peaks and troughs can be obtained by continuous or 20-minute venous sampling for serum GH levels through an indwelling cannula. This so-called GH profile can be performed overnight or for 24 hours. The child must be acclimatized to the ward. GH insufficiency can be diagnosed or excluded by examining the peak GH level reached during sampling. GH insufficiency should be considered if the peak GH value is < 15 mU/L. Unfortunately, GH profiling is too time consuming, labour intensive and expensive to be recommended for routine clinical practice but remains an important technique for research, when sophisticated analyses of GH secretory dynamics can be performed.

Determination of urinary GH concentration in an overnight or 24-hour urine collection has previously been used as a screening test to exclude GH insufficiency but was found to be poorly reproducible and is no longer used.

Serum markers of GH secretion or action. Serum IGF-I and IGFBP-3 reflect the status of GH secretion, provided that the GH receptor is functioning normally. In severe GH deficiency, IGF-I and IGFBP-3 levels are low, whereas in normally growing children they are normal. The problem is that there is a large overlap in both their ranges in normal children and children with less than severe GH deficiency, i.e. most GH-insufficient children, so that while IGF-I and IGFBP-3 measurement is a useful adjunct to the assessment of GH status, it is of limited diagnostic value in isolation.

Pharmacological tests

GH stimulation tests. GH levels are low during much of a 24-hour period. Therefore, GH insufficiency cannot be diagnosed by a random blood test. The GH stimulation test was established to assess the maximum serum GH level which can be released in response to a pharmacological stimulus. There are **many** pharmacological agents which will induce GH release. Those which also stimulate ACTH secretion, causing an increase in serum cortisol, have some theoretical advantage.

A particular test is usually adopted for routine use in a paediatric endocrine unit. Hindmarsh (1998), at the Middlesex Hospital, London, has published widely on the relative advantages of the different tests. Five tests are described in Table 3.9, followed by brief comments on their merits.

Table 3.9 Details of GH stimulation tests. Absolute requirements **before** all GH stimulation tests are to document normal serum T4 concentration and normal serum cortisol concentration (>100 nmol/L). Stilboestrol (priming 1 mg twice daily for 2 days) is performed in some centres before the test in patients with a bone age >10 years.

Glucagon test

Dose	15 µg/kg intramuscularly
Sampling	GH, cortisol, glucose at 0, 30, 60, 90, 120, 150, 180 minutes
Complication	Hypoglycaemia, particularly in young children; nausea
Requirement	Doctor in attendance throughout test
Contraindication	Epilepsy in young children

Clonidine test

Dose	0.15 mg/m^2 orally
Sampling	GH at 0, 30, 60, 90, 120, 150, 180 minutes
Complication	Potential hypotension
Requirement	BP monitoring

Insulin-tolerance test

Dose	0.15 units/kg intravenously
Sampling	GH, cortisol, glucose at 0, 20, 30, 60, 90, 120 minutes
Complication	Hypoglycaemia
Requirement	Doctor at bedside throughout test, blood glucose <2.2 mmol/L
Contraindication	Age <5 years, epilepsy

Arginine test

Dose	0.5 g/kg intravenously over 30 min
Sampling	GH at 0, 30, 60, 90, 120, 150 minutes
Complication	Nausea; irritation at i.v. site

GHRH test

Dose	1 µg/kg intravenously
Sampling	GH at 0, 15, 30, 60, 90, 120 minutes
Complication	Mild facial flushing

Abbreviations: GH, growth hormone; GHRH, GH-releasing hormone.

The two most commonly used tests in paediatric endocrine practice in the United Kingdom are the glucagon and clonidine tests. The glucagon test stimulates cortisol secretion, which can be an advantage if multiple pituitary hormone deficiencies are suspected. As indicated, the glucagon test can cause hypoglycaemia, particularly in young children. The insulin-tolerance test (ITT) is avoided by many centres in the United Kingdom because of the risks of serious hypoglycaemia, and should never be used for children under 5 years, nor should it be performed in a non-specialist environment. However, in the context of an established paediatric endocrine unit the ITT has been found to be safe and probably provides the best validated stimulus for GH secretion. The GHRH test stimulates the pituitary directly and the GH response may not differentiate the GH-insufficient child from the normal short child. Whichever test is used, secure intravenous (IV) access with a good-sized cannula *in situ,* oxygen and suction facilities, and experienced staff **must** be available. If hypoglycaemia occurs the symptoms can be quickly and safely relieved with Lucozade, a readily available glucose drink.

Interpretation
How many GH stimulation tests are required to make a firm diagnosis of GH insufficiency? In the United Kingdom, we usually take the view that one technically satisfactory test, if combined with valid auxological observations, is sufficient. This certainly is not the general view in the rest of Europe or the USA, where at least two tests are usually performed. Confidence in the value of high-quality auxology should remove the need for a second test. What constitutes a normal—or even an abnormal—GH stimulation test? If only paediatric endocrinologists could agree! We suggest the following interpretation of a stimulation test:
• A peak GH level during a satisfactorily performed test (with all samples collected) of <15 mU/L is suggestive of GH insufficiency.
• A peak GH level of 15–25 mU/L may be consistent with GH insufficiency if the auxological criteria are present.
• A peak GH level of >25 mU/L renders GH insufficiency unlikely.

Other endocrine causes of short stature

Hypothyroidism
Unless diagnosed early, congenital hypothyroidism leads to severe stunting of growth. The introduction of neonatal screening has eliminated this cause of short stature. By contrast, acquired hypothyroidism caused by autoimmune thyroiditis may present with short stature and growth failure, hence the need to include thyroid function testing in all short children requiring investigation.

Cushing's syndrome
Hypercortisolaemia suppresses linear growth. Consequently, most patients with Cushing's syndrome, if present for more than several months, will develop subnormal growth. Exceptions are cases where excess adrenal androgens are secreted, which may counteract the growth-suppressive effect of high cortisol. In children and adolescents with Cushing's disease, height may be significantly discrepant with weight being below the 2nd—3rd centile in approximately 50% of patients and, in contrast to simple obesity, below the mid-parental height centile. Cushing's syndrome is discussed in Chapter 8 (adrenal disorders).

GH resistance
GH resistance accounts for a relatively small number of patients with short stature. In its severe form, it presents as Laron syndrome, a very rare and severe autosomal recessive disorder caused by a homozygous mutation of the GH receptor. Growth failure is extreme in this condition, with an untreated final adult height of 120–130 cm. Milder forms of GH resistance may be a cause of short stature, but this has yet to be established.

Idiopathic short stature (ISS)
This is a descriptive rather than a diagnostic category and its definition is controversial. In this chapter, ISS refers to children with significant short stature (< -2.5 SD) in whom the problem is either not attributable to familial short stature/constitutional delay, or associated with marked short stature in one of the parents, and in which other causes of short stature have been excluded. ISS probably includes a range of conditions including partial GH resistance, and skeletal dysplasias which cannot be detected on standard skeletal X-rays.

Treatment of short stature

A great deal of attention is paid in paediatric endocrinology to the treatment of short stature with different hormone preparations. In fact, only a limited repertoire of growth-promoting preparations is available for clinical use. GH is licensed for treatment of GH insufficiency, Turner syndrome, Prader–Willi syndrome, short SGA children and short children with renal failure. Sex steroid therapy is available for stimulation of pubertal growth. Other therapies, such as GHRH and IGF-I, are used in research, but are still far from being available for routine practice.

Consequently, the paediatrician is concerned not so much with which licensed preparation to use, but rather **when** to use it. In this section, guidelines will be discussed for safe and effective use of established hormone therapies.

Constitutional delay of growth and puberty

The physical and psychological well-being of a child or adolescent with delay of growth and puberty can be safely and effectively improved by hormone therapy. In fact, this is one of the most rewarding conditions to treat for the patient, family and paediatrician. By far the majority of patients seen with this problem are boys. Society appears to favour tall individuals at all ages, consequently to be short and physically immature may understandably create psychological stress, particularly during adolescence. The indications for consideration of therapy are summarized in Table 3.10.

The natural history of this has been well documented. The final adult height usually falls short of the mid-parental centile but within the lower end of the parental target range and may be below the predicted mean final adult height, calculated on the basis of height and bone age. However, a Glasgow study reported that almost all boys with delay of growth and puberty attained final heights within the predicted range, when using the RUS(TW2) system of Tanner and Whitehouse. Patients with constitutional growth delay and their parents require regular reassurance and should be followed in the clinic at least until the adolescent growth spurt is firmly established.

Table 3.10 Indications for consideration of endocrine therapy in the patient with constitutional delay in growth and adolescence.

Short stature
Low height velocity (<4 cm per year)
Delayed secondary sexual development
Abnormal body proportions (long legs, short trunk)
Reduced bone mineral density
Psychological distress related to:
• poor self-image
• looking and feeling different or younger than peers
• lack of confidence
• depression
• school refusal
• difficulty participating in sporting activities
• difficulty being admitted to age-appropriate venues (e.g. cinema)
• aggressive behaviour, delinquency
• reduced employment opportunities
Parental concern

Aims of treatment

Males

The aims of treatment depend on the age of the patient. In the boy aged 10–13 years, the aim is to induce growth acceleration. In the boy aged 13 years and over, the aim is to induce growth acceleration together with pubertal development. For the 10–13-year-old boys, the weakly androgenic anabolic steroid Oxandrolone is helpful. Oxandrolone, a non-aromatizable testosterone derivative, is not licensed in the United Kingdom, but can be prescribed on a named patient basis. In the younger age group mentioned above, growth acceleration can be induced using Oxandrolone 1.25 mg orally at night for 3–6 months in boys aged <12 years, 2.5 mg for boys aged >12 years. This regimen will increase height velocity from approximately 4 cm/year to 7.5 cm/year during the first 6 months of therapy. There will be no virilization and bone age will not advance abnormally. If, at the end of the course of treatment, the patient shows evidence of testicular enlargement of >4 mL, linear growth can be expected to continue at greater than the prepubertal rate.

Testosterone

Testosterone therapy will induce growth acceleration and virilization. Its use is therefore indicated in the older age group mentioned above, where growth and secondary sexual development is required. Testosterone esters are licensed as replacement therapy.

Testosterone cypionate (Sustanon) or oenanthate (Primoteston Depot) 25–50 mg 2-weekly to 100–125 mg 4-weekly by intramuscular injection for 3–6 months will induce growth acceleration and virilization. A course of 3- to 6-monthly injections must be terminated to allow re-evaluation of height, puberty stage and bone age. If necessary, particularly if testicular volume is <5–6 mL, indicating that endogenous puberty is still in the early stages, a second course can be given at a later date. Kelly *et al.* in Glasgow, amongst other workers, have shown that final height is not affected when 3 monthly intramuscular injections of 125 mg of testosterone oenanthate were used in boys >13 years.

Females

In girls with delay of growth and puberty, oral ethinylestradiol 2 μg either daily or on alternate days for 6–12 months will induce some growth acceleration, which may be associated with early breast development. However, careful patient selection and evaluation is required in this situation, some specialists electing to 'cover' oestrogen treatment with GH therapy.

GH insufficiency

GH insufficiency can be effectively treated with recombinant GH. Successful treatment is potentially able to normalize height, but this is achieved at a significant economic cost and using invasive therapy in the form of daily subcutaneous injections. A fundamental biological principle needs to be accepted which is that the more severe the GH insufficiency the greater the benefit from replacement therapy.

Every child considered for GH therapy must be assessed in detail so that treatment is reserved for those who will unequivocally benefit by increase in final adult height. Currently in the United Kingdom, the diagnosis of GH insufficiency is made at an average age of approximately 9 years which is relatively late in terms of achieving an optimal long-term result. Early diagnosis and initiation of therapy must be the goal of all those involved in growth assessment.

Guidelines for GH therapy (see Table 3.11)

Before starting treatment, auxological assessment for 12 months is desirable unless the time available for further growth is limited, or the degree of GH insufficiency and short stature is severe. The following conditions should be met:

1 Pubertal assessment and bone age must indicate that growth potential exists.

Table 3.11 Guidelines for GH therapy in children with GH insufficiency.

Early diagnosis and initiation of therapy
Dose 5 mg/m^2 per week (equivalent to 30 μg/kg per day) given subcutaneously in the evening, 7 days a week
4-monthly clinic visits for assessment including auxology and pubertal staging
Enquiry as to the number of injections missed between visits
Home visit from endocrine specialist nurse if growth response disappointing
6–12 monthly IGF-I measurement to monitor dosage and compliance
Annual bone age
Discontinue GH at completion of growth (height velocity < 2 cm per year)
Retest GH status prior to adult transfer (IGF-I and stimulated GH levels)
Transition clinic for adult transfer if permanent GH deficiency confirmed

2 Height velocity must be subnormal before treatment is started.

3 Pre-treatment height velocity assessment should be available so that height velocity after 1 year of treatment can be interpreted.

4 The family must be fully committed after a detailed discussion.

The role of the endocrine nurse specialist is crucial in:

- counselling the families before treatment is started;
- assessing the likelihood of good compliance and the need for support;
- showing the family the various GH brands and devices and helping parents and child to make an informed choice; and
- teaching the technique of daily subcutaneous injection.

It is helpful to explain at the start of therapy that a formal assessment of response will take place after 1 year. At this time, an **increase** in height velocity of >2 cm per year compared with the pre-treatment value is needed to justify continuation of therapy. When no such increment exists, as may occur if compliance is poor, treatment should be stopped. If an unequivocal response occurs, treatment can be continued until final height is reached. We advise 4-monthly rather than 6-monthly clinic visits in order to adequately monitor the response to and compliance with treatment, and to adjust the dose to keep pace with body surface area.

Increasing the dosage of GH during puberty is controversial. Provided normal pubertal growth is occurring, we recommend leaving the dose regimen unchanged at 5 mg/m^2 per week; an alternative if growth is suboptimal is to increase GH to 6.6 mg/m^2 per week. After linear growth is complete, GH secretion should be retested. If GH deficiency is likely or certain (e.g. with craniopharyngioma, or genetically proven GH deficiency), an IGF-I level 6 weeks after stopping treatment is sufficient. Otherwise, a formal GH stimulation test is indicated and many patients with idiopathic GH insufficiency will now have a normal response. Those with proven GH deficiency should be handed over for adult endocrine follow-up. Experience has shown that structured handover at a transition clinic attended by both paediatric and adult endocrinologist improves the quality of transfer, and the chance of compliance with attendance at the adult clinic.

Adverse events

Recombinant GH is remarkably free of side effects. The complication of Creutzfeldt–Jakob disease associated with pituitary-extracted GH was identified in 1985 and from this time only biosynthetic GH should have been used.

Concern over a possible link between GH therapy and the development of leukaemia prompted a number of careful epidemiological studies which have demonstrated that the incidence of leukaemia, at least in Europe and the USA, in patients receiving GH was no greater than in the general population. Moreover, there is no convincing evidence that GH therapy stimulates tumour regrowth in children with cancer.

GH therapy in non-GH-deficient disorders

The availability of recombinant GH, although admittedly at very high cost, has led to its use in a number of non-GH-deficient disorders, where its pharmacological properties might benefit growth. Prominent among these are Turner and Noonan syndromes, short stature related to SGA, renal disease and skeletal dysplasias. Each of these categories will be discussed briefly.

Idiopathic short stature

The use of GH therapy in children with idiopathic short stature remains controversial and often presents the clinician with a moral dilemma. The efficacy of this treatment has been demonstrated, with several clinical studies showing a positive effect on final height. Indeed, GH therapy was approved in the US for children with this indication in 2003. In the United Kingdom, this indication has not found favour, experience showing that many of the families whose children have short stature and borderline growth hormone levels (which do constitute an indication for treatment) become discouraged by the modest increase in height status after 1–2 years, and either openly state their wish to discontinue treatment, or demonstrate their lack of enthusiasm by defaulting from the outpatient clinic.

Turner syndrome

As described above, the mean final height in Turner syndrome is approximately 145 cm. Work from an important Canadian study showed approximately 7 cm of difference between GH-treated and untreated girls. The GH dose required is higher than for classical GH deficiency and in the United Kingdom is 10 mg/m^2 per week (55 μg/kg per day). Recent evidence from a 10-year UK study has shown that the addition of Oxandrolone 0.05 mg/kg per day (maximum dose 2.5 mg daily) from the age of 9 years significantly improves adult height. The same UK study used the following pubertal induction regime at either 12 or 14 years: Ethinyloestradiol 2 μg daily during the first year; 4 μg daily during the second year; and 6, 8 and 10 μg for 4 months each during the third year. Norethisterone

5 mg daily can be added in on days 1–12 of each calendar month once an oestrogen dose of 10 μg daily has been reached, or earlier if breakthrough bleeding occurs. The UK study showed that delaying oestrogen induction to 14 rather than 12 years improved final height outcome but that this benefit was cancelled out by using Oxandrolone. Therefore, we currently recommend starting GH from the age of about 5 years, or sooner if the girl is very short, introducing Oxandrolone at 9 years, and starting pubertal induction at 12 years.

Transfer to a gynaecologist/adult endocrinologist, preferably in the context of an adult Turner clinic, should be arranged on completion of pubertal development and cessation of growth-promoting treatment.

Noonan syndrome

There are few published data on the effect of GH therapy in Noonan syndrome. The group at St. Bartholomew's Hospital, London, published the results of 1 year's treatment using a dosage of 50 μg/kg per day. There was sustained growth acceleration, with height velocity increasing from 3.8 to 10.5 cm per year. No deleterious effects on cardiac muscle thickness were detected. Long-term benefit of GH therapy is not yet established and Noonan's syndrome is not a licensed indication for GH therapy. Patients should be entered into official therapeutic trials, rather than treated on an *ad hoc* basis. Further long-term data are awaited.

Short stature associated with SGA

A number of studies have shown that GH therapy causes a dose-dependent increase in height velocity in this group of patients. De Zegher *et al.* (1998) reported that high-dose therapy for a period of 2 years induced catch-up growth. Catch-down growth has since been reported to occur if treatment is discontinued in childhood. In 2003, a European licence was granted for the treatment of short SGA children. This was based on data showing final adult height in the normal target range. The recommended dose is 33–66 μg/kg per day.

Renal disease

Chronic renal failure is a potent cause of poor growth. Treatment with GH has been extensively studied but this modality is used less often now with the advent of effective strategies which include:
- an aggressive approach to optimizing nutrition;
- meticulous treatment of high blood pressure;
- earlier recourse to transplantation; and
- keeping time on dialysis to a minimum.

GH is occasionally used post-transplantation, but better graft outcomes and reduced steroid use have decreased its role. Since patients are partially GH resistant, pharmacological doses of 0.05 mg/kg per day are required if GH is to be used. The use of GH in renal disease should be monitored in a specialist renal department with experience of this treatment.

Skeletal dysplasias

Patients with skeletal dysplasia have normal GH secretion. GH can improve short-term height velocity in achondroplasia, but the benefit in terms of quality of life (being able to reach objects, self-dress, etc.) are not well documented and there are no data on final height benefit of continuous treatment. One approach is to give GH in childhood to optimise linear growth, followed by limb lengthening from 13 years of age. However, non-intervention is chosen by many families. Data from the Middlesex Hospital, London, suggest that GH may be effective in stimulating pubertal growth, particularly in hypochondroplasia, and patients showing a disappointing early growth response to puberty can therefore be offered GH. The optimal dose is not known, but will be greater than for classic GH deficiency. We recommend a starting dose of 7 mg/m^2 per week (40 μg/kg per day).

Chronic paediatric diseases

As discussed above, the short stature of chronic disease usually results from a combination of pathogenetic mechanisms and it is not reasonable to expect treatment with a growth-promoting agent, such as GH, to overcome or eliminate these processes. The child with chronic disease may have a catabolic state which induces GH resistance, consequently GH therapy is unlikely to be effective.

The most effective treatment of the short stature of chronic illness is the effective treatment of the primary illness itself. This has been dramatically demonstrated in Crohn's disease, where successful resection of the inflamed bowel results in spectacular catch-up growth (Figure 3.10). Growth retardation in chronic inflammatory disease such as Crohn's disease and JIA results from a combination of the inflammatory process itself mediated by proinflammatory cytokines, prolonged use of glucocorticoid and poor nutrition. These factors affect both GH and IGF-I secretion and sensitivity as well as having a direct effect on the growth plate. It is important to optimise nutrition and minimise steroid dosage. Newer treatments including anti-TNFα therapy in Crohn's disease and JIA have led to significant improvements in growth; endocrine

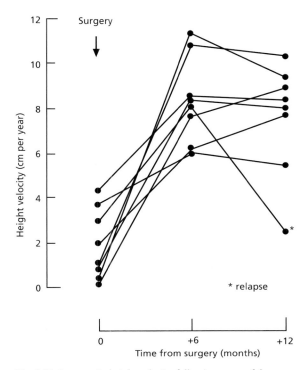

Fig. 3.10 Increase in height velocity following successful resection of inflamed bowel in prepubertal and early pubertal patients with Crohn's disease.

management can then be considered in the minority of patients who continue to grow slowly.

Delayed puberty can be managed with pubertal induction using sex steroid. Use of high dose recombinant GH in Crohn's disease and JIA improves growth rate significantly but not completely, suggesting a degree of resistance at the level of the growth plate.

Psychosocial deprivation

Psychosocial deprivation may also be regarded as a chronic disease state. The best therapy for associated growth failure is to correct or reverse the disadvantageous home setting or, if this is not possible, to remove the child to a supportive environment. GH therapy is not indicated in this context nor is it effective.

IGF-I

Recombinant IGF-I was developed in the late 1980s and is the only therapy available for treatment of severe genetic GH resistance. It is effective in stimulating growth in Laron syndrome and has been shown to improve glycaemic control in adolescent diabetes mellitus. However, a major therapeutic indication for IGF-I is still to be found. A compound which complexes IGF-I with IGFBP-3 has also been developed. This physiological approach is logical; however, its clinical efficacy for treatment of growth disorders remains to be demonstrated.

Use of gonadotrophin-releasing hormone (GnRH) analogue therapy to improve growth

Gonadotrophin-releasing hormone (GnRH) analogues are now an established treatment for central precocious puberty (see Chapter 5). They can suppress gonadotrophin secretion and therefore arrest pubertal development. The possibility of their use in children with short stature has been studied as a way of delaying puberty and hence prolonging prepubertal growth, which might increase final height.

A wealth of literature has emerged on this topic, with the general consensus being that any benefit is marginal. However, the **combination of early puberty and GH insufficiency**, for example after cranial irradiation, constitutes a mandatory indication for combination treatment using GH and GnRH analogue to optimise growth before epiphysial closure. In this situation, puberty should be allowed to continue when an appropriate age is reached, continuing with GH therapy. Controversially, a combination of GH and GnRH analogue can be used to improve final height in children with simple virilizing congenital adrenal hyperplasia when linear growth is poor despite minimal suppressive treatment with glucocorticoids.

Transition

It is now well established that patients with severe GH deficiency, especially if accompanied by other anterior pituitary hormone deficiencies, require adult follow-up to pre-empt and treat the consequences of adult GH deficiency which include incomplete accretion and/or loss of bone mass with increased fracture risk, decrease in muscle mass and increased fat mass (particularly visceral fat), disturbance of insulin and lipid metabolism, and increase in cardiovascular morbidity. Patients with the adult GH deficiency syndrome may experience marked fatigue with reduction in strength and exercise tolerance, and hence reduced quality of life.

For this reason, it is essential that adolescents leaving paediatric care should attend an adult endocrine clinic. The challenge is to convince the patient that this is so,

given that teenagers often view hospital attendance as tedious and non-essential. Experience has shown that the setting up of a transition clinic in the paediatric centre, with quarterly joint clinics attended by the paediatric and adult endocrinologist increases the likelihood of successful long-term follow-up.

Girls with Turner syndrome require surveillance of their reproductive, thyroid, bone, cardiac, and ENT/hearing status, therefore adult follow-up in a specialist clinic is mandatory. The adult Turner clinic can be run by a reproductive endocrinologist, gynaecologist, or adult endocrine physician. Whoever oversees the clinic will need to liaise closely with other disciplines, particularly cardiac and ENT. Again, smooth transition from paediatric to adult care is enhanced by the establishment of a transition clinic.

When to involve a specialist centre

- Short stature whose cause remains uncertain after clinical assessment and baseline investigations.
- GH insufficiency/deficiency states, including those associated with CNS lesion.
- When GH therapy is contemplated.
- Dysmorphic syndromes associated with short stature.
- Management of Turner syndrome.
- Poor postnatal growth with short stature in SGA, particularly if height <2nd centile aged 2 years of more.
- Cranial irradiation associated with GH deficiency.

Future developments

- Alternative methods of GH administration, including a long-acting preparation, are being developed.
- Growth-promoting preparations, such as IGF-I and IGF-I/IGFBP-3, have been tried as an alternative to GH, but are not currently established as being superior, except in severe genetic GH resistance.
- Combination treatment with IGF-I and GH may be a therapeutic option in JIA and Crohn's disease in the future.
- The use of GnRH analogues to delay puberty and possibly increase final height has been tried but this treatment, except in patients with severe GH deficiency, has not been established to give a better long-term outcome.

• Genetic studies to identify the molecular basis of individual growth disorders will develop. The essential clinical component of these studies is to establish the precise clinical phenotype in combination with the genetic analysis. It is likely that children currently diagnosed as idiopathic short stature will gradually be assigned to specific diagnostic categories.

Controversial points

• Treatment of non-GH-deficient children with hGH is an important controversial issue which relates to clinical benefit, risk of therapy and health economics.
• The optimum organization of growth screening in the community is controversial. In general, community paediatricians favour a smaller number of measurements, whereas paediatric endocrinologists and patient support groups, such as the Child Growth Foundation, favour multiple measurements throughout the pre-school period and during school years. The latter view is probably ideal; however, resources are not available for detailed and comprehensive growth screening.
• Genetic analysis of patients with short stature is growing in frequency. The value of this to the patient is evident in certain situations, for example disorders such as multiple endocrine neoplasia. In other situations, genetic

analysis and identification of gene mutations may contribute to the characterization and understanding of the pathophysiology of growth disorders.
• *Treatment of young adults with GH deficiency:* A case can be made for the automatic transition from paediatric to adult GH treatment, the latter being given in the initial dosage of about 0.6 mg daily (far lower than in childhood) and adjusted by titrating against serum IGF-I levels. An alternative approach is to be selective, accepting that compliance with adult GH replacement will be poor in asymptomatic young adults, and to reserve treatment for patients who become symptomatic, or in whom problems such as hyperlipidaemia or reduced bone mass are found in the course of monitoring.

Potential pitfalls

• Over-diagnosis of GH deficiency by focusing on biochemical results rather than the history, examination and auxology.
• Over-reliance on bone age assessment, which is not a diagnostic investigation.
• Reluctance to use testosterone therapy for delayed puberty in males. In short courses, using the appropriate dose, there is no compromising effect on final height and the psychological benefits are great.

Case histories

Case 3.1

A 4-year-old boy was being followed in a joint medical/surgical cryptorchidism clinic and was found to have short stature. He had subtle dysmorphic features with a small mid-face. He was apparently healthy. Both testes were palpable, but the penis was rather small. Height was below the 3rd centile, weight on the 10th centile and height velocity was 3.4 cm per year.

These findings indicated that he was abnormally short (mid-parental height was 75th centile) and that he needed investigation. The results were as follows. Full blood count, erthyrocyte sedimentation rate (ESR), electrolytes, creatinine, liver function tests and endomysial antibodies were normal.

Total thyroxine (T4) 48 nmol/L [NR 58–174]
0.37 μg/dL [NR 4.6–10.5]
TSH 1.8 mU/L [NR 0.3–5.0]
Free T4 6.6 pmol/L [NR 11–25]

[0.53 ng/dL, NR 0.8–2.4]
Cortisol 255 nmol/L [NR 09.00 h, 300–700]
[9.3 μg/dL, NR 8.0–25.0]
Prolactin 286 mU/L [NR up to 360]

Questions
1. What do these baseline results mean?

Answer
1. They show that he has hypothyroidism of central origin because his TSH level is not elevated.

Question
2. What is the next step?

Answer
2. He needs a thyrotrophin-releasing hormone (TRH)stimulation test.

Results of the TRH test (200 mg IV)
0 min TSH 1.1 mU/L
20 min TSH 4.2 mU/L
60 min TSH 4.8 mU/L

Table 3.12 Results of glucagon stimulation test.

Time (min)	GH (mU/L)
0	0.8
60	0.5
90	1.6
120	1.4
150	0.6
180	0.7

Questions

3. Is this test normal?
4. Should he now have assessment of his GH secretion?
5. Are any more investigations needed before he starts his GH therapy?
6. Are there any other pituitary hormone deficiencies?

Answers

3. No, because the rise in TSH is inadequate. In a normal TRH test, the 20 min TSH level should be higher than the 60 min level. This result is indicative of hypothalamic (or tertiary) hypothyroidism.
4. No because, in a child with hypothyroidism, of any cause, GH secretion is suppressed. The next step is to treat his hypothyroidism with T_4 75 µg per day.

Once his T4 level is normal, one can proceed to a glucagon (15 mg/kg intramuscularly (i.m.)) stimulation test to assess his GH secretion. The results are shown in Table 3.12.

All GH values less than 10 mU/L indicate severe GH deficiency.
5. Yes, he needs an MRI scan of the pituitary and hypothalamus to exclude an organic cause of GH deficiency, such as craniopharyngioma. The MRI scan was reported as showing an extremely shallow pituitary fossa with no evidence of pituitary tissue. **The diagnosis is idiopathic hypopituitarism with deficiency of GH and TSH.**
6. He had cryptorchidism and a small penis. This could be caused by gonadotrophin deficiency, which will need investigating at the time of puberty. He started GH therapy in a standard dosage of 0.025 mg/kg per day. His height velocity increased in 6 months from 4.9 to 19.2 cm per year. This was a record for the clinic. At

the age of 9.5 years his height was 139.6 cm, i.e. between the 75th and 90th centiles and within his height target range.

Case 3.2

A 6-year-old girl was referred with growth failure, poor appetite, recurrent abdominal pain, 'thick custard' stools and vomiting.

Question

1. What is the differential diagnosis of this child's short stature?

Answer

1. Look at Table 3.2 and remember that the paediatrician should always approach the problem of short stature as a generalist and not as an endocrinologist. On examination her height was below the 0.4th centile and her weight was on the 2nd centile. Her height velocity was 1.8 cm per year (normal is >4 cm per year). This means that she needs baseline investigations for short stature. The results of these investigations were as follows:

Hb 12.2 g/dL
Ferritin 8.0 µ/L [NR 15–300]
Anti-endomysial positive antibodies
ESR 24 mm/h

Question

2. What is the next investigation needed?

Answer

2. Jejunal biopsy. This showed villous atrophy and lymphocytic infiltrate in the lamina propria with hyperplastic crypts. This confirmed a diagnosis of **coeliac disease.**

Case 3.3

A 7-year-old girl is referred from the cardiac clinic with short stature. She was born weighing 2.73 kg at 40 weeks' gestation (−1.53 SD) and at 9-week check was found to have a heart murmur, echocardiogram showing aortic stenosis. The girl was asymptomatic and the short stature had always been attributed to her parents being short – mother 151.1 cm, father 162.4 cm – but the disparity between her height and that of her school mates seemed to be increasing.

Question

1. What is the differential diagnosis of this child's short stature, and what specific questions should be asked?

Answer

1. Turner's syndrome must be seriously considered in a short girl with aortic stenosis and an enquiry should be made about ear infections, middle ear deafness, difficulty with mathematics, and a history of poor feeding, high activity levels, and sleeplessness in infancy and early childhood.

It is of course possible that this is normal familial short stature compounded by constitutional delay, so the childhood stature and pubertal milestones of the family should be ascertained, together with any history of atopy since asthma can be associated with constitutional delay.

The girl had had a couple of ear infections, otherwise her health was good, and there had been no problems in early childhood with feeding or sleeping. She was doing well at school and had no particular difficulty with mathematics. There was no history of delayed puberty in either parent. Examination showed a normal-looking girl measuring 101.4 cm, (−3.8 SDS, compared with the mid-parental height SDS of −1.7) and weighing 18 kg (−1.7 SDS) with only subtle dysmorphism including slightly puffy fingers and pudgy nail folds, high palate, shield chest, and posteriorly rotated ears. Pulses were normal, blood pressure was 86/56 mm/Hg, aortic stenosis murmur noted with carotid thrill and bruit. Ear examination showed no active inflammation of tympanic membranes.

Question

2. What investigations should be done in this girl?

Answer

2. Chromosomes to confirm the diagnosis of Turner's syndrome, basal LH and FSH to detect evidence of primary ovarian failure, thyroid function and thyroid peroxidase antibodies (since Hashimoto's thyroiditis is common in Turner syndrome), full blood count and ferritin, and IGF-I. Pelvic and renal ultrasound examination to assess ovarian, uterine and renal morphology.

Karyotype showed a 46,XiXq pattern, with duplication of the long arm (q) resulting in an isochromosome and thus loss of the short arm (p). FSH was elevated at 17 U/l consistent with primary ovarian failure, LH normal for age at 0.1 U/l. Thyroid function, and TPO antibodies were normal. Renal ultrasound was normal, uterus slightly hypoplastic, no ovaries identified.

Comment

The clue that the short stature might not be normal genetic (apart from the associated aortic stenosis), was the mismatch between the girl's height and that of her parents, i.e. she was inappropriately short even for her short family. The borderline smallness-for-gestational age is consistent with Turner syndrome. The dysmorphic features were subtle and easily overlooked.

Case 3.4

A boy is referred to the growth clinic aged 10.2 year with short stature. He has been followed up in a general clinic because of the diagnosis of maternal GH deficiency. His height has fallen from the 10th–25th centile at 5.8 years to just below the 3rd centile now. He was born at 39 weeks gestation weighing 6 lb 1 oz to a mother who had received pituitary-derived human GH for 4 years around the age of puberty following the demonstration of low GH levels on stimulation testing. The boy's measurements at the clinic are height 128 cm (−1.80 SDS) and weight 25 kg (−1.68 SDS), mother's height 149.5 cm (−2.09 SDS), father's reported height 6′0″.

Question

What diagnostic possibilities should be considered in this boy?

Answer

This could, of course, be autosomal dominant GH deficiency. However, one would expect more severe short stature from an earlier age if this were the case. Normal variant familial short stature is a possibility, with the mother going through a phase of GH insufficiency, rather than true GH deficiency, when she was tested. A further possibility is an autosomal dominant skeletal dysplasia, the low levels of GH in the mother at the time she was tested being a 'red herring'.

Careful physical examination shows obvious café au lait patches in the boy consistent with neurofibromatosis. These are also present in the mother. Further history reveals that two maternal aunts and two maternal cousins also have café au lait patches. The boy's visual fields and fundi are normal, blood pressure 110/70. He is followed up in the growth clinic and his height continues to be just below the 3rd centile. At 12.5 years dynamic testing shows a GH peak of 10.2 mU/L in response to insulin (partial GH insufficiency), IGF1 117 μg/L (low/normal for age), pubertal LH response to stimulation with GnRH, and normal thyroid function. The boy receives recombinant GH from 12.3 until 17 years, and does well, going through puberty normally and achieving a final height of 169 cm (−0.89 SDS). MRI scans of brain show slight bulkiness of the optic nerves, but normal hypothalamus and pituitary.

Comment

This case illustrates the need to consider a dominant growth disorder when one parent is short. The discovery of café au lait patches was made during careful physical examination, as should always be the case with new patient referrals. The short stature that is frequently seen in subjects with neurofibromatosis is in part related to an accompanying skeletal dysplasia, but subjects may also demonstrate a degree of GH insufficiency. This case reinforces the concept that low GH levels – GH insufficiency – constitute a problem and not a diagnosis.

Useful information for patients and parents

The Restricted Growth Association offers support to a range of short stature conditions, particularly achondroplasia and other causes of disproportionate short stature. Website: http://www.restrictedgrowth.co.uk/
The Turner Syndrome Support Society (TSSS) has excellent information for parents, children and teenagers with Turner syndrome. Website: http://www.tss.org.uk/
The Child Growth Foundation (CGF) offers support to children and adults with growth problems and their families, and also to healthcare professionals with an interest. CGF provides a superb range of 15 booklets on growth and hormone problems including IUGR, GH deficiency, GH deficiency in adults, constitutional delay, Turner syndrome, and craniopharyngioma disorders including GH deficiency. Website: http://www.childgrowthfoundation.org/
European Society for Paediatric Endocrinology Parent and Patient provides pamphlets on a wide variety of growth disorders in English, French, Italian, Spanish and Turkish. Website: http://www.eurospe.org/patient/index.html

Significant guidelines/consensus statements

Short stature
Cohen, P., Rogol, A. D., Deal, C. L. *et al.* (2008) Consensus statement on the diagnosis and treatment of children with idiopathic short stature: a summary of the Growth Hormone Research Society, the Lawson Wilkins Pediatric Endocrine Society, and the European Society for Paediatric Endocrinology Workshop. *The Journal of Clinical Endocrinology & Metabolism* 2008 **93**(11), 4210–4217.

Small-for-gestational age
Lee, P.A., Chernausek, S.D., Hokken-Koelega, A.C.S. and Czernichow, P. International SGA Advisory Board Consensus Development Conference Statement: management of short children born small for gestational age, April 24–October 1, 2001. *Pediatrics* 2003 **111**, 1253–1261.

GH treatment
National Institute for Clinical Excellence (NICE) guidelines Growth hormone deficiency (children) – human growth hormone: http://guidance.nice.org.uk/TA188
Human growth hormone (somatropin) in adults with growth hormone deficiency (TA64); http://guidance.nice.org.uk/TA64/Guidance/Recommendations_1

Consensus guidelines

Consensus Guidelines for the Diagnosis and Treatment of Growth Hormone (GH) Deficiency in Childhood and Adolescence: Summary Statement of the GH Research Society. *The Journal of Clinical Endocrinology & Metabolism* 2000;85 (11):3990–3993

Transitional care of the GH-treated adolescent

PE Clayton, RC Cuneo, A Juul, JP Monson, SM Shalet, M Tauber. Consensus statement on the management of the GH-treated adolescent in the transition to adult care. *European Journal of Endocrinology* 2005;152;165–170

Further reading

Blizzard, R.M. & Bulatovic, A. (1992) Psychosocial short stature: a syndrome with many variables. *Baillière's Clinics in Endocrinology and Metabolism* **6**, 687–712.

Borochowitz, Z.U. & Rimoin, D.I. (1998) Genetic and dysmorphic syndromes of short stature. In: *Growth Disorders: Pathophysiology and Treatment* (eds C.J.H. Kelnar, M.O. Savage, H.F. Stirling & P. Saenger), pp. 297–322. Chapman & Hall Medical, London.

Bourguignon, J.P. (1998) Constitutional delay of growth and puberty. In: *Growth Disorders: Pathophysiology and Treatment* (eds C.J.H. Kelnar, M.O. Savage, H.F. Stirling & P. Saenger), pp. 673– 689. Chapman & Hall Medical, London.

Cowell, C.T. (1995) Short stature. In: *Clinical Paediatric Endocrinology* (ed. C.G.D. Brook), pp. 136–172. Blackwell Science, Oxford.

De Zegher, F., Francois, I., Van Helvoirt *et al.* (1998) Growth hormone treatment of short children born small for gestational age. *Trends in Endocrinology and Metabolism* **9**, 233–237.

Donaldson, M.D.C. & Paterson, W. (1998) Abnormal growth: definition, pathogenesis and practical assessment. In: *Growth Disorders: Pathophysiology and Treatment* (eds C.J.H. Kelnar, M.O. Savage, H.F. Stirling & P. Saenger), pp. 197–224. Chapman & Hall Medical, London.

Freeman, J.V., Cole, T.J., Chinn, S. *et al.* (1995) Cross sectional stature and weight reference curves for the UK. *Archives of Disease in Childhood* **73**, 17–24.

Karlberg, J. (1989) A mathematical model breaking down linear growth from birth to adulthood into 3 components that reflect the different hormonal phases of the growth process. *Acta Paediatr Suppl* **350**, 70–94.

Hagenäs, L. (1998) Skeletal dysplasias. In: *Growth Disorders: Pathophysiology and Treatment* (eds C.J.H. Kelnar, M.O. Savage, H.F. Stirling & P. Saenger), pp. 338–355. Chapman & Hall Medical, London.

Hindmarsh, P.C. (1998) Endocrine assessment of growth. In: *Growth Disorders: Pathophysiology and Treatment* (eds C.J.H. Kelnar, M.O. Savage, H.F. Stirling & P. Saenger), pp. 237–250. Chapman & Hall Medical, London.

Hindmarsh, P.C. (1999) Evidence-based decisions in growth hormone therapy. In: *Current Indications for Growth Hormone Therapy* (ed. P.C. Hindmarsh), pp. 1–12. S. Karger, Basel.

Hintz, R.L. (2005) Growth hormone treatment of idiopathic short stature. *Growth Hormone & IGF Research* **15**, S6–S8.

Johnston, L.B. & Savage, M.O. (2004) Should recombinant human growth hormone therapy be used in short small for gestational age children? *Archives of Disease in Childhood* **89**, 740–744.

Jones, K.L. (1997) *Smith's Recognizable Patterns of Human Malformation.* W.B. Saunders, Philadelphia.

Kelly, B.P., Paterson, W.F., & Donaldson, M.D.C. (2003) Final height outcome and value of height prediction in boys with constitutional delay in growth and adolescence treated with intramuscular testosterone 125 mg per month for 3 months. *Clinical Endocrinology* **58**, 267–272.

Mullis, P.E. (1998) Genetic control of growth. In: *Growth Disorders: Pathophysiology and Treatment* (eds C.J.H. Kelnar, M.O. Savage, H.F. Stirling & P. Saenger), pp. 39–61. Chapman & Hall Medical, London.

Ranke, M.B. (1998) Turner and Noonan syndromes: disease specific growth and growth-promoting therapies. In: *Growth Disorders: Pathophysiology and Treatment* (eds C.J.H. Kelnar, M.O. Savage, H.F. Stirling & P. Saenger), pp. 623–639. Chapman & Hall Medical, London.

Skuse, D., Albanese, A., Stanhope, R. *et al.* (1996) A new stress-related syndrome of growth failure and hyperphagia in children, associated with reversibility of growth hormone insufficiency. *Lancet* **348**, 353–358.

Tanner, J.M. (1986) Normal growth and techniques of growth assessment. In: *Growth Disorders, Clinics in Endocrinology and Metabolism*, **3**, pp. 411–451. W.B. Saunders, London.

Tanner, J.M., Whitehouse, R.H., Cameron, N. *et al.* (1983) Assessment of skeletal maturity and prediction of adult height (TW2 method), 2nd edn. Academic Press, London.

Tanner, J.M., Healy, M.J.R., Goldstein, H. *et al.* (2001) Assessment of skeletal maturity and prediction of adult height (TW3 method), 3rd edn. W.B. Saunders, London.

Website: www.rcpch.ac.uk/Research/UK-WHO-Growth-Charts

Tonshoff, B. & Mehls, O. (1999) Growth retardation in children with chronic renal disease: pathophysiology and treatment. In: *Current Indications for Growth Hormone Therapy* (ed. P.C. Hind-marsh), pp. 118–127. S. Karger, Basel.

Voss, L.D., Wilkin, T.J., Bailey, B.J.R. *et al.* (1991) The reliability of height and height velocity in the assessment of growth (the Wessex Growth Study). *Arch Dis Child* **66**, 833–37.

Tauber, M., Moulin, P., Pienkowski, C. *et al.* (1997) Growth hormone (GH) retesting and auxological data in 131 GH-deficient patients after completion of treatment. *JCEM* **82**, 352–56.

4 Tall Stature

Tall stature is defined as height greater than two standard deviations above the mean (equivalent to >97th or 98th centiles) for the general population. It may be an accompanying feature in disorders such as sexual precocity and simple obesity, and not the prime concern, or the principal reason for referral. In the latter scenario, the family will want an estimate of final height and for possible treatment to be discussed. Tall stature is a much less common cause of referral than short stature, being more acceptable to families than the latter unless the degree of tallness is particularly marked, especially in a girl. The clinician needs to be aware of the pathogenesis, clinical and biochemical associations and potential treatment of tall stature.

Pathogenesis and differential diagnosis

Tall stature is usually associated with one of four broad aetiological categories. In order of frequency these are: familial tall stature/constitutional advance in growth; simple obesity; syndromic tall stature, which has usually been present since infancy; and endocrine causes. The differential diagnosis is shown in Table 4.1. An idea of their relative frequency in the context of tallness being a principal referral feature can be gained from the following breakdown of tall stature referrals to one consultant in Glasgow from 1989–2009: normal genetic tall stature (81); constitutional advance in growth and adolescence (49); tall stature due to simple obesity (70); dysmorphic syndromes: 47,XYY (3), 47,XXY (11), 47,XXX (1), Marfan's syndrome (18),

Sotos (5), Weaver (1), Beckwith–Wiedemann (3), unclassified dysmorphic syndromes (22); sexual precocity (19); thyrotoxicosis (2), growth hormone (GH) excess (2).

Assessment of the child or adolescent with tall stature

The key aspects of clinical assessment of a child or adolescent referred with tall stature are given in Table 4.2. With a combination of auxology, careful history taking and physical examination followed by serial measurement of height the need for laboratory investigations can be excluded in most cases. If there are dysmorphic features, particularly in the context of learning difficulties, a clinical geneticist should be invited to see the child and advise on specific molecular genetic studies. Since the phenotype of Marfan's syndrome (see Table 4.5) can be mild, it is wise to carry out a screening cardiac ultrasound in children who are taller than expected for parental heights, or in whom one parent is particularly tall.

Investigations

Children whose height falls above the parental target range centiles in the absence of a family history of constitutional advance and/or an enhanced growth rate will require investigation as shown in Table 4.3. The combination of

Practical Endocrinology and Diabetes in Children, Third Edition. Joseph E. Raine, Malcolm D.C. Donaldson, John W. Gregory, Guy Van Vliet.
© 2011 Blackwell Publishing Ltd. Published 2011 by Blackwell Publishing Ltd.

Table 4.1 Differential diagnosis of tall stature.

1. Normal familial tall stature
   - Normal genetic tall stature
   - Constitutional advance in growth and adolescence
2. Simple obesity
3. Dysmorphic syndromes associated with tall stature
   - (i) With X or Y aneuploidy
     - 47,XYY
     - 47,XXY (Klinefelter's syndrome)
     - 47,XXX
     - Other aneuploidy syndromes
   - (ii) With metabolic/skeletal abnormality
     - Marfan's syndrome
     - Homocystinuria
     - Total lipodystrophy
     - Other
   - (iii) With symmetrical overgrowth
     - Fragile X syndrome
     - Sotos
     - Weaver
     - Other
   - (iv) With asymmetrical overgrowth
     - Beckwith–Wiedemann
     - Klippel–Trenaunay–Weber
     - Proteus syndrome
     - Other
4. Endocrine causes
   - (i) Sexual precocity (e.g. virilizing congenital adrenal hyperplasia, true central precocious puberty; see Chapter 5)
   - (ii) Thyrotoxicosis
   - (iii) GH excess (very rare)
     - GHRH tumour/dysregulation
     - GH secreting adenoma +/– MEN1, McCune–Albright syndrome
   - (iv) Familial glucocorticoid deficiency
   - (v) Endocrine abnormalities causing delayed epiphyseal closure (e.g. aromatase deficiency and oestrogen receptor defect).

Table 4.2 Clinical assessment of tall stature.

Auxology
Height, weight, height velocity

Heights of parents and siblings

Bone age and (if appropriate) height prediction

History
Pattern of growth including age that tall stature recognized

Birth weight, head circumference and (if available) birth length

Family patterns of childhood growth and puberty

Neurodevelopment, academic performance and behaviour

Examination
Presence of dysmorphic features

Pubertal staging including assessment of testicular volume

Fundoscopy to assess optic discs

Systematic examination

Table 4.3 Baseline investigations for tall stature.

Cardiac ultrasound

Karyotype

FMR1 gene analysis for Fragile X syndrome in boys with tall stature and learning difficulties

DNA for specific syndromes (after assessment by clinical geneticist)

Thyroid function tests

IGF-I

Bone age assessment and (where appropriate) height prediction

tall stature and intellectual delay should always prompt a search for an underlying syndrome but these patients may well have already had investigations. If physical examination is completely normal and the child comes from a tall family, investigations are usually not indicated and regular height measurements will be sufficient. Further investigations will be dictated by the results of the baseline tests. If the diagnosis of excess GH secretion caused by a GH secreting pituitary adenoma is considered, investigation should proceed as shown in Table 4.4.

Table 4.4 Assessment for possible growth hormone excess.

GH suppression test using oral glucose load
MRI of hypothalamo–pituitary axis
Visual fields
9.00 a.m. cortisol
Prolactin
Testosterone, LH, FSH (depending on age)

Protocol for GH suppression test with glucose

This test involves giving 1.75 g/kg carbohydrate orally (up to maximum of 75 g = two glasses of Lucozade) as for the glucose tolerance test, and measuring serum GH at: −30, 0, 30, 60, 90, 120 and 150 minutes together with an IGF-I level at baseline. Normal GH suppression is a value of <4 mU/L at some time during the test.

N.B.: It is wise to put in the request for this test as 'GH suppression test with glucose' rather than 'glucose tolerance test' – if the latter term is used, the day ward is likely to take samples for glucose and not GH!

Causes of tall stature

Familial tall stature and constitutional advance in growth and adolescence

Normal tall stature can be sub-classified into normal genetic tall stature and constitutional advance in growth – the counterpart of normal genetic short stature and constitutional delay (see Chapter 3). As with normal short stature and constitutional delay, there is considerable overlap between familial tallness and constitutional advance. Also, as with short stature the clinician needs to guard against the pitfall of assuming that tallness in one parent is necessarily normal – dominantly inherited tall stature disorders (e.g. Marfan's syndrome) can be mistaken for normal tall stature.

Normal tall stature is the most common cause of referral in tall children and adolescents, and the patient is usually a girl. In this case, it is frequently the mother who, having suffered herself from being tall as a child and adolescent, is concerned about her daughter. In groups of tall children, GH secretion has been shown to be statistically elevated when compared to normal or short statured children. However, in an individual child excess GH secretion is not usually apparent. The tall stature is usually noticeable by primary school entry. It is helpful to ask the parents about their childhood height and onset of puberty. The history of one parent being particularly tall as a child, having an early adolescence, and being relatively less tall as an adult, is indicative of familial constitutional advance, and the diagnosis is supported by bone age advance in the child. Physical examination is normal although advanced adolescence may be noted in girls >9 years. In girls and boys with normal tall stature, prediction of final height from skeletal maturity and current height may be helpful from around 11 years upwards. However, the accuracy of final height prediction in tall stature varies between populations and with the prediction method used, hence should not be used to assess any treatment effect. The likelihood of an earlier than average puberty should be explained to parents whose children are still prepubertal. Reassurance and growth monitoring are the principles of management.

Simple obesity

Children with simple obesity are relatively tall in relation to their parental height centiles, with enhanced height velocity and bone age (Buckler, 1994). This increase in height status may, depending on familial heights, be sufficient to put the child above the 97th or 98th centile for height, or to compound existing tall stature.

Syndromes associated with tall stature

The combination of tall stature and developmental delay should always prompt a search for an underlying dysmorphic syndrome. Boys with learning difficulties should be screened for Fragile X syndrome irrespective of stature. The typical phenotype in this condition includes long face, large and prominent ears, increased head size and (especially after puberty) enlarged testes. Of the aneuploidy syndromes, the 47,XYY syndrome is the most likely to present with tall stature and, in most cases, both phenotype and intelligence are normal. The principal phenotypic features of three important tall stature syndromes which may present to the growth clinic — Marfan, Sotos and Beckwith–Wiedemann syndrome — are given in Table 4.5.

Endocrine causes of tall stature

Sexual precocity, thyrotoxicosis and familial glucocorticoid deficiency (see Chapter 8) do not usually present with tall stature alone, while aromatase deficiency/estrogen receptor defects are extremely rare. Children with suspected GH excess will require hormone investigations to confirm the abnormality; specialist referral at this stage is recommended.

GH secreting pituitary tumour

A GH-secreting tumour causes tall stature and gigantism in childhood and adolescence, and acromegaly in adult life. An association with McCune–Albright syndrome is recognized. Because of its extreme rarity in childhood, this disorder should be managed jointly with an adult endocrinologist, who will have far more experience. Suppression of GH secretion may require pituitary surgery,

Table 4.5 Principal features of Marfan, Sotos and Beckwith-Wiedemann syndromes.

Marfan syndrome
Genetics
- Autosomal dominant; spontaneous mutation in ~ 25%
- Mutations in FBN1 gene (encoding the glycoprotein fibrillin-1)

Clinical features
- Characteristic phenotype – tall thin build, arachnodactyly, long face, high palate
- Joint laxity with hypotonia, kyphoscoliosis, pes planus
- Eye problems – upward lens subluxation, myopia, retinal detachment
- Cardiac problems – aortic root dilatation leading to rupture, mitral valve prolapse

Diagnosis
Clinical, supported by cardiac ultrasound and eye findings, confirmed by genetic studies
N.B.: Phenotype may be mild.

Sotos syndrome
Genetics
- *NSD1* gene (located 5q35) defect in 80%
- Sporadic in 95%, commoner in boys; autosomal dominant transmission

Clinical features
- Accelerated prenatal and infantile growth with large head size
- Tall childhood stature with bone age advance, adult height not excessive
- Variable degree of learning difficulties (50% need learning support)
- Hypotonia and poor coordination
- 'Inverted pear' head shape – long narrow face with high-bossed forehead, prominent jaw, down-slanting eyes

Diagnosis
- Suggested by triad of typical facies, overgrowth, and learning difficulties
- Confirmed by molecular genetic studies

Beckwith–Wiedemann
Genetics
- Two-third patients have demonstrable abnormalities affecting imprinted genes in 11p15.5 region including paternal disomy; abnormal DNA methylation; maternal translocations/inversion with break points
- Sporadic in 85%, autosomal dominant in 15% with incomplete penetrance
- Closely linked with Wilms' tumour gene (*WT2*)
- Imbalance between maternally imprinted IGF-II growth enhancer gene and paternally imprinted H19 growth suppresser gene

Clinical
- Foetal overgrowth with birth weight and length > 90th centile and postnatal overgrowth during first 4–6 years; macroglossia; large kidneys; hemihypertrophy
- Midline abdominal wall defects – omphalocoele, umbilical hernia
- Transient hyperinsulinaemic hypoglycaemia due to pancreatic hyperplasia
- Ear lobe creases and pits
- Predisposition to tumours, especially Wilms' (7%)
- Mild learning difficulties in some patients

Diagnosis
- Presence of 3/5 major criteria (large birth size, abdominal wall defect, macroglossia, ear creases, neonatal hypoglycaemia)
- Genetic studies support rather than exclude diagnosis.

radiotherapy, somatostatin analogue or GH receptor antagonist therapy.

Treatment of familial (constitutional) tall stature

Occasionally, the degree of anxiety surrounding advanced growth, usually in girls, is so great that treatment is indicated to try to slow down growth and therefore reduce final height. Two forms of therapy are currently used:
- High-dose sex-steroid therapy
- GH suppressive therapy using a somatostatin analogue
  In future, GH receptor antagonist therapy may be appropriate.

Sex-steroid therapy
The indication for the use of sex steroids to reduce final height is based on evidence that abnormally high circulating levels will advance skeletal maturation and eventually cause early epiphyseal fusion. De Waal from the Netherlands has published the most extensive results. In girls, ethinyloestradiol 100–300 µg/day orally combined with cyclical progesterone (i.e. norethisterone 5 mg/day for days 1–14 of each calendar month), if used relatively early, reduced final height by up to 7 cm. In boys, testosterone 250–1000 mg monthly caused a similar reduction. An early age of onset of treatment (bone age 10 years in girls, 12.5 years in boys) was associated with the best results. In an extensive inquiry, 10 years after final height, no significant adverse affects were identified. In Glasgow, our experience of tall stature treatment has been virtually limited to selected girls with Marfan's syndrome, using lower doses (50–100 µg daily) of ethinyloestradiol. In boys, high dose intramuscular testosterone therapy (250 mg every 2 weeks) can be given in order to accelerate epiphyseal fusion but in practice few centres employ this strategy.

Somatostatin analogue therapy
Suppression of GH levels should theoretically slow down growth and, if continued on a long-term basis, may reduce final adult height. The short-acting somatostatin analogue octreotide required once or twice daily injections and treatment with long-acting preparations (Carel 2009) are more attractive. Such treatment would be best organized jointly with an adult endocrinologist who has had experience of its use.

GH receptor antagonist therapy
The GH receptor antagonist Pegvisomant, given as a daily subcutaneous injection, is a highly expensive but effective treatment in adults with acromegaly. Pegvisomant, given in doses of 10–30 mg daily, has been shown to normalise IGF-I levels in children with pituitary gigantism but experience is limited to small numbers and final height data are still awaited.

Future developments

- Molecular analysis of tall stature and overgrowth syndromes continues to identify new genetic causes of these disorders.
- Prospective multicentre studies to assess the safety and efficacy of new treatment protocols.
- GH receptor antagonist treatment is likely to become established as the treatment of choice for constitutional tall stature.

When to involve a specialist centre

- Dysmorphic syndromes associated with tall stature.
- Tall stature associated with excess GH secretion.
- Difficult cases of tall stature associated with hyperthyroidism or precocious puberty.

Controversial points

- The treatment of tall stature in girls remains controversial with concerns regarding the long-term safety of high dose oestrogen therapy, which is rarely practised now. Treatment with a somatostatin analogue may be effective, but is invasive and associated with side effects. New therapy using a GH receptor antagonist is promising but not yet established as being beneficial.
- As tall stature is better tolerated by society, there seems to be less indication for therapy.
- Rare conditions, such as GH secreting pituitary tumours, are very infrequently seen in paediatric practice. These patients must be managed jointly with an adult endocrine unit.

Potential pitfalls

• Assuming that tall stature is normal familial in nature when it could be due to a dominant growth disorder such as Marfan's syndrome. This diagnosis has important implications, for these patients need life-long cardiovascular surveillance.

• Failure to consider the diagnosis of, or examine the patient carefully enough for, dysmorphic features suggestive of a syndrome to be appreciated.
• Failure to appreciate that tall stature and delayed puberty are an unusual combination. An important differential diagnosis is Klinefelter syndrome, which should be considered.

Case histories

Case 4.1

A 9-year-old girl was referred because of tall stature. She was in good health with no learning problems. On examination there were no dysmorphic features. Her height was just above the 97th centile and her parents' heights were on the 90th and 97th centiles. Pubertal development was: breast, stage 2; axillary hair, stage 2; pubic hair, stage 3; and no menarche. Baseline investigations (Table 4.3) were all normal. Consequently, an endocrine cause of her advanced growth was not identified. Bone age was 12.4 years and final height prediction was 188 cm. The parents, particularly the mother who had suffered as a result of her own tall stature, enquired about treatment. The child was not particularly concerned. Treatment was not advised.

Question

Are any further investigations indicated?

Answer

Probably not. She had occasional headaches so a magnetic resonance imaging (MRI) scan of the pituitary was performed which showed a pituitary gland with a convex upper border but no suprasellar extension. She also had a height velocity of 9.2 cm per year. She therefore had an oral glucose tolerance test for GH suppression. Her GH levels during the glucose tolerance test suppressed to 0.5 mU/L, indicating that there was no evidence of increased GH secretion. *Diagnosis:* Familial tall stature with constitutional advance.

Case 4.2

A 20-year-old Chinese girl was referred with concern as to her tallness compared with the rest of the family, and lack of secondary sexual development. She had mild to moderate learning difficulties and attended a special needs school in the past. On examination she

measured 167.8 cm (0.96 SDS) whereas the parental height is 154.2 cm (−1.30 SDS) and had some dysmorphic features including triangular, rather concave facies with long mandible, large hands and feet, and claw toes. There was scanty pubic hair (P2) but no significant breast development.

Question

What is the most likely diagnosis?

Answer

An underlying dysmorphic syndrome with overgrowth, learning difficulties, and gonadal impairment would explain the clinical features. Failure of epiphyseal fusion would contribute to the relative tall stature. Investigations showed a bone age of 13.8 years, 46,XX karyotype, elevated FSH and LH – 21.7 and 5.2 units/L, respectively, and hypoplastic uterus with streak ovaries. Treatment with low dose ethinyloestradiol was started to induce puberty, adding in Norethisterone later on. The genetic department was unable to make a specific diagnosis for her underlying syndrome.

Case 4.3

A boy was seen in the dermatology department aged 4 years with a soft tissue swelling in the forehead where he was noted to be very tall and hence referred to the growth clinic. He was born at 40 weeks' gestation weighing 3.75 kg and was noted to be large from the age of 6 months. His mother was 156.8 cm in height (just below 25th centile), father 182 cm (75–90th centiles). On examination at 4.4 years, the child was gigantic – height 128.1 (5.18 SDS), weight 41 kg (5.93 SDS) – and looked more like a 7-year-old than a boy of 4. He was darker-skinned than the rest of the family, prepubertal with 2–3 ml testes, BP 115/70 mm Hg. Fundoscopy showed slight optic nerve pallor on the left.

Question

What is the most likely diagnosis and what investigations should be done?

Answer

Pituitary gigantism is likely. Formal ophthalmology assessment, brain imaging, and an IGF-I level are indicated. The ophthalmologist confirmed the fundoscopic findings, and found slight left visual field constriction with visual acuity 6/9 in the left eye and 6/6 in the right. IGF-I level was elevated at >500 μg/L, GH failed to suppress below 8.6 mu/L after a carbohydrate load, overnight GH profile showed loss of normal pulsatile secretion with failure of GH to fall below 10 mu/L although the highest level was only 55 mu/L, and prolactin was mildly elevated at (600–1300 mu/L). CT scan showed a possible suprasellar tumour. Surgical exploration and biopsy showed that this was in fact a chiasmal and left optic nerve glioma, and histochemistry indicated that it was not secreting any anterior pituitary hormones, including GH.

Question

How could a non-secreting optic nerve glioma result in pituitary gigantism?

Answer

Subsequent MRI scan of brain showed extension of the glioma into the somatostatin-rich temporal lobes, and it was concluded that the GH excess was secondary to loss of somatostatin modulation of GH releasing hormone.

Question

What are the treatment options? What complications of the optic nerve glioma should be pre-empted?

Answer

The lesion could not be removed surgically, and radiotherapy was judged undesirable in child of this age in the absence of progressive visual loss or other pressure effects. The boy was treated with subcutaneous octreotide injections, initially daily, and then monthly when a long-acting preparation became available. His vision was carefully monitored in the ophthalmology clinic and his pubertal status was regularly checked in anticipation of him going into puberty early. Predictably, he developed testicular enlargement (4 ml) at 6.1 years and GnRH test confirmed true puberty, which was treated with long-acting 3 monthly GnRH analogue until 11.5 years following which normal puberty ensued. His vision has fortunately remained stable, and his IGF-I normalized on long-acting Octreotide, remaining normal when this was discontinued at 16.5 years. His final height was 191 cm (2.45 SDS) and at 18 years he was referred to the adult clinic for surveillance. Intracranial neurofibromatosis was suspected but not confirmed, biopsy of the subcutaneous frontal skin lesion showing simple fatty tissue rather than a neurofibroma.

Case 4.4

A 7-year-old girl is referred because of tall stature associated with Marfan's syndrome. Her maternal grandmother, mother and maternal aunt are affected, with eye problems but no cardiac involvement. The mother has suffered from cataract due to previously dislocated lenses but is not especially tall – 171.9 cm (1.65 SDS). The father's reported height is 180 cm (0.80 SDS). On examination, the child has long fingers and toes, and a high palate but does not look particularly Marfanoid. Heart examination is normal, blood pressure 100/60. Her height aged 7.3 years is 137 cm (2.69 SDS) and weight 27.4 kg (0.87 SDS).

Question

Are any genetic or endocrine investigations indicated at this stage?

Answer

Genetic studies confirmed a point mutation in exon 3 of the fibrillin gene on chromosome 15 in the family. Bone age estimation at this age is of limited value in giving a guide as to final height, and formal height prediction is not appropriate in a child with a growth disorder, as opposed to normal tall stature. The girl does of course merit cardiac ultrasound which shows mild aortic root dilatation, requiring surveillance, and follow-up of her growth. At 10.9 years the girl measures 160.4 cm (2.48 SD), the bone age is 12.1 years and her pubertal stage is B2P2A1.

Question

What are the treatment options?

Answer

The options include no treatment, oestrogen therapy to close the epiphyses earlier than usual, and (more recently) somatostatin analogue and GH receptor antagonists. In this case, the family were advised that an adult height of around 5'11" was possible, and they requested treatment. Ethinyloestradiol was given from 11.0 to 16.5 years building up to 100 μg daily during the first year, decreasing the dose to 50 μg during the second year, and giving Loestrin 30 (containing 30 μg of Ethinyloestradiol) thereafter. Blood pressure was monitored 3-monthly and remained normal, cardiac ultrasound was performed annually and was satisfactory. During the first 2 years, Norethisterone 5 mg daily for the first 5 days of each calendar month was also given to induce a monthly bleed. The family were pleased with her final height of 175 cm (2.13 SDS) and she was discharged to long-term cardiac follow-up.

Useful information to patients and parents

Child Growth Foundation (CGF) supports families with tall stature and is the umbrella organisation for the Sotos syndrome support group. Website: http://www.childgrowthfoundation.org/
The Marfan Association UK provides information and support to patients and families, particularly those in whom the diagnosis has been made recently. Website: http://www.marfan-association.org.uk/
High and Mighty (website: http://www.highandmighty.co.uk) and Long Tall Sally (website: http://www.patient.co.uk/support/Long-Tall-Sally.htm) sell clothing and accessories for tall men and women, respectively.

Further reading

Berryman, D.E., Palmer, A.J., Gosney, E.S. *et al.* (2007) Discovery and uses of pegvisomant: a growth hormone antagonist. *Endokrynologia Polska* **58**, 322–9.

Buckler, J.M.H. (1994) Interpretation of weight.. In: *Growth disorders in Children*, pp. 37–46. BMJ Publishing Group, London.

Carel, J-C., Blumberg, J., Bougeard-Julien, M. et al. & Lanreotide in Tall Stature Study Group (2009) Long-acting lanreotide in adolescent girls with constitutional tall stature. *Hormone Research* **71**, 228–36.

De Waal, W.J., GreynFokker, M.H., Stijnen, T. *et al.* (1996) Accuracy of final height prediction and effect of growth reductive therapy in 362 constitutionally tall children. *Journal of Clinical Endocrinology and Metabolism* **81**, 1206–1216.

Drop, S.L.S., de Muinck Keizer-Schrama, S.M.P.F. (2007) Medical management of tall stature. In: Growth Disorders. 2nd Edition. (eds. C.J.H. Kelnar, M.O. Savage, P. Saenger, C.T. Cowell), pp. 655–666. Hodder Arnold, London.

Patten, M.A., Rahman, N. (2007) Genetic and dysmorphic syndromes with increased stature. In: Growth Disorders. 2nd Edition. (eds. C.J.H. Kelnar, M.O. Savage, P. Saenger, C.T. Cowell), pp. 281–290. Hodder Arnold, London.

Venn, A., Hosmer, T., Bruinsma, D. *et al.* (2008) Oestrogen treatment for tall stature in girls: estimating the effect on height and the error in height prediction. *Clinical Endocrinology* **68**, 926–9.

Weimann, E., Bergmann, S. & Bohles, H.J. (1998) Oestrogen treatment of constitutional tall stature: a risk-benefit ratio. *Archives of Disease in Childhood* **78**, 148–51.

5 Puberty

Physiology of normal puberty (see Figure 5.1)

Puberty occurs when the secretion of gonadotrophin-releasing hormone (GnRH) by the hypothalamus, which is largely but not entirely suppressed during childhood, increases so that pulsatile secretion of luteinizing hormone (LH) increases, resulting in sufficient sex steroid production to result in the secondary sexual development.

In boys
• LH stimulates the Leydig cells to produce testosterone which induces the features of secondary sexual development. Human chorionic gonadotrophin (hCG) has similar structure and action to LH.
• Follicle stimulating hormone (FSH) binds to receptors on the Sertoli cells, enhancing spermatogenesis.
• Spermatogenesis depends on the complex interaction of various paracrine factors; qualitatively normal spermatogenesis can occur without FSH and LH but quantitative production requires gonadotrophins.
• Testosterone modulates LH secretion.
• Inhibin B produced by the Sertoli cells exerts a negative feedback effect on FSH secretion.
• Sex hormone-binding globulin (SHBG) levels fall so that free androgen levels rise.

In girls
• LH stimulates proliferation of follicular and thecal cells, and during the follicular phase of the menstrual cycle induces androgen secretion by theca cells.
• FSH induces proliferation of granulosa cells; increases expression of LH receptors on granulosa cells; enhances aromatase activity so that androstenedione is converted to oestradiol (E2); and increases progesterone production.
• E2 acts on FSH receptors on the granulosa cells to cause proliferation of the follicular cells in addition to inducing secondary sexual development.
• Inhibin B is produced by granulosa cells in small antral follicles, inhibin A by large antral follicles and by the corpus luteum. Inhibins may have a role in inhibiting FSH secretion and in dominant follicle selection.
• Ovulation results from interaction of LH, FSH and E2 on the developing primordial follicle (see below).
• SHBG levels decrease only slightly.

In both sexes
• GH and insulin-like growth factor (IGF-I) secretion are enhanced because of increased levels of sex steroids and insulin.
• Insulin secretion rises and is accompanied by an increase in insulin resistance.

Practical Endocrinology and Diabetes in Children, Third Edition. Joseph E. Raine, Malcolm D.C. Donaldson, John W. Gregory, Guy Van Vliet.
© 2011 Blackwell Publishing Ltd. Published 2011 by Blackwell Publishing Ltd.

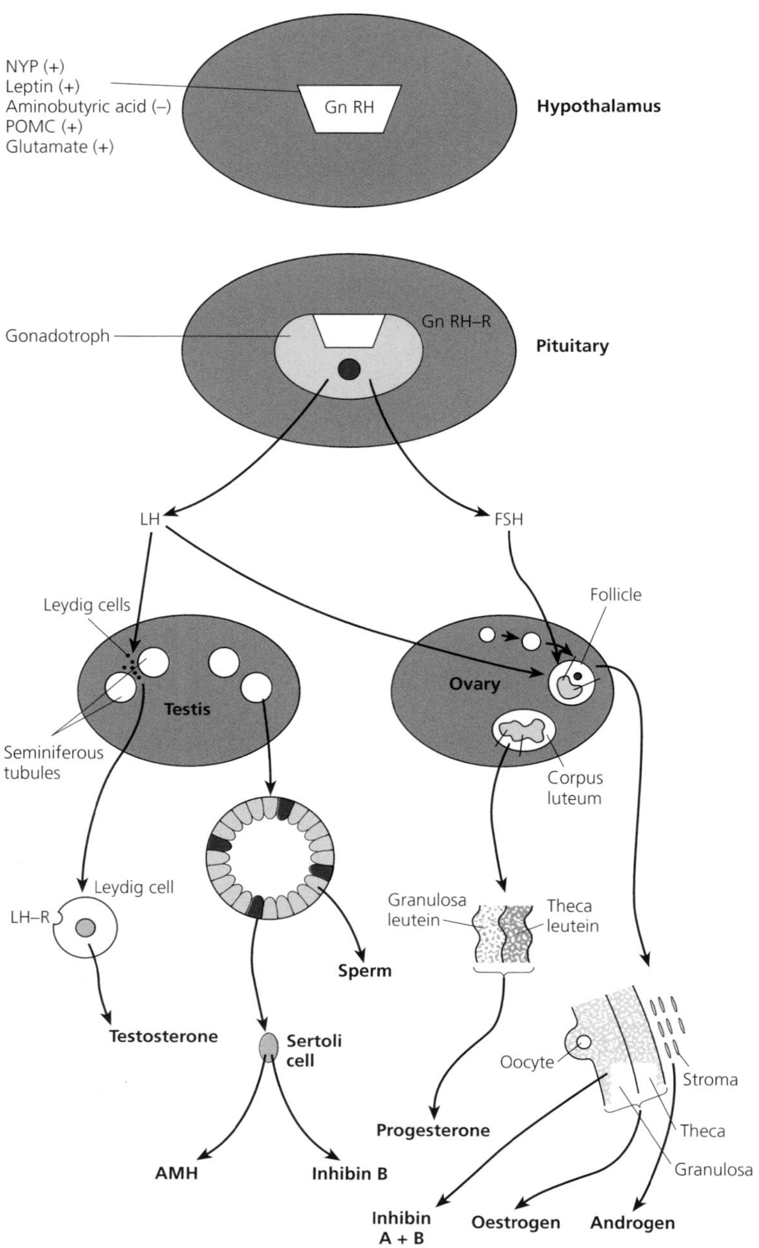

NYP (+)
Leptin (+)
Aminobutyric acid (–)
POMC (+)
Glutamate (+)

Gn RH   **Hypothalamus**

Gonadotroph   Gn RH–R   **Pituitary**

LH   FSH

Leydig cells   Follicle

Testis   **Ovary**

Seminiferous
tubules   Corpus
luteum

Granulosa   Theca
leutein   leutein

Leydig cell

LH–R

Sperm

Testosterone   Sertoli
cell   Oocyte   Stroma

Progesterone   Theca

Granulosa

AMH   Inhibin B

Inhibin   Oestrogen   Androgen
A + B

Fig. 5.1 Schematic representation of
hypothalamic–pituitary–gonadal pathways.
GnRH, gonadotrophin-releasing hormone.

Physiology of the menstrual cycle

During embryogenesis the primordial germ cells migrate
to the ovary and develop into primordial follicles. In the
foetus, the pool of primordial follicles reaches a peak of
around 7 million germ cells at 20 weeks gestation, falling
to 1–2 million at birth, 500,000 at menarche, and about
100 at the menopause. FSH levels reflect the size of the
primordial follicle pool at any given time. Each follicle
contains an oocyte arrested in the prophase of the first
meiotic division.

Follicular phase (approximately 14 days, but variable in duration)

• At the beginning of the menstrual cycle, 15–20 primordial follicles develop of which only one ultimately develops into a Graafian follicle, the rest becoming atretic.

• On day 1 of the follicular phase, FSH levels increase as a result of decreased inhibition from the falling levels of E2 and progesterone (P) at the end of the previous cycle.

• FSH stimulates the follicles to secrete E2 by increasing androstenedione secretion by the thecal cells and inducing aromatase expression in the granulosa cells. Increasing E2 levels causes a decrease in LH and FSH secretion.

• During this time one follicle emerges as dominant, with more FSH receptors than the others; it therefore recruits more of the diminishing supply of FSH, thus secreting more and more E2.

• At this crucial moment E2 feedback on the pituitary changes from negative to positive inducing the pre-ovulatory LH surge.

Luteal phase (always 14 days)

• LH stimulation results in the ovum entering the final phase of 1st meiotic division to become a secondary oocyte. The follicle swells and ruptures, releasing the ovum into the peritoneal cavity, thence into fallopian tube.

• LH induces luteinization of granulosa and thecal cells of the follicle to form the corpus luteum. This results in increased P synthesis; P induces swelling and secretion of the endometrium.

• Progesterone levels peak 5–7 days post ovulation, exerting a negative effect on GnRH and thus causing a decrease in pulse frequency.

• As GnRH pulse frequency falls, FSH and LH secretion decrease, causing the corpus luteum to lose its receptors.

• In the absence of pregnancy, the corpus luteum becomes atretic (corpus albicans), levels of P and E2 fall, and FSH levels start to rise as new cycle begins.

Onset of puberty

The GnRH secreting neurones are under the influence of controlling neurones of both excitatory (glutamate) and inhibitory (GABA) nature. In addition, they are under the control of glial cells which are excitatory. At the time of puberty, changes in trans-synatic neurotransmission and glial inputs (such as that provided by prostaglandins released by astrocytes) result in the pulsatile secretion of GnRH and hence the pubertal cascade.

The following points should be noted:

• In girls, the hypothalamus is more prone to 'break free' of suppression than in boys. Thus, idiopathic precocious puberty is more common in girls, and girls exposed to cranial irradiation and central nervous system (CNS) disorders, such as hydrocephalus, are prone to enter puberty earlier than boys.

• Exposure of the hypothalamus to high levels of sex steroids (e.g. in poorly controlled salt-wasting 21-hydroxylase deficiency) may activate puberty; this phenomenon is known as 'priming'.

Clinical aspects of normal puberty

Pubertal staging

This involves an assessment of breast (B) development in girls, genital (G) development and testicular volume in boys, and pubic (P) and axillary (A) hair development in both sexes. Whenever possible, it is preferable for males to stage boys and for females to stage girls. Male doctors should ensure that a female member of staff is present during the examination of a girl.

Breast staging

  B1 Prepubertal
  B2 Breast budding
  B3 Development of actual breast mound (in obese girls it is difficult to distinguish between B1 and B3)
  B4 Areola projects at an angle to breast mound
  B5 Adult configuration

Genital staging

  G1 Prepubertal penis (unstretched length 2.5–6 cm), scrotum and testes (volume 3 mL)
  G2 Testes 4 mL scrotal laxity, but no penile enlargement
  G3 Penile lengthening with further development of testes and scrotum
  G4 Penile lengthening and broadening, further development of the testes (volume usually 10–12 mL)
  G5 Adult genitalia, testes usually 15–25 mL

N.B.: Testicular volume should be gauged using the Prader orchidometer. Alternatively, length and breadth can be measured using a paper tape measure and assuming that breadth and depth are the same and employing the formula for a prolate ellipsoid, volume can be calculated as 'length × breadth × depth × $\pi/6$'. Penile size (useful for serial staging and important if hypogonadism is suspected) is measured from the base of the penis to tip of the glans (not the foreskin). In obese individuals, it is important to push back the suprapubic fat in order to obtain true penile length.

Pubic hair staging

P1 No pubic hair
P2 Fine hair over mons and/or scrotum/labia
P3 Adult type hair (coarse, curly) but distribution confined to pubis
P4 Extension to near adult distribution
P5 Adult

Axillary hair staging

A1 No axillary hair
A2 Hair present but not adult amount
A3 Adult

Milestones of puberty

Boys enter puberty about 6 months later than girls. Mean ages of breast (B) and genital (G) stages in girls and boys with corresponding height velocities including peak height velocity (PHV) are shown in Table 5.1 (girls) and Table 5.2 (boys).

In girls, breast budding is accompanied by acceleration in growth rate with PHV at B2–3 and usually marked deceleration in height velocity after menarche.

In boys, at G2 growth rate is either the same as or slower than at G1. The increase in growth rate coincides with testicular volumes of 6–10 mL.

In both sexes, the age of onset and duration of pubertal development is subject to marked individual variation. Early puberty is associated with a higher PHV, and delayed puberty with a lower PHV.

The 12.5–14 cm difference in height between adult males and females relates to the following three factors:

Table 5.1 Mean ages of breast (B) stages in girls with corresponding height velocities including peak height velocity (PHV). Data from Tanner et al. 1966.

	Age (years)	Height velocity (cm/year)
B1	Prepuberty	approx 4–7 from 7 years
B2	11.2	7
PHV	12.1	8.3 (6.2–10.4).
B3	12.2	8.2
B4	13.1	5
Menarche	13.5	3.6
B5	15.3	?1

Breast budding is accompanied by acceleration in growth rate with PHV at B2–3 and usually marked deceleration in height velocity after menarche.

Table 5.2 Mean ages of genital (B) stages in boys with corresponding height velocities including peak height velocity (PHV). Data from Tanner et al. 1966.

	Age (years)	Height velocity (cm/year)
G1	Prepuberty	approx 4–7 from 7 years
G2	11.6	5
G3	12.9	6.3
G4	13.8	9.3
PHV	14.0	9.5 (7.2–11.7)
G5	14.9	6.2

At G2 growth rate is either the same as or slower than at G1.
Increase in growth rate coincides with testicular volumes of 6–10 mL.

1 The difference in age of PHV – 12 years in girls and 14 years in boys – means that boys have 2 extra years of 'childhood' growth.
2 The intensity of the growth spurt is greater in boys than girls.
3 Boys are slightly taller than girls during the childhood years.

Pubertal assessment

Clinical

- Height of adolescent
- Mid-parental height and target range
- Height velocity
- Pubertal stage
- Bone age

Pelvic ultrasound

- Assessment of uterine size, shape and endometrial echo reflect the effect of oestrogen.
- Ovarian volumes and the size/number of follicles identified reflect gonadotrophin effect.

Biochemical

This is required where there is diagnostic uncertainty and/or when treatment is contemplated. The biochemical investigation of puberty may include the following tests:

- Karyotype.
- Basal LH and FSH.
- Luteinizing hormone-releasing hormone (LHRH) 100 μg intravenous (IV) with LH and FSH sampling at 0, 30 and 60 minutes.
- Serum testosterone/oestradiol and SHBG.

Table 5.3 Normative data for LH and FSH before (basal) and after (peak) stimulation with 100 μg intravenous LHRH, derived for 85 subjects aged 3–17 years with no evidence of endocrine disease (Tawfik, Galloway and Donaldson). Reference range for testosterone and estradiol is from the Institute of Biochemistry, Glasgow Royal Infirmary.

	LH (units/L)		FSH (units/L)			
Tanner stage	Basal	Peak	Basal	Peak	Testosterone (nmol/L)	Estradiol (pmol/L)
Girls						
B1	0.5 (0.5–2.4)	2.4 (0.5–4.9)	2.0 (0.2–5.0)	12.0 (2.2–26.4)		<50
B2	0.55 (0.5–2.6)	9.7 (1.6–16.4)	3.3 (0.5–8.9)	9.9 (6.8–22.2)		
B3–4	1.6 (0.5–4.8)	23.6 (6.1–50.6)	5.8 (2.5–7.0)	14.3 (12.0–26.7)		
Boys						
G1	0.5 (0.2–0.5)	2.0 (0.5–5.11)	1.0 (0.2–4.7)	4.4 (1.0–11.6)	<0.3	
G2	1.1 (0.5–2.0)	8.3 (4.4–13.8)	1.7 (0.3–4.2)	2.5 (0.9–11.2)		
G3–5	1.9 (1.9–4.0)	16.6 (10.4–21.1)	3.2 (1.8–10.6)	6.3 (2.8–17.0)		
Adult					8.7–35.0	180–1500

- In boys, serum testosterone measurement 4 days after single subcutaneous (sc) injection of hCG 100 units/kg (maximum 1500 units).
- Measurement of serum androstenedione, 17-hydroxy progesterone (17-OHP) and dehydroepiandrosterone sulphate (DHEAS) together with testosterone or oestradiol. In selected cases, this may be done before and after simulation with synacthen together with a 24-hour urine steroid profile.
- Basal gonadotrophins are of limited value in diagnosing puberty, but elevation of FSH (10 units/L) indicates primary gonadal failure.
- Prepubertal LHRH test shows LH peak 5–7 units/L, with LH response less marked than FSH response.
- A pubertal LHRH test shows LH peak 5–7 units/L, LH response usually greater than FSH response.
- A prepubertal LHRH test is indistinguishable from central hypogonadism with GnRH or LH and FSH deficiency.
  Normative data are shown in Table 5.3.

Sexual precocity

Definitions
Sexual precocity: A general term meaning early sexual development of any kind, with no aetiology implied.

True central precocious puberty (TCPP): TCPP is defined in the United Kingdom as normal puberty, resulting from activation of the hypothalamus, and following a normal sequence, but occurring abnormally early—before 8 years in girls and 9 years in boys.

A study in 1997 from the United States demonstrated that signs of early puberty (breast and pubic hair) were present in 25% of black girls and 8% of white girls prior to the age of 8 years. It was therefore suggested that puberty be considered precocious when breast development or pubic hair appeared before the age of 7 years in white girls and before the age of 6 in black girls. This definition would lead to precocious puberty rates of 4–5% in both racial groups. Any girl under the age of 9 years who had started menstruating or who demonstrated rapid pubertal progression would also need to be evaluated.

However, these revised definitions are controversial in the United States and many still use the UK definition. Although most doctors agree that puberty is commencing earlier than in previous generations, the initial definition has not altered in the United Kingdom. This is primarily because there has been no significant change in the average age of menarche which, though slightly earlier than previously, remains at 13 years. Moreover, the assessment of true breast development is difficult in obese girls and the apparent increase in prevalence of early/precocious puberty may reflect the marked rise in obesity prevalence in the West, including the United Kingdom and the United States. Nevertheless, many doctors in the United Kingdom now define early puberty in black girls as that commencing prior to the age of 7 years. Furthermore, there is evidence that 1 in 8 girls start menstruating in primary school. The incidence of precocious puberty in boys is similar in both races.

Precocious pseudopuberty: Sexual precocity caused by the abnormal secretion of sex steroids independent of hypothalamo–pituitary control.

Thelarche: Isolated breast development, commonly in infants and preschool children, in the absence of other symptoms and signs of sexual precocity.

Thelarche variant: A descriptive term for girls in which thelarche is persistent or slowly progressive, often associated with a moderate increase in height velocity and bone age, and sometimes vaginal bleeding, but a prepubertal LHRH test.

Exaggerated adrenarche: In some individuals adrenarche (adrenal puberty occurring between 6 and 8 years) is associated with sufficient androgen secretion to cause symptoms and signs of sexual precocity. This phe-nomenon is often mistakenly referred to as 'premature adrenarche' – a term which should be confined to adrenarche occurring before 6 years of age.

Premature pubarche: A descriptive term simply meaning early onset of pubic hair development which usually occurs in the context of exaggerated adrenarche.

Premature menarche: Cyclical uterine bleeding (confirmed by identifying an endometrial echo on pelvic ultrasound at the time of vaginal bleeding) in the absence of other symptoms and signs of sexual precocity.

Clinical assessment and diagnosis of boys and girls with sexual precocity

Tables 5.4 and 5.5 show the types and causes of sexual precocity in boys and girls. The data illustrate that:

Table 5.4 Types of sexual precocity encountered at Royal Hospital for Sick Children, Glasgow 1989–2009

	Girls	Boys
True central precocious puberty:		
Idiopathic	122	5
Secondary	39	15
Precocious pseudopuberty	10*	9†
Exaggerated adrenarche	251	50
Thelarche	104	
Thelarche variant	44	
Isolated premature menarche	29	

*Feminizing adrenal adenoma (1)
Feminizing ovarian tumour (1)
Virilizing adrenal adenoma (1)
Virilizing ovarian tumour (1)
McCune-Albright syndrome (2)
Simple virilising 21-hydroxylase def (1)
11-hydroxylase def (1)
Cause unknown (2)
†Simple virilising 21-hydroxylase def (3)
Testotoxicosis (1)
Virilizing adrenal adenoma (2)
Oxymetholone (2)
Iatrogenic (accidental absorption testosterone gel) (1)

Table 5.5 Aetiology of true central precocious puberty (onset ≤8 years in girls and ≤9 years in boys) in 189 patients seen at RHSC, Glasgow 1989–2009.

	Girls	Boys
Idiopathic	122	5
Cranial irradiation		
ALL	2	0
Medulloblastoma	1	0
Other tumour	1	0
NHL	0	0
Tumour		
Optic nerve glioma (NF)	6 (4)	5 (3)
Craniopharyngioma	1	1
Hypothalamic hamartoma	3	1
Germinoma	0	1
3rd ventricle cyst	1	1
Neurological disorder		
Learning disability +/– epilepsy	8	4
Hydrocephalus/spina bifida	11	1
Tuberculous meningitis	1	0
Cerebral palsy	5	0
Priming		
11-OHD	1	0
SV 21-OHD	1	3
Oxymethalone	0	2
Testotoxicosis	0	1

Abbreviations: ALL, acute lymphoblastic leukaemia; NF, neurofibromatosis; NHL, non-Hodgkin's lymphoma; 11-OHD, 11-hydroxylase deficiency; SV21-OHD, simple virilizing 21-hydroxylase deficiency.

- TCPP in girls is usually idiopathic (this is the case in >90% of cases);
- idiopathic TCPP is rare in boys;
- precocious pseudopuberty is rare;
- in secondary precocious puberty, the underlying cause is usually self-evident (e.g. known CNS disorder); and
- exaggerated adrenarche is more common in girls than boys.

History

The following two key aspects must be addressed:
1 Symptoms relating to sex steroid production.
2 Features suggesting aetiology of sexual precocity.

Symptoms related to sex steroid production

Androgen-related
- Greasy skin
- Acne
- Greasy hair
- Body odour
- Pubic and/or axillary hair
- Enlargement of penis or clitoris
- Deepening of voice
- Increase in growth rate
- Mood swings/behaviour problems
- Aggression

Oestrogen-related
- Breast tenderness and development (often asymmetrical initially)
- Mood swings/behaviour problems
- Vaginal discharge
- Cyclical vaginal bleeding

Mood swings and behaviour changes; these are important in deciding whether or not to treat precocious puberty, but must be gauged carefully, and where possible, separated as far as possible from 'normal' difficult behaviour!

Features suggesting the cause of sexual precocity
- Family history of early puberty
- Excessive weight gain or obesity in infancy and early childhood
- International adoption
- History of headache, vomiting or visual disturbance (suggestive of intracranial tumour)
- Perinatal problems including: periventricular haemorrhage with hydrocephalus; low birth weight/small for gestational age
- Neurological deficit (e.g. cerebral palsy)

- Cranial irradiation.
- Drug therapy, for example oxymetholone

Physical assessment
- Height.
- Weight.
- Pubertal status, including examination of the genitalia in girls with a history suggestive of androgen excess. Given that it can be difficult to distinguish breast tissue from adipose tissue in overweight girls, examining the patient in the supine position facilitates this distinction.
- Blood pressure.
- Examination of fundi and visual fields.
- Systemic examination.
- Examination for café au lait patches (seen in neurofibromatosis (Figure 5.2) and McCune–Albright syndrome) and axillary freckling (seen in neurofibromatosis).

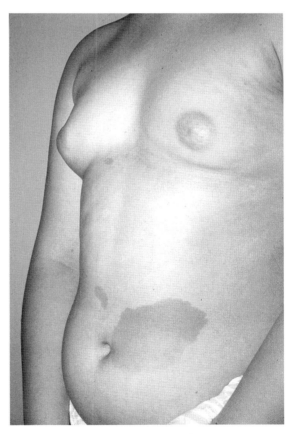

Fig. 5.2 Precocious puberty with B4 development in a 7-year-old girl with neurofibromatosis and optic nerve glioma.

Diagnosis and management of sexual precocity in girls

Oestrogen-mediated sexual precocity

True central precocious puberty (Table 5.5)

Clinical features

In a straightforward case, there will be a history of breast development followed by other features of normal puberty including an increase in growth rate, development of pubic and axillary hair, vaginal discharge, mood swings and sometimes vaginal bleeding. Examination will show a girl who looks older than her chronological age, with a height centile above the parental target range and features of normal puberty.

Investigations

- LHRH test to confirm pubertal response.
- Serum oestradiol.
- In selected cases, thyroid function tests (TFTs), and serum and urine steroid measurements in cases of suspected precocious pseudopuberty.
- Bone age (in TCPP this will often be advanced by ≥ 2 years).
- Pelvic US (in TCPP the ovaries usually enlarge to above 3 mL in volume and contain multiple (>6) follicles that are >4 mm in diameter and the uterus changes from a tubular type structure to a pear-shaped one with the fundal diameter exceeding that of the cervix. Oestrogenization leads to thickening of the endometrium but menarche does not occur until the endometrial thickness is approximately 6–8 mm.
- Pituitary imaging if TCPP confirmed.

Magnetic resonance imaging (MRI) focusing on the hypothalamic–pituitary area and looking for a tumour or hamartoma is the investigation of choice, since resolution is better than with CT scanning.

A French study in 2002 found that the likelihood of finding a tumour or hamartoma in girls with an onset of puberty between the ages of 6–8 years who were otherwise healthy with no neurological symptoms or signs was about 2%. Therefore, an MRI may be unnecessary in this group depending on the clinical situation. The younger the child, the greater the chance of finding a cranial lesion with an incidence of 20% when the onset of puberty is < 6 years.

Management

The object of treatment is to prevent early epiphyseal closure with compromise in final height, and to alleviate psychosocial problems in the girl and her family. In some cases, the pubertal manifestations will remain static or even regress and no treatment will be necessary. In other cases, because the child's age is borderline (i.e. 7–8 years) and the family is coping well or because the progress of puberty is very slow treatment may not indicated. Some families do not wish to have treatment that they perceive as interfering with the natural course of events especially if the TCPP is familial.

If treatment is to be undertaken, the drug of choice is a GnRH analogue which, when given in pharmacological doses, initially leads to stimulation but is then followed by down-regulation of the GnRH receptors, thus inhibiting LH and FSH secretion and leading to a fall in their levels in 2–4 weeks. Available preparations are:

- Goserelin 3.6 mg sc monthly or long-acting preparation giving 10.8 mg s.c. 3-monthly.
- Leuprorelin 3.75 mg sc or intramuscular (im) monthly (half this dose is sometimes used in children <20 kg) or long-acting preparation 11.25 mg sc or im 3-monthly.
- Triptorelin 3.75 mg sc or im monthly (a smaller dose is given in those < 30 kg, an additional single injection is given on day 14 of treatment), or long-acting preparation giving 11.25 mg im. This is the only medication licensed in the United Kingdom for the treatment of TCPP.

In girls with advanced puberty and a thickened endometrium, a withdrawal bleed can occur in the first 4 weeks following the start of treatment due to the fall in the oestrogen levels. This may also occasionally occur in those with less advanced puberty due to the initial stimulatory effect of GnRH treatment. Families should be warned of this possibility. Patients can be treated with cyproterone acetate, starting 3 days before and continuing for 2 weeks after the commencement of GnRH analogue therapy, which usually prevents this problem. However, this drug can cause malaise, weight gain and tiredness, and is therefore only used in selected cases.

Occasionally treatment can be associated with headaches and menopausal symptoms such as hot flushes. Local problems such as erythema and abscesses at the injection site may also sometimes occur.

Rarely, the TCPP is secondary to a tumour in the hypothalamic–pituitary area. In such cases, the histology determines the prognosis. Gliomas tend to be more aggressive than astrocytomas whereas hamartomas are benign. Treatment of the causal lesion usually has no effect on the course of puberty. Hypothalamic hamartomas should not be removed surgically in order to treat the precocious puberty since this can be treated with GnRH analogues. However, hamartomas causing mass effect or gelastic seizures (epileptic fits characterized by laughing) may require surgical management.

Follow-up

Treatment can be expected to prevent or stop menses, to improve mood swings and to decrease height velocity. Usually, treatment maintains the patient at the same pubertal stage as at diagnosis although occasionally there may be a small reduction in breast size. In a minority of girls, puberty continues to progress and in those the monthly preparation of GnRH analogue can be given 3-weekly, or the 3-monthly preparation can be given 9–10 weekly.

The child should be seen 3-monthly initially for clinical assessment and auxology, and then 6-monthly once the symptoms have largely settled and the tempo of puberty is clear. Some centres perform regular pelvic ultrasounds. Bone age should be performed annually.

In girls with very slowly progressive TCPP, there will be little impact on final height. Many girls with untreated TCPP reach a final adult height within the adult reference range. However, these heights may be towards the lower end of the reference range with final heights of 151–155 cm being not uncommon. Final height in treated girls with TCPP will depend on when puberty started and when treatment was commenced. Data on final height suggests that treatment does not fully recover lost height potential and children often do not attain their mid-parental height, possibly because the growth spurt suppressed by treatment does not resume when treatment is stopped. In one study of girls treated till an average age of 11 years, the mean adult height was 160 cm.

The timing of stopping GnRH therapy should be discussed with the family. We have found that menses occurs approximately 12–18 months after discontinuing the injections. This has led us to recommend stopping therapy in the middle to the end of the last year of primary school so that menses usually starts during the first year of secondary school. Families whose girls have learning disabilities may wish to continue treatment for longer but suppressive therapy beyond 11–12 years of age carries the theoretical risk of preventing normal calcium accretion by the skeleton, and so we are reluctant to continue beyond this age.

Precocious pseudopuberty—feminizing (Table 5.4)

The diagnosis is suspected when there is progressive feminizing precocity associated with a prepubertal LHRH test. Causes include adrenal adenoma, granulosa cell tumour of the ovary and McCune–Albright syndrome. The last disorder may present with breast development and vaginal bleeding in a girl with café au lait patches and bony symptoms or signs on X-ray.

Investigations

Serial imaging of the ovaries by pelvic ultrasound, adrenal ultrasound and CT, urine steroid analysis, LHRH test, measurement of the tumour markers – α foetoprotein and β hCG, and a skeletal survey may be required.

Treatment

Surgery is the treatment of choice for adrenal and ovarian tumours. Medical treatment for precocious pseudopuberty is directed at restricting or antagonizing sex steroid production. Useful agents include the following:

- Androgen receptor blockers – cyproterone acetate, flutamide, and spironolactone
- 5α-reductase inhibitors – finasteride
- Testosterone biosynthesis inhibitors – ketoconazole
- Aromatase inhibitors – testolactone, anastrozole

Secondary true puberty resulting from priming of the hypothalamus will require additional GnRH therapy.

Thelarche

Clinical features

Premature thelarche is usually seen in preschool girls (Figure 5.3). Sometimes the breast development has been present from birth. More commonly, the mother notices breast development, often asymmetrical and with a tendency to wax and wane, from the age of 6–12 months. There are no other features of sexual precocity and height velocity is normal. The bone age and pelvic ultrasound are consistent with chronological age.

Investigations

Bone age and pelvic ultrasound may be waived in mild cases of premature thelarche. In more florid cases, these together with an LHRH test should be performed. The FSH response is often pronounced, with 30- or 60-min values of up to 25 units/L while LH values are below 4 units/L. Plasma oestradiol is usually unrecordable using standard assays.

Treatment

None is required.

Follow-up

3- or 4-monthly clinic visits over a 1-year period to confirm that breast development is static or regressing.

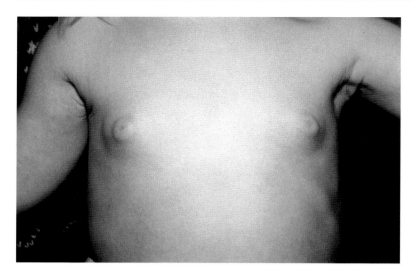

Fig. 5.3 Premature thelarche with stages 2–3 breast development.

Thelarche variant

Girls with thelarche variant are usually between 5 and 8 years of age and present with breast development which persists and may progress slightly in association with slight increase in height velocity and modest advance in bone age. Vaginal bleeding sometimes occurs. Pelvic ultrasound may show an oestrogen effect on the uterus, but is less marked than for TCPP. Ovaries may show some enlargement with an increase in follicular activity.

Diagnosis

Thelarche variant is diagnosed in the context of the clinical and pelvic ultrasound pattern in conjunction with a prepubertal LHRH test, normal imaging of the adrenal glands and an indolent clinical course. Thelarche variant probably includes a variety of conditions including TCPP that is too mild to be detected on the LHRH test, and subtle alterations in responsiveness of the ovaries to normal prepubertal LH and FSH levels.

Management

Usually, no treatment is required but the girls must remain under surveillance and undergo serial auxology, pubertal staging and pelvic ultrasound examination. Rarely, girls may show unacceptable progression of symptoms and signs so that treatment is requested. Under these circumstances, specialist referral is recommended. Peripheral antagonists, such as cyproterone, may be tried.

Premature menarche

This condition occurs in girls usually between 4 and 8 years of age in whom cyclical vaginal bleeding occurs in the absence of other features of sexual precocity. The diagnosis is made by identifying an endometrial echo on pelvic ultrasound when the child is experiencing vaginal bleeding.

Diagnosis

It is essential not to diagnose premature menarche unless the above criteria are satisfied and other causes of vaginal bleeding have been excluded.

These include recurrent vulvovaginitis, foreign body, child sexual abuse, other causes of trauma and vaginal tumours (e.g. rhabdomyosarcoma).

Investigations

Pelvic ultrasound examination is usually sufficient but an LHRH test may be required if there is any suspicion of symptoms other than vaginal bleeding.

Treatment

None required.

Follow-up

3- to 4-monthly review to confirm normal auxology and no development of other features of sexual precocity.

Androgen-mediated sexual precocity

Exaggerated adrenarche

Clinical features
This is by far the most common cause of androgenicity in girls, and presents from 6 years of age with a history of body odour, greasy skin and hair, weight gain and sometimes mood disturbance, usually in association with some pubic and/or axillary hair development.

Diagnosis
Adrenarche must be distinguished from simple virilizing and non-classical 21-hydroxylase deficiency, and androgen secreting tumours of the adrenal glands or ovaries. This is usually easy on clinical grounds as the symptoms and signs of adrenarche are relatively mild and in particular there is no clitoromegaly. Bone age may be advanced by 1 year, sometimes more if obesity is an accompanying feature.

Investigations
In all but the mildest cases, blood should be taken for serum testosterone, androstenedione, 17-OHP and DHEAS (see Chapter 8 for normal values). If baseline androgens are elevated or clinical features are particularly marked, then further investigation with a standard Synacthen test, urine steroid profile and adrenal imaging are indicated to exclude non-classical congenital adrenal hyperplasia (CAH) and an adrenal tumour.

Treatment and follow-up
No treatment is required. If the serum androgens show a mild elevation, particularly of androstenedione and DHEAS, then one further clinic visit in 4–6 months to confirm normal growth rate and lack of progressive virilization is sufficient before discharge. Although a link between exaggerated adrenarche and low birth weight/smallness-for-gestational age and subsequent hyperandrogenism (e.g. polycystic ovary syndrome (PCOS)) has been described, the majority of girls are of normal birth weight and clinical features of androgen excess are mild. We do not, therefore, recommend long-term follow-up in these patients.

Precocious pseudopuberty—virilizing (Table 5.4)
Simple virilizing 21-hydroxylase deficiency is suggested by the combination of advanced growth, clitoromegaly, pubic/axillary hair development and bone age advance, especially if the girl is younger than 6 years. Virilizing

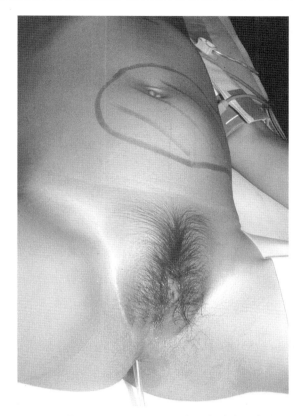

Fig. 5.4 Virilizing ovarian tumour (outline shaded on skin) causing pubic hair and clitoromegaly in a 3-year-old girl.

tumours of the adrenal or ovary are suggested by a shorter history, so that features such as tall stature may not have had time to become manifest (Figure 5.4).

Investigations
Measurement of serum testosterone, 17-OHP, androstenedione and DHEAS under basal conditions and in selected cases after stimulation with Synacthen will demonstrate any abnormalities in serum androgens. A urine steroid analysis may be required to help identify an adrenal enzyme defects. Adrenal MRI or CT may be required as well as careful evaluation of the ovaries on ultrasound. If, despite imaging, a tumour cannot be identified, then selective venous sampling from the adrenal veins should be carried out at a specialist centre.

Treatment and monitoring
Simple virilizing 21-hydroxylase deficiency is discussed in Chapter 8. Virilizing tumours of the adrenal glands and ovaries are treated surgically.

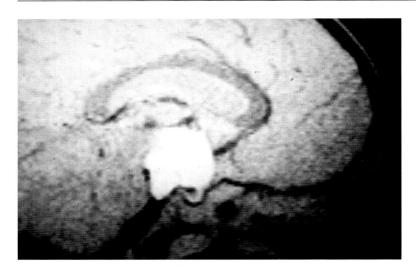

Fig. 5.5 Hypothalamic hamartoma in a 6-year-old boy, causing gelastic seizures and true central precocious puberty.

Follow-up

This involves 3- to 4-monthly assessment to oversee regression of the features of sexual precocity and a normal growth rate. Depending on availability, MRI, CT scanning or ultrasound scanning of the adrenals or ovaries should be performed annually, preferably MRI. Long-term follow-up is needed to pre-empt the development of TCPP because of priming.

Diagnosis and management of sexual precocity in boys

Androgen-mediated sexual precocity

True central precocious puberty (Table 5.5)

This condition is rare in boys, and its occurrence must prompt a search for an underlying cause (Figure 5.5). The prevalence of a brain tumour in boys is 40–90%. Clinical symptoms include rapid growth rate, behaviour disturbances, a deepening of the voice and enlargement of the genitalia. Examination will demonstrate symmetrical enlargement of the testes to volumes 4 mL.

Diagnosis

The combination of sexual precocity with bilateral testicular enlargement makes the diagnosis of TCPP in boys easy. If the testes are prepubertal in volume and/or asymmetrical, the causes of precocious pseudopuberty must be sought (see below).

Investigations

LHRH test to confirm true puberty, with measurement of serum testosterone, followed by imaging of the hypothalamic–pituitary area by MRI. The tumour markers – β hCG and α foetoprotein should be measured to detect germinomas.

Treatment

Treatment is with an LHRH analogue as described for girls with TCPP. Any underlying cause should be treated.

Monitoring

This is as for TCPP in girls. In cases where no brain tumour is found on initial imaging, serial imaging at 6–12-monthly intervals for a 2–3-year period is required to detect an evolving lesion. Testicular size can be expected to diminish and genital development may show some regression. There should also be a reduction in any aggressive behaviour and in the number of erections.

Precocious pseudopuberty (Table 5.4)

Simple virilizing 21-hydroxylase deficiency will result in excessive androgen secretion from the adrenal glands. Adrenal tumours may be androgen secreting. In the testes an activating LH receptor mutation affecting all the Leydig cells (germline) causes a condition known as 'testotoxicosis'. An activating LH receptor mutation affects only a group of cells (somatic) and results in a Leydig cell tumour (Figure 5.6). Precocious pseudopuberty may be seen in boys receiving the anabolic steroid Oxymetholone which exerts a direct androgenic effect (as well as

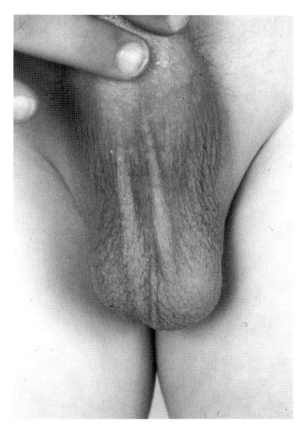

Fig. 5.6 Leydig cell tumour causing slight enlargement of left testis with contralateral atrophy, and precocious pseudopuberty in a 5-year-old boy.

priming the hypothalamus and causing true precocious puberty).

Common to all these rare conditions are testes that are either prepubertal in volume (in the case of adrenal disorders or an exogenous cause), modestly and symmetrically enlarged (i.e. 3–4 mL in testotoxicosis and hCG secreting tumours), or unilaterally enlarged with contralateral atrophy (in Leydig cell tumours). By contrast in TCPP both testes are 4 mL in volume.

Investigations

The LHRH test will show suppressed LH and FSH values in precocious pseudopuberty unless the primary disorder has activated the hypothalamus. Investigations of the underlying cause may include β hCG and α foetoprotein measurement; serum testosterone, 17-OHP, androstenedione and DHEAS before and, in selected cases, following Synacthen stimulation; urine steroid analysis; testicular ultrasound; and adrenal MRI or CT.

Treatment

Surgery is the treatment of choice for tumours. Medical treatments include ketoconazole, cyproterone, testolactone and flutamide.

Adrenarche

Adrenarche is less common in boys than girls, but is still the most common cause of androgenicity. The clinical diagnosis, investigations and management are as for girls.

Oestrogen-mediated sexual precocity

Feminizing tumours of the adrenal glands and testes are extremely rare. Gynaecomastia, caused either by enhanced oestrogen production from aromatization of testosterone at puberty, or by increased tissue sensitivity to normal circulating oestrogen levels, is a relatively common problem in boys and is discussed below.

Delayed puberty and pubertal failure

Definitions

Delayed puberty: This is arbitrarily defined as absence of signs of secondary sexual development in a girl aged 13 years or a boy aged 14 years. A more practical definition is delay in the onset, progression or completion of puberty sufficient to cause concern to the adolescent, parents or physician.

Pubertal failure: Puberty that either fails to begin, or having begun, fails to complete (in which case the term 'mid-pubertal arrest' is often used).

Delayed menarche: First period after 15 years.

Primary amenorrhoea: Failure to start periods.

Secondary amenorrhoea: Cessation of established menses.

Oligomenorrhoea: Infrequent periods (6 per year).

Classification

Delayed puberty is described as **central** or **peripheral**, depending on whether the site of the problem lies in the hypothalamo–pituitary axis or in the gonads. Central delayed puberty can be further subdivided into delay with intact hypothalamo–pituitary axis, and delay caused by impairment of the axis. Table 5.6 gives a working classification of delayed puberty and its causes.

Table 5.6 Classification of delayed and abnormal puberty (including delayed/absent menarche).

Central (both sexes)

Intact H–P axis	CDGA Chronic systemic disease Poor nutrition (including anorexia nervosa) Psychosocial deprivation Steroid therapy Hypothyroidism	

Impaired H–P axis	Tumours adjacent to H–P axis
	    Craniopharyngioma
	    Optic glioma
	    Germinomas, astrocytomas
	Congenital anomalies
	    Septo-optic dysplasia
	    Congenital panhypopituitarism
	Irradiation
	    Pituitary tumour/optic glioma
	    Craniospinal axis for medulloblastoma
	Trauma
	    Surgery, e.g. for craniopharyngioma
	    Head injury
	GnRH/LH/FSH deficiency
	    Congenital idiopathic
	    Kallmann's syndrome
	    Prader–Willi syndrome
	    Laurence–Moon–Bardet–Biedl syndrome	

Peripheral	*Boys*	*Girls*

	Bilateral testicular damage
	    Cryptorchidism
	    Failed orchidopexy
	    Atresia
	    Torsion
	    Syndromes associated with cryptorchidism
		Gonadal dysgenesis
		    Turner's syndrome
		    Pure gonadal dysgenesis

Irradiation/chemotherapy	Noonan's
	Prader–Willi
	Laurence–Moon–Bardet–Biedl
	
	Gonadal dysgenesis
	    Klinefelter's
	    Other XY aneuploidy syndromes
	    XO/XY
	Irradiation/chemotherapy
	    Testicular irradiation
	    Total body irradiation
	    Cyclophosphamide
		Abdominal irradiation
		(for Wilms' tumour)
		Total body irradiation
		Cyclophosphamide, busulphan
		Intersex disorders
		    Including CAIS
		
		Polycystic ovary syndrome
		Toxic damage
		    Galactosaemia
		    Iron overload (thalassaemia)

Abbreviations: CAIS, complete androgen insensitivity syndrome; CDGA, constitutional delay in growth and adolescence; FSH, follicle-stimulating hormone; GnRH, gonadotrophin-releasing hormone; H–P, hypothalamo–pituitary; LH, luteinizing hormone.

Clinical assessment of boys and girls with delayed puberty

Almost all boys and most girls with delayed puberty have simple constitutional delay in growth and adolescence (CDGA). In pathological delayed puberty, the cause may be obvious from the past medical history. The challenge is to diagnose the occasional case of pathological delay in puberty in which the cause is not evident and also the more complicated cases with a multifactorial aetiology (e.g. constitutional, nutritional, social).

History

- *Growth pattern:* The history of long-standing short stature followed by a widening gap in height status between the patient and peer group from secondary school entry onwards is suggestive of CDGA.
- *General health:* An enquiry should be made for any symptoms of chronic ill health. Asthma may be associated with delayed puberty, especially when inhaled steroids have been used.
- *Features/associations with gonadal impairment:* These include a previous history of cryptorchidism, orchidopexy, and gonadal irradiation. An idea of sense of smell can be determined by asking if the adolescent can smell toast burning or unpleasant odours such as rotten eggs.
- *Family patterns:* An enquiry should be made concerning age at menarche in the mother and delayed growth spurt/voice breaking in the father. Where applicable, the pubertal milestones of siblings should be sought.
- *Social and educational aspects:* A tactful enquiry as to the occupation and lifestyle of the family may indicate whether or not there is social disadvantage. The presence of learning disability is established by asking about the need for learning support in mainstream or special education. Learning disability may be a component of dysmorphic syndromes associated with delayed puberty (e.g. Noonan's syndrome).

Examination

- Height, weight
- Measured or (much less reliable!) reported parental heights
- Measured or reported sibling heights
- Pubertal staging
- Nutrition
- Dysmorphic features
- General examination with particular attention to:
  - clubbing;
  - blood pressure; and
  - fundi.

Investigations
(If indicated.)
- Bone age
- Chromosomes
- Basal FSH and LH and serum oestradiol/testosterone
- Pelvic ultrasound in girls
- LHRH test
- Serum testosterone 4 days after hCG 100 units/kg (max 1500 units)
- Urinalysis for blood and protein
- Test of sense of smell

Causes of delayed puberty and pubertal failure

Central delay with intact axis

Constitutional delay in growth and adolescence in boys
By far the most common cause of delayed puberty, CDGA is usually easily diagnosed by the history of long-standing short/borderline short stature during childhood. Following secondary school entry at 11 years, there is a decline in height status so that the boy becomes progressively shorter for age. Commonly, there is a family history of delayed puberty. Frequently, the boy expresses distress to his parents, sometimes related to teasing, but more often because of discomfort at being small and young-looking for age. There is frequently embarrassment about taking showers at school. In boys of 13 years and over, the testes usually show some enlargement (4 mL), but no penile enlargement.

Diagnosis
CDGA should usually be a positive diagnosis and not one of exclusion. However, the presence of possible contributory factors such as poor nutrition, socio-economic and psychological difficulties, and chronic ill health (e.g. severe asthma) can render assessment difficult. Endocrine disturbance is suggested when the short stature and delayed puberty are out of context with the family pattern, when the testes are undescended or abnormal, when there are symptoms and signs such as headache or optic atrophy suggestive of craniopharyngioma, or when penis and testes are hypoplastic, especially in association with impaired sense of smell (Kallmann's syndrome).

Investigation

None is necessary in CDGA except for bone age estimation which usually shows delay.

Management

The boy should be reassured that he is normal, simply a late developer. Prediction of adult height is helpful providing that a single experienced observer performs the bone age assessment. In the United Kingdom, the RUS (TW3) method of Tanner and Whitehouse is preferred. The following medical treatments can be offered in order to enhance growth rate and expedite the features of puberty without affecting final height outcome:
• In boys aged 11.5–13.5 years, oxandrolone 1.25–2.5 mg at night for 3–6 months may be helpful in maintaining a reasonable prepubertal height velocity (4–6 cm per year). Occasionally, such treatment may increase the height velocity to 6–7 cm per year.
• In boys over 13.5 years of age, testosterone therapy may be offered. This can be given as Sustanon 100 mg intramuscularly once a month for 3 months, or as testosterone undecanoate 40 mg orally daily for 3 months. Such treatment should only be given if the clinician is confident that the delay in puberty is physiological, and not a manifestation of underlying disease (e.g. Crohn's disease).

Follow up

Six-monthly visits to the clinic may be helpful in reassuring untreated boys. Boys treated with oxandrolone or testosterone should be seen 6-monthly for two visits following treatment to ensure satisfactory progress. Occasionally, a repeat course of testosterone is indicated. If there is any doubt about the diagnosis of CDGA, it is prudent to keep the boy under observation until testicular volumes are 10 mL.

Constitutional delay in growth and adolescence in girls (Figure 5.7)

CDGA in girls is less common than in boys but remains the most common cause of delayed puberty. Characteristically, the tempo of puberty, when it starts, is slower and a gradual increase in height rather than a discernible adolescent growth spurt is observed (Figure 5.7).

Diagnosis

CDGA in girls must be distinguished from Turner's syndrome as well as other pathological causes of delayed puberty. In doubtful cases, the chromosomes and basal gonadotrophins should be checked and a pelvic ultrasound performed. It should be noted that failure to iden-

tify one, and occasionally both, ovaries may occur in normal girls.

Treatment

In contrast to boys, who can be given a sizeable dose of testosterone with no ill effect on final height, oestrogen therapy in girls is both less effective and more likely to cause premature epiphyseal closure.

Occasionally, pubertal delay is so marked and growth rate so slow that there is a need for treatment. In these circumstances, growth hormone (GH) levels should be measured. Daily ethinyloestradiol 2 µg for a 1–2-year period can be given, with concurrent GH administration if stimulation testing shows GH insufficiency.

Delayed puberty caused by chronic disease

Sometimes the chronic disease is obvious, and the child is referred simply to confirm that no other pathology is responsible and to advise as to possible treatment. The clinician must assess the severity of the chronic disease and confirm that the severity of the delay in growth and adolescence matches the severity of the chronic condition. If this is not the case, then further investigation is indicated.

A small proportion of girls and boys presenting with delayed puberty will be found to have chronic disease as the underlying cause. Gastrointestinal conditions, such as coeliac disease and Crohn's disease, can be notoriously silent. The following screening investigations are of value in selected cases:
• Chromosomes.
• TFT, LH and FSH, cortisol, prolactin (screening for endocrine disease).
• Full blood count (FBC), ferritin, red cell folate, erythrocyte sedimentation rate (screening for gastrointestinal disease).
• IgA Tissue Transglutaminase antibodies (screening for coeliac disease).
• Creatinine, urea and electrolytes, calcium, phosphate, alkaline phosphatase, urinalysis and culture, renal ultrasound (screening for renal disease).

Impairment of the hypothalamo–pituitary–gonadal axis in boys

Central (Table 5.6)

Some adolescents have clear evidence of damage to the hypothalamo–pituitary axis (e.g. craniopharyngioma) and will clearly not enter or complete puberty without

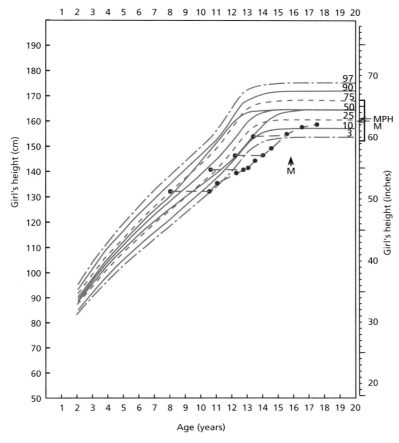

Fig. 5.7 Growth chart of girl with delay in growth and adolescence showing attenuated and late growth spurt with menarche at 15 years of age. Final height is equal to the mid-parental height (MPH). M, menarche.

treatment. Adolescents with delayed puberty who do not fulfil the criteria of CDGA pose some difficulty, for the LHRH test cannot distinguish between physiological central delay and true GnRH or gonadotrophin deficiency.

A history of impaired sense of smell, testicular maldescent and/or surgery and assessment of academic performance must be sought. Examination includes a search for dysmorphic features, systemic examination and detailed examination of the external genitalia. Investigations are detailed above.

Management

In doubtful cases, it is best to induce puberty with testosterone from the age of 13–14 years onwards until either full secondary sexual development has occurred or spontaneous testicular development to 10 mL has taken place (indicating intact endogenous gonadotrophin secretion).

If spontaneous testicular enlargement has not occurred by the age of 16–18 years, replacement therapy should be discontinued and the gonadal axis fully re-evaluated.

Peripheral (Table 5.6)

Primary hypogonadism is suggested by the combination of:

• history compatible with testicular injury (bilateral cryptorchidism, testicular surgery, testicular irradiation, total body irradiation, bilateral torsion);

• behaviour and learning difficulties (evocative of a chromosomal disorder, such as Klinefelter's syndrome);

• abnormal genital examination with one or both testes cryptorchid or abnormally small; and

• testicular volumes which are inappropriate for genital and pubic hair stage (e.g. 4 mL testes in the context of G4, P4).

Investigations

These will show elevated FSH (above 10 units/L) with exaggerated LH and FSH responses to LHRH (FSH often above 50 units/L). Human chorionic gonadotrophin test may show impaired testosterone rise, or no rise in severe cases.

Management

Anorchic subjects will clearly require therapy, as will individuals with poor progression of secondary sexual development, particularly if testosterone levels are low with poor response to hCG. By contrast, boys with low testicular volumes but normal genital and pubic hair development and acceleration of linear growth will not require treatment. As with central hypogonadism, it is best to treat doubtful cases pre-emptively rather than waiting, which carries the risk that development may not progress satisfactorily, resulting in distress to the patient.

Treatment of hypogonadism

The following regimen will bring about satisfactory secondary development in hypogonadal boys:
• Sustanon 100 or 125 mg (half a 250 mg ampoule) every 6 weeks for the first year.
• Sustanon 100 or 125 mg every 4 weeks for the second year.
• Sustanon 250 mg every 4 weeks for the third year, then 250–500 mg every 3–4 weeks depending on clinical factors and serum testosterone levels. Testosterone enanthate, in similar doses, can be used instead of sustanon.

Alternatives include oral testosterone undecanoate 40 mg per day for the first year, 80 mg per day for the second year and 120 mg per day thereafter. Transdermal testosterone in the form of Testogel, 50 mg in 5 mL, can be used, beginning with the application of one sachet weekly and increasing at appropriate intervals by 1 day per week to mimic normal pubertal development is another option which is likely to become more popular in the future. Testosterone pellets implanted every 3–6 months can be used once secondary sexual development is established, but are not currently used to induce puberty.

Impairment of the hypothalamo–pituitary–gonadal axis in girls

Central

The causes of hypothalamic and pituitary gonadotrophin deficiency in girls are similar to boys, although isolated GnRH and gonadotrophin deficiency are rarer. Investigations will show low LH and FSH levels and management is as for boys.

Peripheral

Gonadal dysgenesis as a result of Turner's syndrome or iatrogenic damage from total body irradiation are the main causes of primary gonadal failure in girls.

Investigation

Basal FSH and LH will be elevated in frank ovarian impairment. An LHRH test may be required to demonstrate milder germ cell damage. Pelvic ultrasound may show a less developed uterus than would be expected from the pubertal stage, while ovaries may be small or unidentifiable.

Management

In doubtful cases, pubertal induction should be offered from 12–13 years.

Treatment

It is important for oestrogen replacement to be gradual, not only to avoid premature fusion of the epiphyses, but also to prevent unsightly overdevelopment of the areolae of the breast. The 3-year oral induction regime most commonly used in the United Kingdom is as follows:
• Ethinyloestradiol 2 μg per day for 1 year followed by 4 μg per day for a further year.
• Ethinyloestradiol 6, 8 and 10 μg per day during the third year, in 4-monthly steps.
• Norethisterone 5 mg/day for the first 12 days of each calendar month once the ethinyloestradiol dosage reaches 10 μg per day, or sooner if breakthrough bleeding occurs.

More recently, transdermal oestrogen induction has been used in some centres. A possible regimen is as follows:
• Evorel '25' as a $^1/_4$; patch (6.25 μg per 24 hours) applied twice weekly for 1 year
• Evorel '25' $^1/_2$ a patch (12.5 μg per 24 hours) applied twice weekly for 1 year
• Evorel '25' $^3/_4$ patch (18.75 μg per 24 hours) applied twice weekly for 6 months, then whole patch (25 μg per 24 hours) applied twice weekly for 6 months during the third year, giving Norethisterone 5 mg orally for the first 12 days of each month during the final 4 months.

Following successful pubertal induction:
• low-dose combined contraceptive pill, e.g. Loestrin 20 (21 days on and 7 days off) or ethinyloestradiol 20 μg

daily with Norethisterone 5 mg during the first 12 days of each calendar month may be given; and
• a gynaecologist should be consulted so that further modes of oestrogen replacement (including transdermal patches) can be discussed.

Other pubertal disorders

Menstrual problems

The most common complaint is that of irregular, prolonged and heavy uterine bleeding, sometimes associated with considerable discomfort. This is related to immaturity of the hypothalamic–pituitary–ovarian axis and to anovulatory cycles after onset of menses, and should be considered a normal phenomenon during the first 2 years following menarche. Maintaining a menstrual diary will help assess the severity of the problem. Usually, no treatment is required other than simple analgesia such as mefenamic acid. The antifibrinolytic drug, tranexamic acid, can also be used during episodes of bleeding to diminish blood loss. However, the symptoms may be severe and affect schooling and further treatment may be required.

The following strategies may help:
• Medroxyprogesterone 10 mg per day for the first 5–10 days of menstrual bleeding. This medication may not stop the acute bleeding episode but should produce a normal bleeding episode following withdrawal. It acts by stopping endometrial cell proliferation and allowing organized sloughing of the cells following withdrawal. It will lead to regular cyclic withdrawal bleeding until the hypothalamic—pituitary–ovarian axis has matured.
• Low-dose contraceptive pill such as Loestrin 20 for a 6–12 month period.

Prior to prescribing the above two medications, hypertension and a family history of deep vein thrombosis should be excluded. Caution should also be exercised in patients with epilepsy and liver dysfunction.

In cases of severe and frequent dysfunctional uterine bleeding and when bleeding is so heavy that it is accompanied by clots, one should consider undiagnosed underlying causes such as von Willebrand's disease. An FBC to exclude anaemia and thrombocytopaenia, and iron and coagulation studies may be required. Dietary advice and iron supplements may also be required.

If there is no improvement in the dysmenorrhoea, alternative diagnoses such as endometriosis or obstruction of the lower genital tract should be considered and discussed with a gynaecologist.

Amenorrhoea and oligomenorrhoea are commonly seen as part of normal delayed puberty, and are particularly likely to occur in the context of a low body mass caused by extreme physical training, poor nutrition and eating disorders such as anorexia nervosa. It is rare for girls to start their periods if their body weight is <40 kg. A minimum of 3 to 4 periods a year are required to ensure adequate oestrogenization and to minimize the risk of osteoporosis. If the patient has a completely normal physical examination with secondary amenorrhoea, consider administering medroxyprogesterone, 10 mg once daily for 5 to 10 days to diagnose anovulation as the cause of the amenorrhoea and to see if a withdrawal bleed will occur (progesterone challenge test). If bleeding occurs, then adequate levels of endogenous oestrogen and a normal anatomy have been demonstrated.

Primary amenorrhoea is seen in girls with pubertal failure, anatomical disorders of the reproductive tract (e.g. imperforate vagina or Rokitansky syndrome in which there is congenital absence of the uterus and some or all of the vagina) and in the syndrome of complete androgen insensitivity (see Chapter 7).

Investigation

None is required where the history and examination indicate the diagnosis. Pelvic ultrasound assessment and blood samples for chromosomes, gonadotrophins and sex steroids are helpful in selected cases.

Hirsutism and hypertrichosis

There is an overlap between hirsutism (inappropriate/excessive hair growth in androgen-dependent sites such as moustache and beard area, chest, etc.) and hypertrichosis (generalized increase in body hair).

Hirsutism may be seen in the following instances:
• Certain ethnic groups, for example Mediterranean, Indian subcontinent.
• Caused by androgen secretion by ovarian or adrenal tumours and adrenal enzyme disorders.
• As part of the PCOS.
• Idiopathic, presumably caused by increase in end organ sensitivity.
• Hypertrichosis may be seen in:
• Certain ethnic groups as for hirsutism.
• Primary hypothyroidism.
• Cushing's syndrome, especially iatrogenic.
• Certain dysmorphic syndromes.
• Secondary to drugs such as diazoxide and cyclosporin A.
• Idiopathic.

Diagnosis and management

Androgen excess can be gauged by accompanying features such as tall stature, bone age advance, clitoromegaly, etc. PCOS is suggested by accompanying oligomenorrhoea and/or obesity.

Investigations

These are unnecessary if the hirsutism is mild and the cause obvious (e.g. racial). In selected cases, investigations should be performed as for PCOS.

Treatment

Treatment is directed at the underlying cause, and where this is not possible, cosmetic strategies include bleaching of facial hair, removal of hair by electrolysis and referral to a dermatologist for consideration of laser treatment.

Polycystic ovary syndrome

PCOS has been recently defined by the 'Rotterdam criteria' as the presence of two of the following three criteria:

- Oligo-ovulation or anovulation.
- Hyperandrogenism (clinical or biochemical).
- Polycystic ovaries (defined as an ovary with 12 or more immature follicles measuring 2–9 mm in diameter) with the exclusion of other causes of androgen excess or related disorders.

PCOS may occur in postmenarcheal teenagers and, very occasionally, in premenarcheal girls. The clinical features of PCOS include obesity, hirsutism, greasy skin and hair, acne, oligo/amenorrhoea and subfertility.

In addition to having multiple follicles, polycystic ovaries are often bilaterally enlarged (>9 cm in diameter) and have an increased stromal density.

Polycystic ovaries are not a prerequisite for the diagnosis of PCOS, and are found in approximately 25% of normal women. Laboratory features include elevated serum androgens (particularly testosterone and androstenedione), LH hypersecretion (with an LH to FSH ratio of 3:1 or more), and hyperinsulinism with low SHBG levels. Frequently, only some of the clinical and laboratory features are present.

The cause of PCOS is controversial. Insulin resistance and consequent hyperinsulinaemia in association with obesity are considered key to the pathophysiology but are clearly not essential in slim women who develop PCOS. Nevertheless, even if insulin resistance and hyperandrogenism are not the primary aetiology they do amplify hyperandrogenism in women who put on weight. Moreover, the frequent association of PCOS and obesity has a cumulative deleterious effect on glucose homeostasis and can worsen the hyperandrogenism and anovulation.

Insulin by binding to its own receptor and to IGF-I receptors can increase ovarian androgen production in response to stimulation by LH. Hyperinsulinaemia can also decrease the synthesis of SHBG leading to an increase in circulating free testosterone. Genetic and environmental factors also contribute to the development of PCOS. For instance, South Asian women have the worst symptoms with an increased risk of developing type 2 diabetes.

Diagnosis and management

In a girl with a history suggestive of PCOS, investigations are directed at confirming the diagnosis and excluding conditions such as non-classical CAH and other causes of hyperandrogenism. The full investigation of PCOS with the exclusion of CAH consists of:

- pelvic ultrasound;
- basal LH, FSH and oestradiol;
- serum testosterone, SHBG, androstenedione and DHEAS
- 17-OHP (if 8.00 a.m. 17-OHP is raised a standard Synacthen test (250 µg) is indicated to exclude non-classical CAH due to 21-hydroxylase deficiency)
- Fasting glucose, insulin, HbA1, cholesterol and triglycerides
- TFTs

Testosterone levels are elevated in PCOS but levels of >5.0 nmol/L are unusual and suggest an androgen secreting tumour of the adrenal gland or ovary. An MRI should rule out adrenal pathology and the pelvic ultrasound should have ruled out an ovarian tumour. DHEAS and androstenedione levels are also often elevated. Thyroid dysfunction can lead to amenorrhoea and hirsutism.

Treatment

Mild cases do not require treatment, nor do girls with polycystic ovaries but who are not showing any features of the condition. The cornerstone of non-medical management in obese individuals is weight reduction (by dietary measures and exercise) which reduces the hyperinsulinism and the risk of type 2 diabetes.

Medical treatment is directed at the hyperinsulinaemia and hyperandrogenism. Metformin is used in hyperinsulinaemic girls, especially in the context of obesity. It increases insulin sensitivity and may help to regulate periods. Periods can be regulated with the oral contraceptive pill which will also aid the skin problems. In those with hirsutism, the combination of an oestrogen with an anti-androgen will help combat signs of androgen excess as well as regulating periods. Dianette which contains the anti-androgen cyproterone and ethinyloestradiol and the newer combined contraceptive pill Yasmin which contains drosperidone and ethinyloestradiol can help in this regard. It is important to manage PCOS in collaboration with an adult endocrine physician or a gynaecologist experienced in the field. PCOS is associated with psychological morbidity and an impaired quality of life, and referral to a psychologist or psychiatrist may be indicated.

Breast problems

Breast problems can be divided into gynaecomastia in boys and either asymmetrical or symmetrical smallness or largeness of breast size in girls.

Boys with gynaecomastia

An unfortunate emphasis in fat distribution towards the breast area in simple obesity causes apparent gynaecomastia. Exaggerated breast development at puberty is the most common cause of true gynaecomastia in boys. Normal genital and testicular development should be verified. In severe or doubtful cases, chromosomes for Klinefelter's syndrome, basal gonadotrophins and serum oestradiol should be checked. Occasionally, drugs such as spironolactone will cause gynaecomastia.

Treatment

If gynaecomastia is severe and causing distressing problems (Figure 5.8), for example the boy will not participate in physical activities or have showers in front of his peers, then plastic surgery referral is indicated with a view to mammary reduction by either liposuction or subareolar incision and removal of excess tissue.

Girls with asymmetrical or symmetrical smallness or largeness of breasts

Symmetrical enlargement

Occasionally, breast size is unacceptably large to the girl and family, in which case referral to a plastic surgeon for consideration of reduction mammoplasty is indicated.

Symmetrical smallness

Girls with delayed puberty will have smaller breasts than their peers and can be reassured accordingly. Poor breast growth may occur in girls who have received chest irradiation for cancer (e.g. lung metastases). Once optimal breast size has been achieved by waiting for endogenous puberty to complete, or by oestrogen administration in girls with gonadal failure, referral for augmentation mammoplasty should be discussed with the family. If there is reluctance to inject foreign material, such as silicone, into the breasts of teenage girls on the part of the plastic surgeon, then reconstructive surgery should be considered.

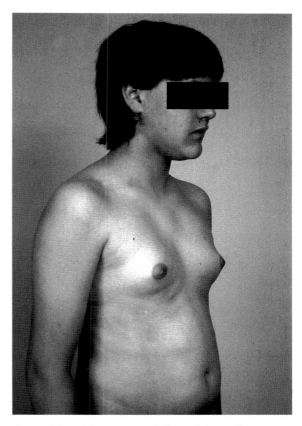

Fig. 5.8 Idiopathic gynaecomastia in an adolescent boy.

Asymmetrical largeness or smallness

Asymmetrical breast development is very common in the early stages of puberty, particularly in girls with sexual precocity. Occasionally, postpubertal girls present with an unacceptable discrepancy in breast size. Investigation is unhelpful and referral to a plastic surgeon is indicated for either reduction mammoplasty on one side or augmentation mammoplasty on the other.

Future developments

- More physiological approaches to the delivery of sex steroids is required both in the context of pubertal induction and hormone replacement. Transdermal regimens are likely to become more widely used although a recent UK survey has shown that the oral contraceptive pill is still the most common form of maintenance replacement in adolescents and young adults with Turner's syndrome.

• Measures of the adequacy of sex steroid replacement in adolescents and young adults will include bone mineral density, cardiovascular risk factors and, in females, uterine morphology.
• There is interest in offering males with central hypogonadism, who have completed pubertal induction with testosterone, therapy with LH and FSH to increase testicular volume and thereby facilitate fertility at a later stage.
• The psychological assessment and counselling of adolescents and young adults with hypogonadism and infertility is an important area for further development.

Potential pitfalls

• Girls with apparent breast development in association with weight gain, tall stature, and pubic hair may be considered to have precocious or early puberty when the actual diagnosis is that of exaggerated adrenarche in association with simple obesity (causing increased growth rate) and giving the impression of true breast development. Pelvic ultrasound is useful in showing a prepubertal uterus, but a GnRH test may be required to clarify the diagnosis in some cases.
• The diagnosis of puberty should not be made by measurement of basal gonadotrophins alone, particularly when GnRH analogue treatment is contemplated, and an LHRH test should be performed.

Controversial points

• What is the preferred option for the hormonal treatment of CDGA in boys?
• What hCG regimen (dose, number of injections, and time scale) should be used in the gonadal assessment of boys?
• What hormonal treatment can be offered to girls with CDGA?
• There is no consensus as to the most physiological and acceptable methods of long-term sex steroid replacement in boys and girls with hypogonadism.

When to involve a specialist centre

• Girls with sexual precocity when
  (a) diagnosis unclear; or
  (b) treatment contemplated.
• All boys with sexual precocity.
• Hypogonadism.
• PCOS.

Useful information for parents and patients

Premature Sexual Maturation Group (part of the Child Growth Foundation) 2 Mayfield Avenue, Chiswick, London W4 1PW, UK. Tel: 02089950257. Fax: 02089959075. Website: www.heightmatters.org.uk
Serono/Child Growth Foundation booklets. Websites: http://www.bsped.org.uk/patients/serono/04_Premature_Sexual_Maturation%20.pdf
http://www.bsped.org.uk/patients/serono/03_Puberty_and_the_Growth_Hormone_Defficient_Child.pdf
European Society of Paediatric Endocrinology leaflets (available in a number of languages) Websites: http://www.eurospe.org/patient/English/easy/Precocious%20puberty%20easy%20readability.pdf
http://www.eurospe.org/patient/English/average/puberty%20and%20the%20GHD%20child%20average%20readability.pdf

Significant guidelines/consensus statements

Carel, J.C., Eugster, E.A., Rogol, A. *et al.* Consensus statement on the use of gonadotropin-releasing hormone analogs in children. *Pediatrics Apr* 2009 **123**(4), e752–62.

Case histories

Case 5.1

A 7-year-old girl presents with breast enlargement and slight vaginal discharge, together with moodiness and body odour. There is no relevant past history and she is well with no headaches, visual disturbance or polydipsia. Mother and two elder sisters had early menarche at 10–11 years. At the age of 7.8 years, the girl looks more like an 11-year-old and bone age is advanced at 10.8 years. Height is on the 90th centile and mid-parental height 50th centile. Examination shows Tanner stage B3, P2, A1. Pelvic ultrasound shows heart-shaped uterus with 4-mm endometrial echo, uterine length 5 cm. Ovaries are 3.5 mL in volume with 5–6 6-mm follicles in each. GnRH test shows basal/stimulated values of 2.6/20 units/L for LH, and 3.2/15 units/L for FSH.

Question

What is the diagnosis, what further investigations should be carried out, and what treatment should be offered?

Answer

This girl has true precocious puberty—onset of pubertal development before the age of 8 years in a girl with a pubertal LHRH test. Idiopathic TCPP is the likeliest cause but it is now regarded as good practice to carry out pituitary imaging with MRI in girls as well as boys with TCPP. Given the age of the girl, the intensity of pubertal tempo and the behaviour disturbances, most clinicians would recommend suppressive therapy with an LHRH analogue but this must be carefully discussed with the family.

Case 5.2

A boy of 14 is referred with short stature and concern over pubertal development. He is a somewhat reticent historian but systematic inquiry reveals a fall-off in school attendance and performance over the past year. Further questioning indicates that he has been experiencing some diarrhoea and abdominal pain. On examination, the boy does not look unwell, but weight has dropped from 42 kg at clinic 3 months ago to 39.2 kg now. Height at 138 cm is below the 3rd centile (mid-parental height 25th centile). There is mild finger clubbing. The testes are enlarged (4 mL) with scrotal laxity but prepubertal penis and no pubic or axillary hair. Examination is otherwise unremarkable, blood pressure 110/70. Bone age is delayed at 11.2 years.

Questions

What is the pubertal stage in this boy? What is the clinical diagnosis? What (if any) investigations should be carried out. What treatment should be offered?

Answers

The pubertal stage is G2, P1, A1. While physiological delay in puberty is by far the most common cause of short stature and delayed puberty in boys, the vague abdominal symptoms, poor school performance, and finger clubbing suggest that the boy should be investigated for chronic disease. Barium meal and follow through showed extensive abnormality in the small bowel, particularly the terminal ileum and the diagnosis of Crohn's disease was subsequently confirmed.

This case illustrates the importance of history taking and general examination in endocrine practice. It would be inappropriate to carry out a height prediction on this boy, whose delayed puberty was caused by illness. Successful treatment of the underlying disease, rather than testosterone therapy, is indicated here.

Case 5.3

A girl of 14 years is seen in the joint oncology/endocrine clinic with concern over delayed menarche. She developed acute lymphoblastic leukaemia aged 10 years, relapsed 18 months after treatment and was successfully managed with autologous bone marrow transplantation. Total body irradiation in the dose of 1400 cGy and cyclophosphamide were given as part of her conditioning pre-transplant. On examination, she is on the 25th centile for height (mid-parental height 75th centile), Tanner stage B3, P3, A2. Pelvic ultrasound shows a cylindrical uterus measuring 3.2 cm with no endometrial echo, ovaries 1.2 and 1.8 mL in volume with no follicles seen. Basal FSH is 58 units/L, LH 20 units/L, oestradiol <50 pmol/L.

Questions

What is the diagnosis, what further data are required, and how should this girl be managed?

Answers

This girl has primary ovarian failure caused by total body irradiation, resulting in mid-pubertal arrest. Pelvic ultrasound shows reduced uterine size and immature configuration attributable to oestrogen insufficiency. She will require oestrogen replacement, but before instituting this, her bone age and stimulated GH level should be tested. Bone age was 11.6 years and peak GH level 14 mU/L following insulin hypoglycaemia. Treatment with GH therapy was declined by the girl and her family but she agreed to starting low-dose ethinyloestradiol aiming for a full replacement dose within 18 months.

Case 5.4

A 15-year-old girl presents to the emergency department with heavy periods. Her general practitioner (GP) has done an FBC which has shown haemoglobin of 5.2 g/dL with a normal white cell and platelet count. Her periods started at the age of 11 years and are regular at 4 weekly intervals but are heavy with some clots. She says she feels a little tired. She has no bleeding or bruising elsewhere and there is no family history of heavy periods or bleeding disorders. She is otherwise well. The family are vegetarians. On examination, she looks pale. Respiratory rate is 20/min and her chest is clear. Pulse rate is 96/min and there is a grade 2/6 ejection systolic murmur heard loudest to the left of the sternal edge. There is no hepatomegaly and there are no other cardiac signs.

Questions

1. What is the likeliest cause of the heart murmur?
2. What investigations should be performed?
3. What treatment should be instituted?

Answers

1. The likeliest cause of the heart murmur is anaemia which can lead to a hyperdynamic circulation and a subsequent flow murmur. In the absence of any cardiological symptoms and any other cardiac signs, it could be kept under review as it is likely to disappear once anaemia has resolved.
2. A ferritin, and in the appropriate racial groups, a haemoglobinopathy screen, should be performed. This girl's ferritin was low at 12 ng/mL (normal range 20–300 ng/mL) due to heavy bleeding (the presence of clots denotes heavy bleeding) and her vegetarian diet. A clotting screen should also be done to try and rule out conditions such as von Willebrand's disease. However, the absence of heavy periods in her mother and bleeding disorders in the family makes this diagnosis unlikely. A pelvic ultrasound would also be useful to confirm that the reproductive organs are normal. A gynaecological opinion would also be helpful.
3. Although she is severely anaemic, she has no significant symptoms. Her respiratory and pulse rate are within normal limits and she is not in heart failure. The onset of anaemia is likely to have been slow over several months. A blood transfusion is therefore not indicated and iron tablets should be prescribed. She does not eat meat which is the best dietary source of iron, but green vegetables and cereals are also good sources. Tranexamic acid (an antifibrinolytic agent) can also be used on the days when there is bleeding to diminish the blood loss. If heavy periods persist, then a low dose contraceptive pill could be used to decrease the bleeding.

Further reading

Carr, B.R. (1998) Disorders of the ovaries and female reproductive tract. In: *Williams Textbook of Endocrinology* (eds J.D. Wilson, D.W. Foster, H.M. Kronenberg & P.R. Larsen), 9th edn., pp. 751–818. W.B. Saunders, Philadelphia.

Chalumeau, M., Chemaitilly, W., Trivin, C. *et al.* (2002) Central precocious puberty in girls: an evidence-based diagnosis tree to predict central nervous system abnormalities. *Pediatrics Jan 2002* **109** (1), 61–7.

Gault, E.J. & Donaldson, M. (2009) Oestrogen replacement in Turner syndrome: current prescribing practice in the UK. *Clinical Endocrinology 2009* **71**, 752–755.

Griffen, J.E. & Wilson, J.D. (1998) Disorders of the testes and male reproductive tract. In: *Williams Textbook of Endocrinology* (eds J.D. Wilson, D.W. Foster, H.M. Kronenberg & P.R. Larsen), 9th edn., pp. 819–876. W.B. Saunders, Philadelphia.

Griffin, I.J., Cole, T.J., Duncan, K.A. *et al.* (1995) Pelvic ultrasound measurements in normal girls. *Acta Paediatrica* **84**, 536–543.

Herman-Giddens, M.E., Slora, E.J., Wasserman, R.C. *et al.* (1997) Secondary sexual characteristics and menses in young girls seen in office practice: a study from the Pediatric Research in Office Settings network. *Pediatrics Apr 1997* **99** (4), 505–12.

Kaplowitz, P.B. & Oberfield, S.E. (1999) Reexamination of the age limit for defining when puberty is precocious in girls in the United States: implications for evaluation and treatment. Drug and Therapeutics and Executive Committees of the Lawson Wilkins Pediatric Endocrine Society. *Pediatrics Oct 1999* **104** (4 Pt 1), 936–41.

Kelly, B.P., Paterson, W.F. & Donaldson, M.D.C. (2003). Final height outcome and value of height prediction in boys with constitutional delay in growth and adolescence treated with intramuscular testosterone 125 mg per month for 3 months. *Clinical Endocrinology* **58**, 267–272.

Marshall, W.A. & Tanner, J.M. (1969) Variations in pattern of pubertal changes in girls. *Archives of Disease in Childhood* **44**, 291–303.

Marshall, W.A. & Tanner, J.M. (1970) Variations in the pattern of pubertal changes in boys. *Archives of Disease in Childhood* **45**, 13–23.

Paterson, W.F., Hollman, A.S., McNeill, E. *et al.* (1998) Use of long acting goserelin in the treatment of girls with precocious and early puberty. *Archives of Disease in Childhood* **79**, 323–327.

Tanner, J.M. (1962) *Growth at Adolescence*, 2nd edn. Blackwell, Oxford.

Tsilchorozidou, T., Overton, C. & Conway, G.S. (2004) The pathophysiology of polycystic ovarian disease. *Clinical Endocrinology* **60** (1), 1–17.

6 Thyroid Disorders

Embryology, anatomy and physiology of the thyroid gland

Embryology and anatomy

The thyroid gland develops from the floor of the pharynx at 4 weeks gestation in the form of a diverticulum which travels inferiorly leaving the thyroglossal tract in the neck. The latter normally disappears but cystic remnants may remain and form a thyroglossal cyst. The diverticulum becomes bi-lobed and fuses with the ventral aspect of the fourth pharyngeal pouch. Our understanding of the genetic mechanisms controlling thyroid organogenesis is incomplete but three transcription factors TTF1, TTF2 and Pax8 are known to have a crucial role in activating thyroid specific genes such as thyroglobulin and thyroid peroxidase. The thyroid gland has a butterfly-shaped structure with its two lobes connected by the isthmus and is situated below the Adam's apple (larynx) between C5 and T1 overlying the 2nd–4th tracheal rings. In an adult, each lobe is about 5 cm long and 1.5 cm wide.

Physiology

The main function of the thyroid gland is to synthesize thyroxine (T4) and triiodothyronine (T3).

Control of thyroid metabolism

The hypothalamus secretes thyrotropin-releasing hormone (TRH), which stimulates the anterior pituitary to secrete thyroid-stimulating hormone (TSH). TSH acts on the thyroid cell by binding to a specific receptor (TSH-R) as shown in Figure 6.1. The occupied receptor activates the G stimulatory protein which then stimulates thyroid metabolism via the adenylate cyclase, calcium and phospholipase C pathways.

T4 synthesis

Figure 6.2 shows the main steps in T4 synthesis. Dietary iodine is actively taken up by the thyroid follicular cells by the sodium iodide transporter (NIS) and transported within the thyrocyte to the colloid by the protein Pendrin. Iodine is oxidized to iodide by hydrogen peroxide, which is generated by the thyroid oxidase genes *THOX-1* and *THOX-2*, and controlled by the enzyme thyroid peroxidase (TPO). Tyrosyl residues on the thyroglobulin molecule are then iodinated to form monoiodotyrosine (MIT) and diiodotyrosine (DIT). These iodinated tyrosine molecules are coupled to form the iodothyronines, again under TPO control, followed by cleavage of the residues from the thyroglobulin molecule to release MIT, DIT, T3 and T4. The redundant tyrosine molecules then undergo deiodination by iodotyrosine dehalogenase to

Practical Endocrinology and Diabetes in Children, Third Edition. Joseph E. Raine, Malcolm D.C. Donaldson, John W. Gregory, Guy Van Vliet.
© 2011 Blackwell Publishing Ltd. Published 2011 by Blackwell Publishing Ltd.

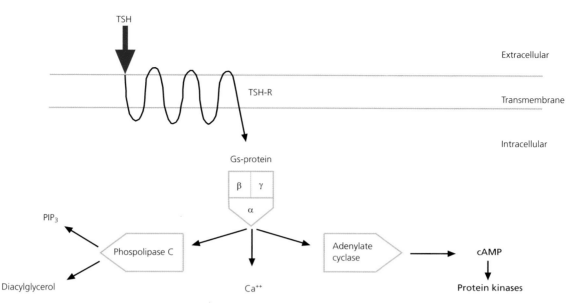

Fig. 6.1 Schematic representation of TSH receptor, TSH-R, and intracellular pathways. Gs-protein, G stimulatory protein; PIP$_3$, phosphatidyl inositol triphosphate.

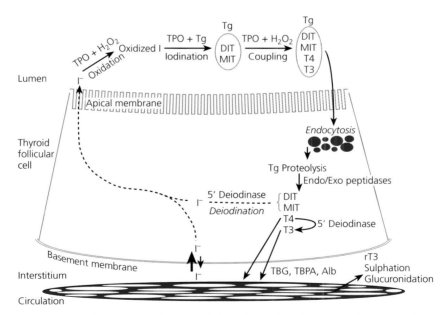

Fig. 6.2 Schematic representation of thyroxine (T4) and triiodothyronine (T3) synthesis. TPO, thyroid peroxidase; H$_2$O$_2$, hydrogen peroxide; Tg, thyroglobulin; MIT, monoiodo-tyrosine, DIT, diiodotyrosine; TBG, thyroxine-binding globulin; TBPA, thyroid binding pre-albumin; Alb, albumin; rT3, reverse T3.

salvage the iodide. The thyroid gland is the sole pro-
ducer of T4 and produces 20% of T3. Most T3 is produced by deiodination in the peripheral tissues. T3 is
3–4 times more potent than T4 and is responsible for
most thyroid activity. Gene mutations encoding various
thyroid enzymes, for example thyroid peroxidase, may
occur resulting in dyshormonogenesis. These mutations
are inherited in an autosomal recessive manner.

T4 metabolism

After T4 is secreted by the thyroid gland, it is metabolized by the tissue enzymes deiodinase type I, II and III.
Type II deiodinase catalyses T4 to T3 conversion by outer
ring deiodination (ORD) (Figure 6.3). Type III deiodinase converts T4 to the inactive reverse T3 (rT3) by inner
ring deiodination (IRD) while type I deiodinase catalyses
both ORD and IRD. Seventy per cent of circulating T4 and
50% of circulating T3 is bound to thyroxine-binding globulin (TBG), the remainder to other proteins, primarily
albumin. Only 0.03% of circulating T4 and 0.3% of T3 is
unbound. Thus, total T4 and T3 concentrations reflect the
TBG concentration, while free hormone measurements
represent the active hormones and are therefore a more
accurate assay of thyroid function.

Action of the thyroid hormones

The thyroid hormones have profound effects on growth,
neurological development, metabolism, and cardiovascular function. T4 and T3 bind to α, β1 and β2 receptors in
the target tissues, for example pituitary and hypothalamus (β2), liver (β1 and β2), heart (α), and brain (α and
β1). This results in an increase in oxygen consumption,
altered protein carbohydrate and lipid metabolism and
potentiation of the action of catecholamines.

Foetal and neonatal thyroid metabolism

Foetal thyroid metabolism

During the first trimester the foetus is largely dependent
on small amounts of maternal T4 and T3 that cross the
placenta. Levels of TSH start to rise from the second
trimester onwards. Total T4 rises in response to this and
also to increasing TBG levels. However, plasma T3 and
T4 levels are low in foetal life compared with high inactive
rT3 levels because of the foetal predisposition to inactivation of the thyroid hormones. Although plasma T4 and
T3 are low, these hormones are present in relatively high
concentrations in target tissues, such as the brain. Furthermore, while only small amounts of maternal T4 and
T3 cross the placenta, the quantities are significant so

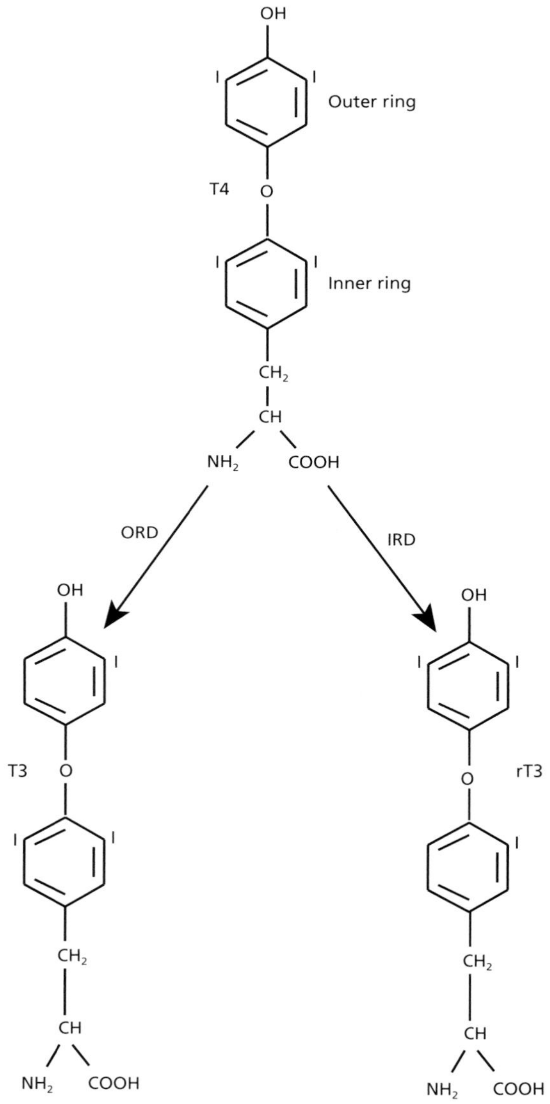

Fig. 6.3 Conversion of T4 by outer ring deiodination (ORD) to
T3 and inner ring deiodination (IRD) to reverse T3 (rT3).

that T4 is measurable in babies with thyroid agenesis
shortly after birth. Maternal iodine deficiency and maternal hypothyroidism are both associated with intellectual
impairment in the child, proof of the vital importance of
the maternal contribution to foetal thyroid function.

Thyroid function in term neonates

At birth there is an acute release of TSH. This TSH surge
results in high T4 and T3 levels (Figure 6.4). The ratio of
T4 and T3 to rT3 rises corresponding to preferential ORD

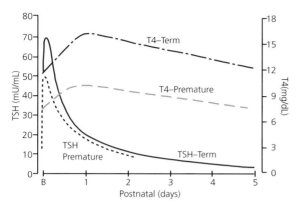

Fig. 6.4 Changes in serum TSH and T4 concentrations in full term and premature infants during the first 5 days of life. (From Fisher & Klein 1981, copyright 1981 Massachusetts Medical Society. All rights reserved.)

Table 6.1 Normal values for the common thyroid function tests.

Free T4	10–26 pmol/L	0.8–2.4 mg/dL
Free T3	2.5–5.3 pmol/L	2.0–4.0 pg/mL
Total T4	58–140 nmol/L	4.6–10.5 μg/dL
Total T3	1.1–2.2 nmol/L	80–185 ng/dL
TSH	0.5–6.0 mU/L	
Thyroglobulin		
• Cord blood	150 pmol/L	100 μg/L
• Newborn period	50–256 pmol/L	33–170 μg/L
TPO antibodies	<50 mU/L	
TSH receptor antibodies	<15 U/L	

Abbreviations: T3, triiodothyronine; T4, thyroxine; TSH, thyroid-stimulating hormone; TPO, thyroid peroxidase.

of T4 and decreased thyroid hormone inactivation. Levels of T4 and T3 are high by 7 days, falling thereafter so that by 14 days of age concentrations are similar to those found in infancy and childhood.

Thyroid function in preterm neonates

The preterm infant, especially below 34 weeks gestation, shows the foetal pattern of low plasma T3 and T4 with high rT3. Factors contributing to this pattern include immaturity of the hypothalamic–pituitary axis, premature cessation of the small but significant maternal contribution to circulating thyroid hormone levels, persistence of the foetal tendency towards inactivation of T4 and T3 and a negative iodine balance. It is uncertain whether or not the preterm thyroid state should be regarded as physiological, or pathological and requiring intervention. The situation is complicated by the knowledge that concentrations of thyroid hormones in the tissues may be substantially different to those found in the plasma. The issue of low T4 levels in preterm infants is discussed further below.

Thyroid function tests (TFTs)

Table 6.1 shows the normal values for the commonly measured TFTs. Free T4 (FT4) or T4 and TSH measurements are the mainstay of assessment in hypothyroidism, with TSH the most sensitive indicator of primary disease. In primary hyperthyroidism, TSH is suppressed and there is preferential conversion of T4 to T3, so that the latter should be measured in suspected cases. TBG measurement is helpful in distinguishing between spurious and true hypothyroxinaemia but is redundant if FT4 is measured.

Measurement of TPO antibodies (previously antimicrosomal and antithyroglobulin antibodies were measured) is used in the diagnosis of autoimmune thyroiditis. Stimulatory TSH receptor antibodies are positive in Graves' disease. Thyroglobulin is a 660 kDa protein synthesized exclusively in the thyroid gland so that the presence of thyroid tissue can be inferred if it is detectable in the serum. Thyroglobulin can be useful in diagnosing the cause of congenital hypothyroidism (see below) and in the monitoring of patients following thyroidectomy or radioiodine for thyroid cancer. In pituitary and hypothalamic diseases, TSH levels will be inappropriately low for the low FT4 (or T4) level. The TRH test has traditionally been used to help differentiate secondary and tertiary hypothyroidism. Recent improvements in the quality of hypothalamic and pituitary magnetic resonance imaging (MRI) have provided a further means of assessment.

TRH test

TRH test is no longer available in North America but this test is still sometimes used in the United Kingdom and in other countries.

Preparation: Non-fasting.

Precautions: May cause mild flushing and desire to micturate.

Protocol: T = 0: 7 μg/kg TRH (protirelin), 200 μg max., intravenously over 1 min.

T = 0, 20, 60 min: serum TSH.

Interpretation: Normally TSH peaks at 10–30 mU/L at 20 min with a fall by 60 min. With dysfunction in the thyroid gland itself, basal TSH is > 6 mU/L and the peak is >30 mU/L. In pituitary disease, TSH levels fail to rise normally in response to TRH. In contrast, in hypothalamic disease basal TSH is high/normal and there is a delayed TSH response to TRH, with TSH higher at 60 min than at 20 min.

Definition and classification of thyroid disorders

The term **hypothyroxinaemia** describes the phenomenon of low T4 levels in the context of normal plasma TSH levels. It is encountered in the preterm infant, in acute non-thyroidal illness (e. g. during malnutrition, trauma and diabetic ketoacidosis when it is sometimes termed the 'sick euthyroid syndrome') and in association with certain drugs. During recovery, thyroid hormone levels spontaneously return to normal.

Hyperthyrotropinaemia is a purely descriptive term which refers to a mild elevation of TSH (e. g. 7–15 mU/L) in the context of normal FT4 (or T4) concentrations.

Hypothyroidism is a state in which the hypothalamic–pituitary–thyroid axis is failing, or is in danger of failing, to produce sufficient T4. Hypothyroidism can be classified according to:
- *site of abnormality:* thyroid (primary), pituitary (secondary), hypothalamus (tertiary);
- *timing of abnormality:* prenatal (congenital) or postnatal (acquired); and
- *severity:* thyroid axis jeopardized but able to produce normal T4 levels (compensated hypothyroidism); thyroid axis unable to maintain normal T4 levels (decompensated hypothyroidism).

Hyperthyroidism refers to overproduction of T4 and is almost invariably primary.

The term **goitre** refers to thyroid gland enlargement. A goitre is best inspected with the child's neck slightly extended. Asking the child to swallow will make a goitre more obvious. The gland is best palpated with the examiner standing behind the child and can be described in terms of size, texture (e. g. smooth or nodular), consistency and symmetry. Goitres may be sub-classified according to thyroid function—hypothyroid, hyperthyroid or euthyroid goitre.

Neonatal hypothyroxinaemia, hyperthyrotropinaemia and transient neonatal hypothyroidism

Neonatal hypothyroxinaemia
Preterm infants commonly have hypothyroxinaemia which may become more marked during acute ill-

ness (e. g. respiratory distress syndrome). The hypothyroxinaemia may be secondary to immaturity of the hypothalamic–pituitary axis and the T4 level may be normal for the infant's gestational age. TSH levels are usually normal. TFTs should be repeated after 2 weeks and kept under surveillance. If the T4 level remains low with an elevated TSH than treatment is indicated.

There is some evidence that mortality and neurodevelopmental outcome is worse in preterm infants who have been hypothyroxinaemic, prompting interest in giving thyroid replacement. However, T4 administration is ineffective, FT4 and T4 levels rise but T3 remains low and it is likely that the administered T4 is converted to rT3. Preliminary data suggest that T3 administration is also ineffective. Moreover, the safety of exposing preterm infants to thyroid hormones is unknown. A Cochrane review concluded that there is insufficient evidence at present to support the use of thyroid hormones in preterm infants.

Hyperthyrotropinaemia
This non-specific label should only be used once mild compensated primary congenital hypothyroidism (e. g. due to thyroid ectopia) has been excluded by thyroid imaging. Neonatal hyperthyrotropinaemia may reflect the physiological TSH surge or be caused by delayed maturation of the hypothalamic–pituitary–thyroid axis. It is commoner in preterm infants. No treatment is required but the infant should be kept under surveillance until the TSH normalizes.

Transient neonatal hypothyroidism
(Table 6.2)
Transient TSH elevation, with or without a low FT4 (or T4), accounts for roughly 25% of cases referred by the screening laboratory if TSH is measured on day 5. It is strongly associated with sick and/or preterm newborns

Table 6.2 Causes of transient neonatal hypothyroidism.

Chronic iodine deficiency
Acute iodine excess (e. g. following antiseptic administration for sterile procedures)
Perinatal stress (e. g. birth asphyxia, respiratory distress, sepsis)
Down's syndrome
Transplacental transfer of maternal antibodies
Maternal drugs (e. g. carbimazole, amiodarone)

and those suffering from congenital malformations. More rarely, it is caused by transplacental transfer of maternal medication, transplacental transfer of maternal TSH receptor blocking antibodies, or iodine deficiency or excess. If TSH elevation is >10 mU/L then treatment should be started (see section 'Congenital hypothyroidism').

Congenital hypothyroidism

Permanent congenital hypothyroidism is one of the most common disorders in paediatric endocrinology with an incidence of approximately 1 in 3500 births. It is the commonest treatable cause of learning difficulties. The commonest worldwide cause is iodine deficiency. In areas with severe iodine deficiency, congenital hypothyroidism is endemic and leads to learning difficulties, short stature, deafness and neurological abnormalities.

Aetiology (Table 6.3)

Thyroid dysgenesis accounts for approximately 70–80% of congenital hypothyroidism. The most common form is an ectopic thyroid, followed by thyroid agenesis (undetectable thyroid gland on thyroid imaging) which may be subdivided into true (undetectable thyroglobulin) and apparent (thyroglobulin detectable) thyroid agenesis. The third form of thyroid dysgenesis, hypoplastic gland *in situ*, is much less common – an important cause being a TSH receptor mutation which can cause severe thyroid hypoplasia or even apparent thyroid agenesis. Inherited or *de novo* gene mutations affecting the transcription factors TTF1, TTF2 and PAX8 may be responsible for a small number (probably <2%) of cases of thyroid dysgenesis. Thyroid dyshormonogenesis due to autosomal recessive defects in thyroid hormone synthesis account for 10–15% of congenital hypothyroidism in the United Kingdom. A number of gene mutations responsible for these defects have been discovered, most commonly mutations in the TPO and thyroglobulin genes. Mutations in the iodotyrosine dehalogenase gene result in iodine wasting with a goiter, similar to the pattern seen with dietary iodine deficiency. Pendred's syndrome – sensorineural deafness with or without dyshormonogenetic goitre – is due to a mutation in the Pendrin gene.

Sodium iodine symporter and *THOX* gene defects also occur. In contrast to infants with thyroid dysgenesis, infants with synthetic defects will show a normal or enlarged thyroid gland *in situ*, provided that the defect is distal to the TSH receptor.

Table 6.3 Causes of congenital hypothyroidism.

Thyroid dysgenesis
Thyroid agenesis
• True (thyroglobulin undetectable)
• Apparent (thyroglobulin detectable)
Hypoplastic gland
Ectopic (usually sublingual) gland

Synthetic defects
TRH and TSH deficiency
TSH receptor defect
G-protein defect (as part of Albright's hereditary osteodystrophy)
Defects in T4 synthesis (dyshormonogenesis)
• Iodide transport defect
• Organification defect
• Peroxidase deficiency
• Thyroglobulin defect
• Dehalogenase deficiency
Pendred's syndrome

Maternal disease
Thyroid disease with transplacental transfer of thyroid peroxidase antibody or thyrotropin receptor blocking antibody
Maternal drugs, for example propylthiouracil

Miscellaneous
Down's syndrome

Abbreviations: T4, thyroxine; TRH, thyrotropin releasing hormone; TSH, thyroid stimulating hormone.

Other causes of congenital hypothyroidism are rare. TSH or TRH deficiency accounts for hypothyroidism in approximately 1 in 100,000 births and usually occurs in the context of disorders causing multiple pituitary deficiencies, for example septo-optic dysplasia.

Screening

The combination of difficulty in achieving an early clinical diagnosis and the severe neurodevelopmental consequences of a late diagnosis, especially beyond 3 months of age, led to the establishment of screening programmes in the late 1970's and early 1980's in most developed countries. In the United Kingdom, screening is usually performed between days 5 and 7 of life. In North America, babies are usually tested between 48 hours and 4 days, but may be tested before 48 hours of age if they are discharged from the hospital prior to that time. These early measurements may lead to false positive results and it is very

important that the TSH reading is assessed in the light of age appropriate normal values. Capillary blood is collected from the baby's heel. Screening options include TSH measurement only (which will miss secondary and tertiary hypothyroidism), T4 measurement only (which will miss compensated hypothyroidism) and measurement of both T4 and TSH (the ideal method). In the United Kingdom and in most of North America, TSH measurement is used. Practices vary in different centres, but the following is fairly standard:
• If TSH ≥25 mU/L, the laboratory notifies the paediatrician.

Notification should be by day 14 of life.

The infant should then be examined, TFT's urgently repeated for confirmation and treatment should be started within 24 hours of notification.
• If TSH is 6–24 mU/L, a repeat capillary sample is requested by the laboratory and the paediatrician notified if the repeat value is > 6mU/L. Formal TFT's will then be performed. If the TSH is > 10 mU/L after 2 weeks of age then it is wise to begin treatment with a view to re-investigating the child at the age of 3 years. The management of babies with TSH levels of 6–10 mU/L that persist at 1 month of age is controversial. A normal range for TSH of 1.7–9.1 mU/L has been reported in infants aged 2–20 weeks. Thus, treating all babies with TSH values of 6–10 mU/L will result in treating some euthyroid infants. The authors advocate not treating automatically in those circumstances but carrying out thyroid imaging to identify mild thyroid dysgenesis or dyshormonogenesis, measuring maternal TSH receptor antibodies and maternal and infant TPO antibodies and monitoring TFT's at monthly intervals in the first instance. If treatment is started, then a trial off treatment can be conducted at 3 years of age to assess if the hypothyroidism was transient or permanent.

A recent study has suggested that preterm babies <1500 g and acutely ill babies >1500 g should undergo re-screening for capillary TSH elevation since the initial screening test may have been negative due to an intervention, for example iodine exposure, a blood transfusion or a dopamine infusion. This retesting could be performed at 2 and 4 weeks in babies <1500 g and also at discharge. Several cases of delayed thyrotropin elevation were detected in the study with some infants also having low T4 levels. Though most were due to transient, rather than permanent disorders, detection of thyroid dysfunction was considered important due to the critical role of thyroid hormones in neurodevelopment. Retesting may be particularly important in term infants with cardiac disease due to the association of congenital heart disease and congenital hypothyroidism. In addition, in the case of monozygotic twins, a second specimen should be taken at 2 weeks of age as foetal blood mixing may have masked the screening test result.

Some centres routinely retest all newborns at 2–6 weeks of age or selected groups of patients (e. g. patients in the neonatal intensive care unit). In the United Kingdom, preterm infants (born at <36 weeks) have a second blood spot sample taken at the equivalent of 36 weeks gestation.

However, these practices are not universal and further data is required before re-screening can be regarded as mandatory.

It is important to note that no screening programme is perfect and occasional errors will occur. For example, missed patients, mislabelling and loss of samples. Furthermore, rarely infantile hypothyroidism can develop after newborn screening.

Clinical features

Awareness of the clinical symptoms and signs is required for the detection of infants missed on the screening programme and for the assessment of infants with high TSH values.

History
• Sleepiness
• Poor feeding
• Prolonged jaundice
• Constipation
• Hoarse cry
• Family history of congenital hypothyroidism/parental consanguinity
• Maternal history of thyroid disease

Signs
• Lethargy
• Jaundice
• Large tongue
• Goitre
• Coarse facies
• Umbilical hernia
• Dry skin
• Wide posterior fontanelle
• Hypothermia
• Cold peripheries
• Peripheral cyanosis
• Oedema

There is a slightly increased prevalence (5%) of non-thyroidal malformations, particularly cardiac, and a thorough examination is therefore indicated.

Investigations

If hypothyroidism has been diagnosed on neonatal screening then an urgent venous sample for FT4 (or T4) and TSH measurement should be taken to confirm the diagnosis. In most laboratories the result can be obtained on the same day. In a well term baby with unequivocal TSH elevation (>30 mU/L), the likelihood of permanent congenital hypothyroidism is such that treatment should be started immediately. If the TSH <30 mU/L and there are no clinical features of hypothyroidism, then treatment can be deferred until the results of the venous sample are known (see 'Transient neonatal hypothyroidism', page 120). Thyroglobulin measurement is helpful in selected cases, being undetectable (<2 μg/L) in true agenesis, detectable in apparent agenesis, usually elevated (>150 μg/L) in thyroid ectopia, undetectable with thyroid gene mutations and elevated in *TPO* gene mutations. In cases where the mother has a history of autoimmune thyroid disease or if there has been a previously affected infant, TPO antibodies or TSH receptor blocking antibodies can be measured in the infant and/or mother and may identify this as the cause of a transient hypothyroidism.

The role of isotope and ultrasound scanning of the thyroid gland as part of the assessment of babies with congenital hypothyroidism is controversial. Sceptics point out that a marked TSH elevation in an otherwise normal term infant is virtually diagnostic of congenital hypothyroidism and that, providing cord TSH is measured in all subsequent offspring, the precise diagnosis is unimportant. Advocates of scanning report that the establishment of a precise diagnosis during the newborn period, which can be achieved in over 80% of infants, is greatly valued by parents in confirming and thus helping them to come to terms with the need for lifelong T4 treatment, reassuring them (in most cases) of the very low recurrence risk or (in cases of dyshormonogenesis), helping to provide sound genetic counselling. Thyroid imaging is also useful in identifying infants in whom genetic studies may be helpful. It is our view that diagnostic imaging should be performed in newborn infants as the benefits outweigh the disadvantages, and that such imaging should also be carried out in infants with mild but persistent TSH elevation-hyperthyrotropinaemia- to try and reach a more precise diagnosis.

^{99m}Tc-pertechnetate or ^{123}I-labelled sodium iodide scans will, if performed before or within a few days of starting T4 treatment (while the TSH level is high), provide information about the presence and site of the thyroid gland, thus helping distinguish between thyroid ectopia, agenesis and an *in situ* gland which may be normal, hypoplastic or enlarged as a result of dyshormonogenesis. The disadvantage of isotope scanning is that uptake may be decreased or absent in babies with anatomically normal thyroid glands following exposure to iodine, in the presence of maternal TSH blocking antibodies, in the case of TSH receptor or iodine transport defects, or if the scan is performed after T4 treatment has led to TSH suppression.

Ultrasound scanning of the thyroid is superior to isotope scanning in defining thyroid size and morphology, but has the disadvantage that thyroid ectopia is often undetectable. However, recent studies have suggested that colour Doppler is useful in detecting ectopic thyroid tissue and if confirmed, ultrasound may take the place of isotope scanning as the preferred initial imaging option. In some centres, both isotope and ultrasound scanning are performed. An important pitfall in ultrasound scanning of the thyroid has recently been highlighted by Jones *et al.* (2010). This group and others have shown that ultrasound in infants with proven thyroid ectopia on radioisotope scanning often shows non-thyroidal tissue in the thyroid fossa which can be easily mistaken for thyroid hypoplasia (Figure 6.5), and that experience is needed in order to interpret the ultrasound correctly. It is possible that the true incidence of thyroid hypoplasia has been overestimated by thyroid ultrasound in the past by the misdiagnosis of non-thyroidal thyroid fossa tissue.

In cases where scans have shown normal or high uptake of isotope and normal thyroid position and anatomy, the likely diagnosis is dyshormonogenesis or occasionally transient hypothyroidism. In suspected dyshormonogenesis, specific gene mutations can be sought and the thyroglobulin value is helpful in targeting these. In cases of suspected or confirmed dyshormonogenesis, parents should be counselled concerning the '1 in 4' recurrence risk.

Patients who have not undergone thyroid imaging can have an ultrasound performed at 3 years of age. If this demonstrates a normally sized and sited thyroid gland, and the patient is on a small dose of T4 with normal TFT's, then T4 treatment can be discontinued for 4 weeks without impairing neurodevelopment. The repeat TFT's after 4 weeks should clarify whether the hypothyroidism was transient or permanent.

All infants with congenital hypothyroidism should have their hearing tested due to the association of congenital

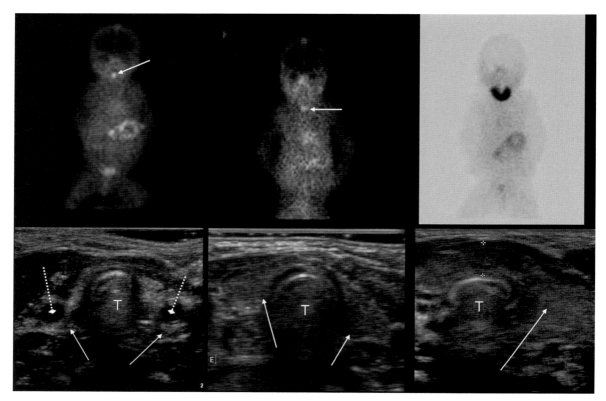

Fig. 6.5 Isotope (top row) and ultrasound (bottom row) images from infants with thyroid ectopia (left), thyroid hypoplasia due to a TSH receptor defect (centre), and dyshormonogenesis (right). The isotope scans show lingual ectopia, a normally sited small gland, and avid uptake into an enlarged gland, respectively. The ultrasound scans show non-thyroidal tissue in the thyroid fossa of the infant with thyroid ectopia, reduced thyroid volume in the infant with thyroid hypoplasia and a bulky gland in the infant with dyshormonogenesis. Note that the non-thyroidal tissue has a hyperechoic and heterogeneous texture (arrowed), compared with that of the true thyroid tissue shown in the two other infants (arrowed), and that it also wraps around the major vessels (broken arrows). T, trachea.

hypothyroidism and sensorineural hearing loss. In countries with universal neonatal hearing screening, this will be routinely done. Where there is no such programme a hearing assessment should be arranged.

Treatment

Ideally, treatment should be started by 14 days of age. The initial dose of T4 should be 10–15 μg/kg per day depending on the severity of the hypothyroidism, equating to 37.5–50 μg daily in most term infants. The aim of treatment is to normalize FT4 (or T4) and TSH within 2 weeks if possible, given the evidence of a better neurodevelopmental outcome if this is the case. The FT4 (or T4) should be maintained in the upper half of the normal range with a low normal TSH. The fall in the TSH is sometimes delayed due to relative pituitary resistance. In those cases in which the FT4 (or T4) level is near the top of the normal range with an inappropriately raised TSH level, the FT4 (or T4) level should be used to determine the dose. It is important to exclude poor compliance as the cause of a persistently raised TSH level. Untoward symptoms due to high FT4 (or T4) levels such as tachycardia, irritability and diarrhoea are rare. The T4 dose should be adjusted according to the infant's clinical response and TFT's. If there are clinical or biochemical signs of over-treatment, the dose can be reduced by 12.5 μg.

The normal range of TFT's is higher in neonates than in older children and many laboratories will have slightly different normal ranges for the different age groups.

The dosage of T4 is increased as the infant grows and in line with the TFT's. Often a dose of 50 μg per day is required from 6 months to 1 year of age and 75 μg per day by 2 years of age. The dosage of T4 is approximately 100 μg/m^2 per day and doses of up to 200 μg once daily may be required in adulthood. T4 in infants can be administered as crushed tablets and mixed with a few millilitres of water or milk (smallest tablet 25 μg, but this can be halved and dose changes of 12.5 μg can be made). T4 can also be administered in the form of a relatively new liquid preparation, Evotrox. This is a particularly attractive option in infants, especially preterm babies. However, Evotrox has not yet been formally tested in children and infants. Furthermore, if Evotrox is used the doctor, pharmacist and family should be aware that there are three different strengths – 25, 50 and 100 μg/5 mL – to ensure that the correct dose of T4 is administered.

Soya milk formulas, iron medication, calcium and fibre administered in close time proximity to T4 can interfere with T4 absorption. Disorders associated with malabsorption, for example coeliac disease, may effect T4 levels and certain medications, for example anticonvulsants, can increase T4 degradation. Such infants may require more frequent follow-up and higher doses of T4.

Information leaflets and visual aids are very useful, as is contact with a similarly affected child and family or a support group.

Follow-up

Developmental progress, growth and thyroid function should be checked at the following intervals:
1 Weekly after the start of T4 for the first month of life, to ensure that the family are appropriately counselled and compliant with T4 treatment.
2 Every 1–2 months up to 6 months of age.
3 Every 3–4 months between 6 months and 3 years.
4 Every 6–12 months until growth is completed.
Follow-up should be more frequent if there are concerns about compliance, if TFT's are abnormal or if the dose has been altered. Some children will have TSH concentrations of 10–20 mU/L despite FT4 (or T4) values in the upper half of the normal range. This is most commonly due to problems with compliance or the method of administration but rarely may be due to a resetting of the pituitary–thyroid feedback threshold.

Failure to comply with treatment, especially during the first 3 years of life, may impair normal brain development. Conversely, over-treatment may cause features of T4 excess. If the TSH is >6 mU/L and the T4 level is in the lower half of the normal range or below the normal range, then the dose should be raised by 12.5–25 μg per day and the TFT's should be repeated in 4–6 weeks. Conversely, the dose should be reduced by a similar amount if the TSH level is <0.5 mU/L.

A period off treatment for 4 weeks with measurement of FT4 (or T4) and TSH before and after stopping treatment is indicated in selected cases at about 3 years of age to exclude transient hypothyroidism. This is unnecessary in infants shown to have an unequivocal cause of congenital hypothyroidism such as agenesis or thyroid ectopia on scanning performed in the newborn period, and in cases with a TSH >10 mU/L on treatment after 12 months of age. If, after 4 weeks off treatment, the TSH is >10 mU/L with a low or normal FT4 (or T4) then permanent hypothyroidism is confirmed and treatment is re-started. If the TSH is borderline (>6 but <10 mU/L) then the child can be followed up and re-tested after a few months. If the TFT's are normal after 4 weeks off treatment, then the child can be discharged with a presumed diagnosis of transient hypothyroidism. Parents should know the symptoms of hypothyroidism and TFT's can be repeated if clinically indicated.

Outcome

Neonatal screening programmes have revolutionized the outlook for babies with congenital hypothyroidism and the prognosis is now excellent. However, there is still controversy as to whether very early treatment can completely reverse the effects of hypothyroidism. A large American retrospective study of pregnant mothers with thyroid disease demonstrated a 4 IQ points deficit in infants of mothers with a high TSH and a normal FT4 and a 7 IQ points deficit in infants of mothers with a low FT4 level (a small number of whom were treated in pregnancy) compared to the control group of infants (none of the babies had congenital hypothyroidism). This suggests that some of the prenatal effects of hypothyroidism may be irreversible.

The infants at greatest risk of neurodevelopmental impairment are those with thyroid agenesis and low initial FT4 levels. Delay in starting treatment, poor compliance and sub-optimal dosing are further exacerbating factors. There are only minor differences in IQ, school achievement and neuropsychological testing in adults with congenital hypothyroidism treated early compared to controls. Neurodevelopmental impairment is subtle and selective and can affect a wide range of areas including sensorineural hearing and speech, visuospatial abilities, memory and sensorimotor defects. A 1996 meta-analysis performed on seven major follow-up studies demonstrated that children with congenital hypothyroidism had

IQ levels that were, on average, 6 points lower than in the control group. Clearly, the parents' IQ and environmental factors will also play a part in the child's neurodevelopment and achievement. It is possible that the more recently used higher dose initial T4 regimens may improve neurodevelopmental outcome, but further studies are needed to substantiate this.

In the rare cases when both maternal and neonatal hypothyroidism are present, for example due to iodine deficiency or potent TSH receptor blocking antibodies, there can be a significant impairment in neurodevelopment even with prompt and optimal T4 therapy.

Acquired hypothyroidism

This condition can be difficult to recognize as its onset may be very insidious and it has often been present for a number of years prior to diagnosis.

Aetiology

Causes of acquired hypothyroidism

Primary
- Iodine deficiency
- Autoimmune (Hashimoto's) thyroiditis
- Thyroid surgery
- Following irradiation to neck (e. g. craniospinal irradiation, total body irradiation)
- Radioiodine therapy
- Antithyroid drugs (e. g. carbimazole)
- Goitrogens

Secondary and tertiary
- Craniopharyngioma and other tumours impinging on the hypothalamic–pituitary axis
- Neurosurgery
- Cranial irradiation

Iodine deficiency
Although this is the most common worldwide cause of hypothyroidism, it more commonly results in a euthyroid goitre. Clinical iodine deficiency is extremely rare in the United Kingdom but is more common in other European countries, such as Poland. As migration increases the incidence of this condition in the United Kingdom may rise. The condition is suspected in cases of goitre, a family history of iodine deficiency and from a knowledge of the regional iodine status. It is diagnosed by urinary iodine measurements and treated with trace amounts of iodine.

The iodination of salt is reducing the prevalence of this problem.

Autoimmune (Hashimoto's) thyroiditis
This is the most common cause of acquired hypothyroidism in the Western world. It is more common in girls, particularly in adolescence, and there is a family history in approximately a third of cases. Presentation may be with euthyroid goitre, goitre with compensated hypothyroidism, goitre or an atrophic gland with decompensated hypothyroidism or during screening because of the presence of another autoimmune condition. Autoantibodies are present in 95% of cases. Autoimmune thyroiditis may be associated with other autoimmune diseases, such as diabetes mellitus, coeliac disease and Addison's disease, as well as with skin disorders, such as alopecia areata and vitiligo.

It is particularly common in Down's syndrome, affecting around 7% of school-aged children. Regular screening is indicated, one method being annual capillary blood spot TSH screening from 1 year of age onwards. If the TSH is raised then venous TFT's and a TPO antibody measurement should be performed. Clearly, TSH screening will not detect Hashimoto's disease if it goes through a hyperthyroidism phase (see page 133) but this condition should be clinically obvious. Girls with Turner's syndrome are also at increased risk.

Miscellaneous causes
These include the hypothalamic–pituitary disorders in which other anterior pituitary hormone deficiencies will almost invariably be present. Dietary goitrogens, such as iodide, cabbage and soya beans, have also been reported to cause hypothyroidism. Obesity can lead to slight TSH resistance with a TSH sometimes ≤ 2 mU/L above the upper limit of the normal range but with normal FT4 levels. A reduction in weight can lead to a fall in the TSH level.

Clinical features (Figure 6.6)

History
- Weight gain
- Tiredness
- Constipation
- Cold intolerance
- Slowing of linear growth ± short stature
- Delayed puberty (occasionally sexual precocity)
- Menstrual irregularity
- Presence of other autoimmune disorders

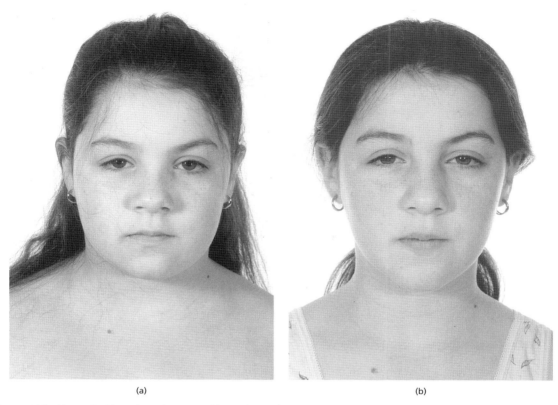

(a)   (b)

Fig. 6.6 Girl with acquired hypothyroidism caused by Hashimoto's disease (a) before and (b) after treatment.

- History of slipped upper femoral epiphysis
- Family history of thyroid or other autoimmune disorders

Signs
- Myxoedematous facies
- Short stature
- Goitre
- Obesity
- Dry skin
- Increase in body hair
- Pallor
- Vitiligo
- Proximal muscle weakness
- Delayed relaxation of ankle reflexes
- Delayed puberty (occasionally precocious puberty)

This condition can be very insidious and in retrospect it may become apparent that it has been present for several months or even 2 to 3 years. The principal symptoms of hypothyroidism are tiredness and weight gain, while the key signs are pallor, myxoedematous facies and short stature relative to the mid-parental height. If previous heights are available it may be possible to pinpoint the start of the hypothyroidism. The goitre is usually diffuse and non-tender, but may be nodular and is occasionally tender. Usually puberty is delayed, but occasionally cross-stimulation of FSH receptors by TSH may lead to incomplete sexual precocity with enlarged ovaries on ultrasound scan in girls and testicular enlargement with low testosterone in boys. Paradoxically, in all but the most severe cases of acquired hypothyroidism, children do well at school, methodically doing their homework until it is completed.

Investigations
These will depend on the cause of the hypothyroidism. FT4 (or T4) and TSH measurements are required to confirm the diagnosis. In acquired hypothyroidism, TPO antibodies should always be measured. A bone age is sometimes performed and usually shows delay. A thyroid

ultrasound should be done if a nodule is palpable or if there is clear asymmetry but is rarely necessary. If there is no goitre and the autoantibody screen is negative then an isotope or ultrasound scan should be performed to exclude a late presentation of thyroid dysgenesis. Inappropriately low or normal TSH values in the face of a low FT4 (or T4) suggests pituitary or hypothalamic disease which can be further investigated with the TRH test. Proven secondary and tertiary hypothyroidism should be investigated by further pituitary testing and MRI.

Treatment

Treatment is with T4 100 μg/m² per day given as a single daily dose. Children with clinical hypothyroidism should start on a small dose of T4, 25–50 μg once daily. TFT's should be measured every 2–4 weeks and the dose adjusted in 25 μg steps as necessary until TFT's have normalized. Catch-up growth with increased height velocity will occur. Unfortunately, the majority of children with hypothyroidism do not loose weight following treatment though a few with severe hypothyroidism may loose a small amount of weight. Treatment for severe hypothyroidism, even if gradual, may be associated with marked adverse symptoms including fatigue, irritability, poor concentration and emotional lability, particularly in children with learning difficulties. School performance may also deteriorate. In those with compensated hypothyroidism, adverse symptoms are much less likely and treatment can be increased more quickly.

There is controversy as to whether euthyroid patients with compensated autoimmune thyroiditis should be treated. A pragmatic approach is to give T4 replacement if the TSH value is >15 mU/L, or if the TSH is > 6 mU/L in the presence of goitre. The presence of elevated TPO antibodies may also influence the decision and there is some evidence that in those with goitre there will be a reduction in thyroid volume. Occasionally, treatment may be associated with the development of a slipped upper femoral epiphysis or Perthes' disease, both of which cause leg pain and a limp. However, the former is more likely to be seen as a presenting feature of hypothyroidism. Families should be told that in the unlikely event of the child developing leg pain or a limp they should attend the emergency department that day.

Follow-up

Considerable surveillance and reassurance may be required by some families during the first few months following diagnosis. Thereafter, clinic visits and TFT's should take place 6–12-monthly. The TSH level is a sensitive marker of under- or over-replacement. In the case of non-compliance, FT4 (or T4) will be normal if T4 was taken on the day of the clinic visit but the TSH level will be raised.

Outcome

The prognosis for autoimmune thyroiditis is very good and the outlook partly depends on whether the child will develop other autoimmune diseases. Most patients need treatment for life, but very occasionally spontaneous remission occurs. Complete catch-up growth following treatment can be expected in mild to moderate cases. However, complete catch-up may not occur in severely affected children with prolonged hypothyroidism. Parents of children with severe hypothyroidism should be warned that it may take several months before their child is completely back to normal.

Hyperthyroidism

The causes of hyperthyroidism are the following:
- Graves' disease
- Neonatal thyrotoxicosis
- Autoimmune (Hashimoto's) thyroiditis
- Syndrome of selective T4 resistance
- Autonomous nodules
- TSH-dependent hyperthyroidism (rare):
  - TSH-secreting adenoma
  - Activating mutations of the TSH receptor

Graves' disease (Figure 6.7)

Graves' disease is rare, with an incidence of 0.8 per 100,000 children per year. It usually occurs in the second decade, is six times more common in girls and in up to 60% of cases there is a family history of thyroid disease. It occurs more commonly in children with other autoimmune disorders and there may also be a family history of non-thyroidal autoimmune disease. It is caused by stimulation of the TSH receptor by immunoglobulins. The associated exophthalmos is because of infiltration of the orbit and surrounding structures with lymphocytes, mucopolysaccharides and oedema.

Clinical features

The onset of Graves' disease is usually insidious, over several months, but may be acute.

History
- Anxiety
- Irritability and hyperactivity

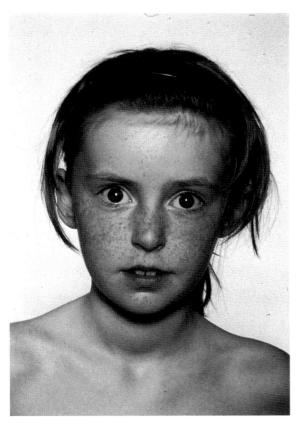

Fig. 6.7 Girl with Graves' disease.

- Tiredness
- Deteriorating school performance and handwriting
- Weight loss in spite of increased appetite
- Rapid height increase
- Palpitations
- Heat intolerance
- Sleep disturbance
- Diarrhoea
- Menstrual irregularities or amenorrhoea
- Family history

Examination
- Goitre (usually diffuse)
- Exophthalmos (rarely associated with ophthalmoplegia)
- Tachycardia
- Hypertension
- Facial flushing
- Tremor

- Sweatiness
- Relative tall stature (height centile usually above parental target range centiles)
- Thyroid bruit
- Heart murmur
- Choreiform movements

Thyroid crisis or storm is a form of thyrotoxicosis characterized by an acute onset which may be precipitated by surgery, infections, drug withdrawal/non-compliance and radioiodine treatment. The patient develops hyperthermia, severe tachycardia and restlessness and may become delirious, comatose or die. It is rare in childhood.

Diagnosis

The diagnosis is usually obvious and is confirmed by finding elevated FT4 (or T4) and FT3 (or T3) concentrations, with TSH suppression. Rarely, FT4 (or T4) levels are normal but FT3 (or T3) levels are elevated, so-called 'T3 toxicosis'. TSH receptor antibodies (TRAb) are elevated and in most cases TPO antibodies are also positive. Bone age is usually advanced.

Treatment

The majority of patients do not require admission. If symptoms are severe, for example marked tachycardia and hypertension, then admission may be necessary till the propranolol has taken effect and the patient can then be reviewed in clinic the following week.

The three modalities of treatment in Graves' disease are medical, radioactive iodine and surgery.

Medical treatment

Carbimazole or methimazole (carbimazole is the prodrug of methimazole), initial dose 0.25 mg/kg (maximum 10 mg) three times a day in children up to 12 years of age and 10 mg three times a day in children aged 12 to 18 years. Higher initial doses are occasionally required. The maximum total daily dose is 40 mg a day. It may take 2 weeks to become euthyroid.

The most serious side effect of these drugs is agranulocytosis and neutropenia. It is idiosyncratic and not predictable from regular blood tests but may be commoner with higher drug doses. Routine monitoring of the full blood count (FBC) is not indicated. Neutropenia occurs in approximately 0.3% of patients, usually within the first 3 months. A slightly greater percentage may develop mild to moderate leucopoenia. Patients should be asked to report symptoms of infection, especially sore throat, mouth ulcers and bruising. In such instances, treatment should be stopped and an urgent FBC performed. Whenever possible, written information should be provided to back up the verbal advice. Stopping the medication nearly always leads to resolution of the problem after 1–2 weeks. In severe cases, granulocyte colony stimulating factor may be used. A further side effect is itchy rashes which occur in 2–5% of patients. These are usually transient, can be treated with antihistamines and rarely necessitate stopping therapy. Hepatotoxicity, nausea, headaches and myalgia may also occur.

Propylthiouracil has also been used to treat thyrotoxicosis. However, carbimazole and methimazole are more effective in severe hyperthyroidism, have better compliance rates and fewer side effects. Carbimazole and methimazole can cause liver injury characterized by cholestatic dysfunction (rather than hepatocellular inflammation or liver failure). However, there is recent evidence that in children on propylthiouracil there is a '1 in 1000' risk of liver failure, a percentage of whom may require liver transplantation or die. In view of this, propylthiouracil should be restricted to the very few patients in whom carbimazole or methimazole have led to a toxic reaction and in whom both radioiodine and surgery are not considered an option.

Propranolol (dose 250–750 μg/kg per dose three times a day, dose adjusted according to response) is also required during the first few weeks in most cases to help control the signs of sympathetic over-activity, such as tachycardia and tremor. Propranolol can be reduced and stopped once thyroid function has returned to normal and should not be used in patients with asthma or heart failure.

After 4–8 weeks of starting antithyroid drugs, FT4 (or T4) and FT3 (or T3) will fall to within the reference range but the TSH will remain suppressed for several more weeks. The rapidity of the response is usually proportional to the size of the gland. When the FT4 (or T4) and FT3 (or T3) fall to within the lower half of the reference range (usually after 6–12 weeks of treatment), there are the following two possible approaches:

1 Approximately half the previous total dose of carbimazole or methimazole is administered as a single daily dose. The dosage is titrated to maintain normal thyroid hormone concentrations (titration regimen).

2 The initial antithyroid dosage—sufficient to cause hypothyroidism—is continued, and a small replacement dose of T4, initially 25 μg once daily, is commenced (block and replace regime). The dose of T4 may need to be increased subsequently to 50–75 μg daily, depending on the patient's size and TFT's.

Both methods have their advocates. The advantages of the more popular dose titration regime are that there are fewer side effects on the lower drug doses and that compliance is better on one rather than two drugs. The advantages of the block and replace regimen are improved stability with fewer episodes of hyperthyroidism and hypothyroidism, a reduced number of blood tests and clinic appointments and possibly an improved remission rate following a larger antithyroid drug dose, although this remains to be proven.

Eye disease is milder in children than in adults. If the patient develops symptoms such as dry or painful eyes hypromellose eye drops, one drop to each eye up to four times a day may be indicated. In the case of significant symptoms or impaired eye movements, early referral to an ophthalmologist will be required.

Attempts to stop antithyroid medication after 24 months are usually unsuccessful, particularly in prepubertal children, in those with a high T4 level at presentation and in those with a moderate or large goitre at presentation. Therefore, a cautious reduction in treatment rather than sudden discontinuation of antithyroid drugs is recommended. In the majority of cases, approximately 75%, the patient relapses.

In such cases the options are further medical treatment, radioactive iodine or surgery. Further medical treatment is often opted for, but this does not increase the likelihood of long-term remission. Poor compliance with drug treatment and drug side effects may also lead to consideration of radioiodine treatment or surgery.

Radioactive iodine

Radioiodine therapy should be conducted in collaboration with a nuclear medicine specialist or an adult endocrinologist with a special interest in thyroid disorders.

Radioiodine is administered orally and is given with the aim of ablating the thyroid gland and inducing hypothyroidism. Antithyroid medication should be stopped 5 days prior to treatment. Symptoms of hyperthyroidism can be treated with β-blockers if necessary. When children are treated with >150 μCi of ^{131}I per g of thyroid tissue, hypothyroidism is achieved in the vast majority of cases. Following treatment, patients should be reviewed after a few days as thyroid hormone concentrations can rise transiently 4–10 days after treatment due to their release from the damaged gland. β-blockers may be necessary. Analgesia may be needed to treat the neck pain of radiation thyroiditis and rarely nausea may occur. A therapeutic effect is usually observed within 3 months and the patient should be closely monitored so that T4 treatment can pre-empt the onset of severe hypothyroidism. In the rare cases when hyperthyroidism persists beyond 6 months then patients can be retreated.

Traditionally, there has been a reluctance to give radioiodine treatment to children because of concerns about cancer. The relatively high dose of radioiodine used should lead to thyroid gland ablation and the risk of a subsequent thyroid malignancy should therefore be extremely low. However, there have been cases of thyroid cancer in children who received radioiodine treatment which presumably occurred in a remnant of the gland. However, this is very rare and thyroid cancer is commoner in patients with Graves' disease who have not had radioiodine treatment. Long-term follow-up studies of both thyroid and extra-thyroid cancer risk in patients who received radioiodine have been very reassuring. Furthermore, studies to date have not shown an increased risk of congenital abnormalities in children born to mothers treated with radioiodine. Nevertheless, further long-term follow-up data of children and adolescents treated with the currently used doses of radioiodine is required. For this reason in the United Kingdom radioiodine treatment is generally only considered in children over 10 years of age. However, in North America it is also administered in children ≥ 5 years.

In the minority of children with severe eye disease radioactive iodine should be used with caution as it may exacerbate the ophthalmopathy. Steroid treatment for several weeks may be helpful. Alternatively, surgery may be required.

Thyroid surgery

The main advantage of this treatment is the rapid cure of the thyrotoxicosis. It is particularly useful in young children (under 10 and particularly under 5 years of age) in whom definitive treatment is required and in those with a very large thyroid gland. Euthyroid status must be induced prior to surgery. Ten to 14 days prior to surgery, iodides (e.g. Lugol's solution, see Table 6.4, 0.1–0.3 mL, three times a day (tds), orally) should be administered to decrease the vascularity of the gland.

Most surgeons favour performing a total thyroidectomy. Hypothyroidism results and standard T4 treatment is administered. It is very important that surgery is carried out by an experienced thyroid surgeon to minimize the risk of complications. These include recurrent laryngeal nerve palsy with a resultant hoarse voice, hypoparathyroidism causing hypocalcaemia, unsightly keloid scar formation and haematoma.

Table 6.4 The emergency management of neonatal thyrotoxicosis

1. Carbimazole (or methimazole) 250 µg/kg tds oral
2. Sympathomimetic effects can be suppressed by propranolol 250–750 µg/kg tds oral (monitor pulse, blood pressure and possible side effect of hypoglycaemia)
3. Lugol's solution (5% iodine, 10% potassium iodide = 130 mg iodine/mL) can be used in severe cases. It produces the most rapid response with effects within 48 hours. 0.05–0.1 mL, tds oral.
4. Sedatives may be required, for example chloral hydrate 30 mg/kg/dose, 8 hourly as necessary, orally
5. In severe cases, prednisolone, which inhibits the conversion of T4 to T3 and inhibits thyroid hormone secretion can also be used, 2 mg/kg/day, oral
6. Heart failure may require treatment with diuretics

Neonatal thyrotoxicosis

This rare condition is caused by the trans-placental transfer of maternal TSH receptor antibodies which stimulate the foetal and neonatal thyroid. The higher the thyroid stimulating immunoglobulin level in pregnancy, the greater the risk that the infant will develop thyrotoxicosis. This disease may occur in infants of mothers with active hyperthyroidism who are on treatment and in those with inactive hyperthyroidism. Only a very small minority of infants of mothers with Graves' disease are affected.

The degree of thyroid dysfunction will depend on the net effect of maternal thyroid stimulating and blocking TSH receptor antibodies, maternal hyperthyroxinaemia and maternal antithyroid drugs. A scheme for the investigation of babies of mothers with Graves' disease and hypothyrodism is outlined in Figure 6.8. TSH and T4 levels rise in the first few days of life and the assessment of the infant's thyroid status should be made with reference to the normal TSH and FT4 (or T4) levels at that postnatal age. Babies at high risk of thyrotoxicosis (e. g. thyroid stimulating immunoglobulin level raised or not measured in pregnancy, clinical thyrotoxicosis or drug therapy in third trimester, evidence of foetal thyrotoxicosis) may need to be observed in hospital for a few days following delivery. Infants at low risk, for instance those whose mothers had normal (or negative) thyroid stimulating immunoglobulin levels, may be discharged immediately, but parents should be aware of the possible symptoms and the infant should be reviewed at 5–10 days. Symptoms usually develop at 24–48 hours of age, but may

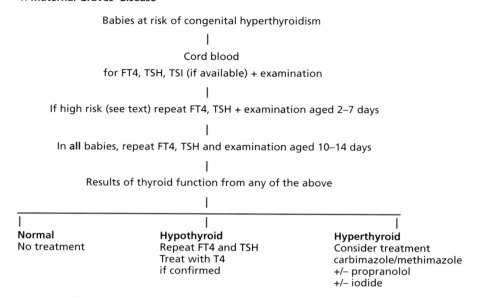

1. **Maternal Graves' disease**

Babies at risk of congenital hyperthyroidism

|

Cord blood

for FT4, TSH, TSI (if available) + examination

|

If high risk (see text) repeat FT4, TSH + examination aged 2–7 days

|

In **all** babies, repeat FT4, TSH and examination aged 10–14 days

|

Results of thyroid function from any of the above

|

Normal
No treatment

Hypothyroid
Repeat FT4 and TSH
Treat with T4
if confirmed

Hyperthyroid
Consider treatment
carbimazole/methimazole
+/– propranolol
+/– iodide

2. **Maternal hypothyroidism**
This is usually secondary to autoimmune thyroiditis and the mother may be producing thyroid inhibiting or rarely thyroid stimulating antibodies, so the baby may develop transient hypothyroidism or, very rarely, hyperthyroidism. These babies should be reviewed at 10 days to 2 weeks and thyroid function (TSH and FT4) measured.
    If the maternal hypothyroidism is secondary to congenital aplasia or hypoplasia of the thyroid gland, there is only a slightly increased risk to the baby of hypothyroidism and the Guthrie test should suffice.
    If the hypothyroidism is secondary to treatment (surgery or radioiodine) for Graves' disease, the baby is at risk of neonatal thyrotoxicosis and will need to be managed as in the flow diagram above.

Fig. 6.8 Investigation of babies of mothers with thyroid disease. TSI, thyroid stimulating immunoglobulin. (Amended and reproduced from A. L. Ogilvy-Stuart (2002) *Archives of Disease in Childhood* **87**, 165–171 with permission from the BMJ publishing group.)

be delayed for up to 10 days in babies whose mothers are on antithyroid drugs which cross the placenta. Most infants have biochemical thyrotoxicosis with no or few symptoms but a minority will be severely affected with goitre, tachycardia, arrhythmias, hypertension, cardiac failure, increased appetite, weight loss, diarrhoea, irritability and exophthalmos. Cord bloods may be normal, especially in infants of mothers on antithyroid drugs, but subsequently FT3 (or T3) and FT4 (or T4) levels will rise, while TSH concentrations will fall below the lower limit of normal. The half-life of thyroid stimulating immunoglobulins is approximately 12 days and resolution of the disease corresponds to their degradation so that the disorder is self-limiting over 3–12 week.

Treatment is as shown in Table 6.4. Whether one should treat biochemical thyrotoxicosis in the absence of symptoms is controversial. Treatment with carbimazole or methimazole with the addition of propranolol in those with sympathomimetic symptoms is usually sufficient, but iodine may also be required and occasionally a sedative such as chloral hydrate is also helpful. In severe cases prednisolone may also be needed. The clinical features should significantly improve within 48 hours. After 1 week of treatment the iodine can be stopped and the propranolol reduced. Babies should be reviewed weekly until stable. Subsequently, visits can be extended to 2 weekly. The antithyroid drug may be needed for 6 weeks to 3 months with the dose being gradually reduced to keep the baby euthyroid. Mortality rates of up to 20% have been reported usually from arrhythmias and/or heart failure but occasionally from tracheal compression or infection. There is little data on the long-term sequelae of neonatal thyrotoxicosis. Documented long-term side effects include an increased risk of intellectual impairment and of craniosynostosis, and these babies should therefore be followed up in clinic.

Other causes of hyperthyroidism

Hashimoto's thyroiditis

Hashimoto's thyroiditis may cause initial thyrotoxicosis in a very small proportion of patients. TPO antibodies are present and TRAb antibodies are usually absent. Treatment is as for Graves' disease but as the condition is milder and remits more readily; neither radioactive iodine nor surgery is indicated. The patient may subsequently become hypothyroid.

Thyroid hormone resistance syndrome

This rare congenital and genetic disorder has been described in over 1000 people in the world. In approximately 75% of cases there is evidence of a family history. There are mutations in the β-thyroid hormone receptors so tissues fail to respond to thyroid hormones. This results in the body trying to compensate by the thyroid secreting increased amounts of T4 and T3. Thus, the blood level of these hormones is high although the TSH level is not suppressed. Because the abnormality in the thyroid hormone receptors may vary from one tissue or organ to another, the responsiveness of the cells to the excess thyroid hormones also varies. There may be retardation of growth and a delay in the way the bones mature. Some of the cells in the brain may be relatively unresponsive so that the person has learning difficulties and an attention deficit when concentrating, although the IQ is usually normal. Other tissues continue to respond to the increased amounts of thyroid hormone and this may manifest itself as hyperactivity and tachycardia. A goitre is nearly always present.

Most people with this condition have few symptoms and treatment is not usually required. The diagnosis is important as it allows appropriate family counselling. Symptoms of thyrotoxicosis, particularly tachycardia, can be treated with a β-blocker. The person may be given high doses of T3, which will increase the blood level of this hormone even more above the normal range and this may help to surmount the resistance of the tissues and reduce the size of the goitre.

Autonomous nodules

Very rarely an autonomous nodule or nodules, due to an activating somatic TSH receptor mutation, may cause hyperthyroidism. McCune–Albright syndrome is associated with autonomous thyroid adenomas. The nodule(s), which are follicular adenomas, can be diagnosed clinically and by isotope scanning and are very rarely malignant. Treatment is generally surgical.

TSH-dependent hyperthyroidism

TSH-dependent hyperthyroidism is a very rare condition which is caused by a pituitary TSH-secreting tumour (a 'TSHoma'). Thyroid hormone levels are elevated and the TSH is normal or raised. Neurological signs, for example visual changes, are often present. Neuro-radiological evaluation is required.

Activating mutations of the TSH receptor

Rarely activating germline mutations of the TSH receptor can be responsible for familial and sporadic cases of non-immune hyperthyroidism. These patients may present in the neonatal period or in childhood with a goitre and suppressed TSH levels. Hyperthyroidism with a multinodular goitre occasionally occurs in patients with the McCune-Albright syndrome as a result of an activating mutation of the α subunit of the G protein.

Thyroid neoplasia

Solitary or multiple thyroid nodules are very rare in childhood. Over 50% of isolated thyroid nodules are cysts or benign adenomas, 30–40% are malignant while hyperfunctioning adenomas are very rare. Of the malignant nodules, over 90% are papillary or follicular carcinomas. The classification of neoplastic thyroid nodules is shown in Table 6.5.

Children with thyroid neoplasia may have a history of head and neck irradiation, a painless rapidly enlarging nodule, hoarseness or dysphagia. Examination may reveal a hard nodule, lymphadenopathy or evidence of metastases (e. g. lung). Of patients with autoimmune thyroiditis, 10–15% will have nodules and these are nearly always benign. Patients with thyroid nodules are usually euthyroid and autoantibody-negative. An ultrasound may identify a cystic lesion which is nearly always benign. Patients with non-cystic lesions may require a radioisotope scan.

Table 6.5 Classification of neoplastic thyroid nodules.

Follicular tumours
   Follicular adenoma
   Follicular carcinoma
   Papillary carcinoma
   Anaplastic carcinoma

Non-follicular tumours
   Medullary carcinoma
   Lymphoma
   Teratoma
   Metastatic
   Miscellaneous

Nodules which concentrate iodide are usually benign. If there is *any* doubt following the above investigations then a fine needle biopsy, if feasible, should be performed.

If the clinical picture is suggestive of malignancy, or if the needle biopsy is positive or suspicious then surgery is indicated. Surgery consists of removal of the affected lobe followed by total thyroidectomy if frozen sections confirm malignancy. Postoperative T4 therapy should lead to complete suppression of TSH so as not to stimulate tumour regrowth. Radioactive iodine treatment is also given if there is evidence of metastatic disease or distant lymph node involvement. Follow-up consists of regular clinical assessment and measurement of TFT's to ensure TSH suppression. Thyroglobulin is also measured as it indicates the presence or absence of functioning thyroid tissue. Ultrasound is also useful in detecting neck recurrences. The prognosis in the papillary and follicular carcinomas is very good, even in those with metastases, and life expectancy is normal. The prognosis in the much rarer cancers, for example anaplastic carcinoma, is much poorer and more aggressive treatment is necessary.

Medullary thyroid carcinoma (MTC) arises from the parafollicular C cells and usually secretes calcitonin and occasionally other hormones, such as adrenocorticotrophic hormone (ACTH). It is related to spontaneous or dominantly inherited mutations in the *REP* proto-oncogene which may be isolated or associated with other tumours in one of the multiple endocrine neoplasia (MEN) syndromes. The three phenotypes are:
• Medullary thyroid carcinoma which may be familial or sporadic (75% of cases).
• MEN 2 A: Medullary thyroid carcinoma, pheochromocytoma and hyperparathyroidism. A mutation in codon 634 of the *RET* gene is commonly found in MEN 2A.

• MEN 2B: Medullary thyroid carcinoma, pheochromocytoma and multiple mucosal neuromata. A mutation in codon 918 of the *RET* gene is found in 97% of patients.

In children with a family history of MEN 2 A or 2B in whom genetic studies have shown that the child is affected, complete thyroidectomy is now recommended before the age of 5 years for MEN 2 A and before 1 year in MEN 2B to try and pre-empt the inevitable development of medullary thyroid cancer, which has a poor prognosis once it has become clinically evident. Follow-up includes calcitonin and thyroglobulin monitoring.

Miscellaneous disorders

Colloid (simple) goitre
During adolescence the thyroid gland may become diffusely enlarged. TFT's and an autoantibody screen should be performed and, if both these are normal, the diagnosis—by elimination—is that of a colloid goitre. The goitre usually resolves spontaneously. However, in some cases the goitre can fluctuate in size and in a minority of cases results in a large nodular goitre in later life. There is no evidence that T4 treatment to suppress the TSH is helpful in colloid goitre, but this is sometimes tried if the goitre is large. Rarely, surgery is required for cosmetic reasons.

Subacute thyroiditis
In this condition the thyroid gland is acutely inflamed because of a viral infection. There is often evidence of a recent or intercurrent upper respiratory tract infection. The patient may be febrile and the gland may be enlarged, tender and painful. The inflammation results in leakage of preformed thyroid hormones into the circulation. TFT's may be normal but are usually elevated with symptoms and signs of hyperthyroidism. Inflammatory markers such as the ESR are raised whilst TPO antibody levels may be weakly positive. A radioiodine scan is sometimes performed to confirm the diagnosis and will demonstrate reduced or absent radioiodine uptake (unlike Graves' disease).

Treatment is with analgesics and non-steroidal anti-inflammatory drugs but, in severe cases, steroids may be needed. Propranolol may also be necessary. Antithyroid medication is not indicated. Hyperthyroidism usually lasts for 1–4 weeks and may be followed by a period of hypothyroidism as the gland recovers. The total course of the illness is 2–9 months with most patients making a complete recovery but occasionally, permanent hypothyroidism may occur.

Transition

Transitional clinics specifically for children with thyroid disorders are rare. More commonly the patient may be seen in an adolescent endocrine clinic.

After the age of 16 years most children with congenital and acquired hypothyroidism can be discharged to the care of their general practitioner (family doctor). Most will just require annual reviews with annual TFT's.

Children with thyrotoxicosis are best followed up in hospital and a detailed referral letter to the adult endocrinologist should be written. Following definitive treatment with radioiodine or surgery the patient can be referred back to their general practitioner once the patient has been stabilized on T4 and has normal TFTs.

Children with a history of thyroid neoplasia should remain under hospital follow-up.

When to involve a specialist centre

- Neonatal thyrotoxicosis.
- Investigation of familial and/or goitrous congenital hypothyroidism.
- Graves' disease that is difficult to control or is relapsing.
- A thyrotoxic crisis.
- Suspected thyroid neoplasia and MTC, MEN 2 A and MEN 2B.
- Hypothyroidism secondary to pituitary disease.
- Multinodular goitre.

Future developments

- Advances in molecular genetics are likely to lead to a better understanding of the aetiology of congenital hypothyroidism together with clearer guidelines on the investigation, treatment and prognosis of congenital hypothyroidism.
- It is likely that there will be an increase in the use of radioactive iodine in thyrotoxicosis.
- Further insight into the effect of maternal thyroid dysfunction on foetal development may lead to thyroid screening in pregnancy.

- Further research should determine whether preterm infants with hypothyroxinaemia should be treated with T4.

Controversial points

- Should preterm neonates <1500 g or acutely ill neonates >1500 g have repeat TFT's and if so, when?
- Should imaging be performed on all infants with congenital hypothyroidism? If so, should an isotope scan, an ultrasound, or both be performed?
- Should first-degree relatives of children with autoimmune thyroiditis or Graves' disease have their thyroid function checked?
- What initial dosage regimen should be administered to infants with congenital hypothyroidism?
- Should patients with Graves' disease who have relapsed after 2 years of medical treatment be offered further medical treatment, radioactive iodine or a thyroidectomy?
- Should all pregnant women have their TFT's measured to avoid possible adverse effects on their infants?

Common pitfalls

- A normal T4 with a high TSH level may indicate that T4 has been taken on the day of the blood test but irregularly prior to that. Diplomatic questioning should help determine if the problem is non-compliance or if a higher T4 dose is needed.
- Children with congenital hypothyroidism who at the age of 3 years are on a small dose of T4 and in whom investigation has shown a normally located thyroid gland may require re-evaluation. They may have had transient hypothyroidism and may not require lifelong treatment.
- In children with acquired decompensated hypothyroidism T4 treatment should be started in a stepwise fashion to diminish the risk of behavioural problems (especially in children with learning difficulties).
- Children with thyrotoxicosis with a normal FT4 (or T4) and a suppressed TSH level who still have symptoms should have their FT3 (or T3) measured. The FT3 may be elevated and the cause of their symptoms and the suppressed TSH.
- A low FT4 (or T4) level with a normal or only slightly elevated TSH level (TSH < 10 mU/L) should prompt consideration of the possibility of secondary or tertiary hypothyroidism.

Significant guidelines/consensus statements

Rose, S.R., Brown, R. S., Foley, T. *et al.* (2006) Update of newborn screening and therapy for congenital hypothyroidism. *Pediatrics* 117 (6), 2290–2300.

Useful information for patients and parents

Serono/Child Growth Foundation booklet. Website: www.bsped.org.uk/patients/serono/15_Hypothyro-idism.pdf. Good booklet for parents and patients on paediatric thyroid disease.
London Institute of Child Health fact sheet on congenital hypothyroidism. Website: http://www.ich.ucl.ac.uk/gosh_families/information_sheets/congenital_hypothyroidism. Good booklet for parents on congenital hypothyroidism.
European Society for Paediatric Endocrinology patient pamphlets. Website: http://www.eurospe.org/patient/index.html. Booklets on hypothyroidism including congenital and acquired hypothyroidism and hyperthyroidism for parents and patients in easy and average readability formats in English, French, Italian, Spanish and Turkish.
The Thyroid Foundation of Canada. Website: www.thyroid. ca. Contains educational material on paediatric thyroid disorders in English and French.
The British Thyroid Foundation, PO Box 97, Clifford, Wetherby, West Yorkshire LS23 6XD UK. Website: www.btf-thyroid.org. Contains educational information about the thyroid gland. Educational material mainly relates to adult thyroid disease.

Case histories

Case 6.1

A 13-year-old girl presented at clinic having been diagnosed as having hypothyroidism by her family doctor who had confirmed the diagnosis with TFT's. She also had a 2-year history of a limp in her left leg. On examination, she was short and obese with a goitre and other signs of hypothyroidism. She had limitation of movement of her left hip and a limp.

Questions
1 What is the most likely diagnosis?
2 What investigations should be done?
3 What is the treatment?

Answers
1 Slipped upper femoral epiphysis and Hashimoto's disease.
2 Frontal and lateral hip X-rays (a frontal X-ray alone may not demonstrate the slipped epiphysis) and thyroid autoantibodies.
3 In spite of the long history, urgent referral to an orthopaedic surgeon and urgent surgery are necessary. An acute or chronic slip of the epiphysis may cause avascular necrosis of the femoral head. Prophylactic pinning of the other femoral head is advocated by some surgeons. T4 treatment should also be started.

Case 6.2

An endocrinological opinion was sought about the following series of TFT's. They were taken from a boy with congenital hypothyroidism caused by an ectopic gland who had been treated with T4 from day 15 of life. At 5 years of age, he was in a mainstream school but had speech delay and behavioural problems (Table 6.6).

Table 6.6 Thyroid function tests.

Age	FT4 (normal 12–26 pmol/L)	TSH (normal 0.5–6.0 mU/L)
10 months	20.9	2.5
1.5 years	22.9	3.7
2.1 years	9.0	53.8
2.2 years	10.6	79.6
2.3 years	32.7	0.91
2.6 years	9.3	44.2
3.1 years	22.8	32.5
4.7 years	23.9	34.5
5.1 years	18.5	29.3

Abbreviations: FT4, free thyroxine; TSH, thyroid stimulating hormone.

Questions
1 What is your interpretation of these results?
2 Are there any measures you could have taken or would take now to alter the situation?

Answers
1 These results indicate poor compliance. The FT4 values are normal as a result of the tablets having been taken in the few days prior to the blood test. However, the half-life of TSH is longer and the elevated TSH values point to a lack of compliance.
2 Earlier recognition and action may well have reduced this boy's poor compliance, developmental delay and behavioural problems. If, despite full explanations and maximum support, the situation did not improve then there would be grounds for considering child protection proceedings.

Case 6.3
A 13-year-old boy was referred to the regional endocrine clinic for consideration of growth hormone (GH) treatment. He also had delayed puberty and intermittent headaches. On examination, his height was > −4.0 SD with evidence of growth failure for at least 4 years. His weight was −1.0 SD and he was entirely prepubertal. A recent GH stimulation test at the referring hospital showed a maximum response to a diethylstilbestrol primed clonidine test of 5 mU/L. He was said to have had normal TFT's 2 years previously with a FT4 = 9.2 pmol/L (9–24) and a TSH of 1.2 mU/L (0.4–4.0).

Questions
1 Are these TFT's normal?
2 What is the likely overall diagnosis?
3 Is there a problem in interpreting his clonidine test?

Answers
1 Highly suggestive of secondary or tertiary hypothyroidism.
2 Panhypopituitarism secondary to a pituitary tumour.
3 Yes, one can get a low GH level in any form of untreated hypothyroidism. However, he is likely to be GH deficient and in fact had a large cystic craniopharyngioma.

Case 6.4
An 11-year-old girl with Down's syndrome is referred with tiredness, mild diarrhoea and a TSH of 9.2 mU/L (0.4–4.0) and a FT4 of 14.1 pmol/L (9–24). She also has a raised TPO antibody titre.

Questions
1 Would you treat this child with T4?
2 What other investigations would you consider doing?
3 What is the likely diagnosis?

Answers
1 The thyroid function is only mildly deranged with a normal FT4 and a slightly raised TSH. This slight abnormality is unlikely to cause any symptoms. Most children with Down's syndrome have an atrophic thyroiditis with no goitre. TSH levels sometimes rise transiently and can fluctuate. If the TSH rises to above 10 mU/L the child should have TFT's 6 monthly. If the TSH rises above 15 mU/L the child should have TFT's 3 monthly and is likely to eventually require T4. In the above situations the family should be told of the symptoms to look out for. If the TSH ≥ 20 mU/L with a normal FT4 the patient should be treated with T4.
2 A general paediatric approach should be taken looking for the large number of causes of tiredness and diarrhoea in a child with Down's syndrome. The two most important investigations are a FBC looking for anaemia and a coeliac screen.
3 The likeliest diagnosis is coeliac disease. The anti-transglutaminase antibodies were positive and a jejunal biopsy confirmed coeliac disease. Coeliac disease is an immunological disorder and is commoner in Down's syndrome. The tiredness and diarrhoea resolved on a gluten-free diet.

Further reading

Birrell, G. & Cheetham, T. (2004) Juvenile thyrotoxicosis; can we do better? *Arch Dis Child* **89**, 745–750.
Brown, R. S. (2009) The thyroid gland. In: *Brook's Clinical Paediatric Endocrinology* (ed. C.G.D. Brook, P. Clayton & R. S. Brown), 6th edn., pp. 250–282. Wiley-Blackwell, Oxford.

Djemli, A., Van Vliet, G., Belgoudi, J. *et al.* (2004) Reference intervals for free thyroxine, total triiodothyronine, thyrotropin and thyroglobulin for Quebec newborns, children and teenagers. *Clinical Biochemistry* **37**, 328–330.

Haddow, J.E., Palomaki, G.E. *et al.* (1999) Maternal thyroid deficiency during pregnancy and subsequent neuropsychological development in the child. *New England Journal of Medicine* **341**, 549–555.

Jones, J.H., Attaie, M., Maroo, S. *et al.* (2010) Heterogeneous tissue in the thyroid fossa on ultrasound in infants with proven thyroid ectopia on isotope scan – a diagnostic trap. *Pediatr Radiology* **40**, 725–731.

LaFranchi, S. (2007) Disorders of the thyroid gland. In: *Nelson's Textbook of Pediatrics* (ed. R.M. Kliegman, R.E. Behrman, H.B. Jenson & B.F. Stanton), 18th edn., pp. 2316–2340. Saunders Elsevier, Philadelphia.

Larson, C., Hermos, R., Delaney A. *et al.* (2003) Risk factors associated with delayed thyrotropin elevations in congenital hypothyroidism. *J Pediatr* **143**, 587–591.

Oakley, G.A., Muir, T., Ray, M. *et al.* (1998) Increased incidence of congenital malformation in infants with TSH elevation detected on newborn screening. *J Pediatr* **132**(4), 726–730.

Ogilvy-Stuart, A.L. & Midgley, P. (2006) *Practical Neonatal Endocrinology*. Cambridge University Press, Cambridge.

Rovet J. (2003) Long-term follow-up of children born with sporadic congenital hypothyroidism. *Ann Endocrinol* **64**(1), 58–61.

7 Disorders of Sex Development and Common Genital Anomalies

Introduction

In 2006, the term 'disorders of sex development (DSDs)' was proposed to replace 'intersex', which was felt to be derogatory. It may be that, in the future, even the word 'disorder' might be considered so and be replaced by the term 'variant'. In the restricted sense, patients with DSDs present with external genitalia that are sufficiently ambiguous to cause uncertainty as to which gender should be assigned and this is the major focus of this chapter. However, in the broader sense, DSDs encompass all situations when the karyotype is at partial or complete variance with the primary or secondary sexual characteristics. Understanding normal sexual differentiation and its genetic and hormonal control is a prerequisite to properly understanding and managing patients with DSDs.

Normal sexual differentiation and its genetic and hormonal control

Basic concepts of the embryology of sexual differentiation

An essential concept is that the human embryo is bipotential until 40 days gestation. Regardless of whether they are derived from a 46,XX or a 46,XY zygote, the gonads and the internal (Müllerian and Wolffian ducts) and external genitalia (genital tubercle and urethral and genital folds) have a similar appearance. After 40 days, the gonads differentiate into either testes, which start producing anti-Müllerian hormone (AMH), a glycoprotein, at about 6–8 weeks and then testosterone, or into ovaries, with germ cell meiosis at 11–12 weeks. Recent studies have shown that the differentiation of both the ovaries and the testes require activation of specific gene cascades, thus challenging the long-held concept of 'female development by default'. However, this concept still applies to the differentiation of the internal and external genitalia and of the urogenital sinus (see below).

Genetic control of gonadal sex determination

A detailed discussion of this complex process is beyond the scope of this chapter. With few exceptions, the presence of a Y chromosome containing a normal SRY (sex determining region of the Y chromosome) gene will result in the differentiation of the bipotential gonad into a testis. However, a number of other genes, acting up- or downstream of SRY, are required for normal testicular development. Table 7.1 lists some of these genes and their characteristics. As indicated above, ovarian differentiation also requires activation of specific gene pathways, notably the WNT-4 (Wingless Type, member 4) pathway.

Practical Endocrinology and Diabetes in Children, Third Edition. Joseph E. Raine, Malcolm D.C. Donaldson, John W. Gregory, Guy Van Vliet.
© 2011 Blackwell Publishing Ltd. Published 2011 by Blackwell Publishing Ltd.

Table 7.1 Selected genes involved in development of the testes and effects of mutations in humans

Gene	Full name	Function	Effect of mutations in humans
SRY	Sex determining region of the Y chromosome	Testis determination	46, XY with pure gonadal dysgenesis (46, XY PGD)
SOX	SRY-like HMG Box	Family homologous to SRY	46, XY PGD with camptomelic dysplasia (SOX-9)
DAX-1	Dosage sensitive sex reversal, adrenal hypoplasia congenita on the X chromosome, gene 1	Development of: -gonadotrophs, -adrenals -gonads	-Adrenal hypoplasia -Gonadotrophin deficiency -46, XY PGD (duplication)
WT-1	Wilms' tumour-1	Testis determination	-Testicular dysgenesis -Urogenital malformations -Malignancy (Dennis-Drash, Frasier, WAGR syndromes)
SF-1	Steroidogenic Factor-1	Testis determination	Testicular dysgenesis Primary adrenal insufficiency in severe cases
RSPO1	R-Spondin-1	Antagonizes testis determination	46, XX testicular DSD (formerly "46,XX male")

Internal genitalia (see Figure 7.1)

From 6–8 weeks, in the presence of a testis, the Müllerian system involutes under the influence of the AMH secreted by the Sertoli cells, while the Wolffian system is stabilized by testosterone secreted by the Leydig cells, which are stimulated by placental human chorionic gonadotrophin (hCG), into the epididymis, vas deferens, seminal vesicles and ejaculatory ducts. It is important to note that AMH exerts its effect in a paracrine fashion (i.e. a local effect near its site of production), while testosterone acts both locally (to stabilize the Wolffian ducts) and in a classical endocrine way (to masculinize the urogenital sinus and the external genitalia) after being transported through the bloodstream. In the absence of a testis, the Wolffian system involutes and the Müllerian system develops into the Fallopian tubes, uterus and the upper third of the vagina.

Urogenital sinus

Under the influence of testosterone, the sinus narrows to form the posterior urethra and the prostate and the glands of Cowper develop from outgrowths of the sinus. In the absence of testosterone, the sinus forms the lower two-thirds of the vagina and the urethra and its outgrowths form the para-urethral glands of Skene and the vestibular glands of Bartholin.

External genitalia (see Figure 7.2)

From 8 weeks onwards in the male, under the influence of dihydrotestosterone (DHT, converted from testosterone in genital skin by 5-α reductase type 2), the genital tubercle will grow to form the penis, the urethral folds will develop into the corpus spongiosum surrounding the urethra and the genital folds will fuse in the midline to form the scrotum and ventral part of the penis. In the female, the same structures will form the clitoris, the labia minora and the labia majora.

Classification of DSDs

Historically, individuals with ambiguous genitalia had been classified according to the histology of their gonads. Thus, those with both ovarian and testicular tissue were called 'true hermaphrodites', those with only ovarian tissue 'female pseudohermaphrodites' and those with only testicular tissue 'male pseudohermaphrodites'. Since the discovery of the human sex chromosomes in 1956, gonadal biopsies are only required to establish a diagnosis of true hermaphrodism, a very rare occurrence. On the other hand, the somewhat monstrous connotation of the term (pseudo)hermaphrodite has led to a proposed new nomenclature (Table 7.2). Of note, mixed gonadal

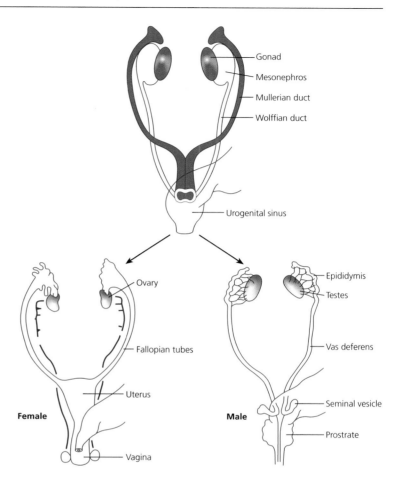

Female

Male

Gonad
Mesonephros
Mullerian duct
Wolffian duct
Urogenital sinus
Ovary
Epididymis
Testes
Fallopian tubes
Vas deferens
Uterus
Seminal vesicle
Prostrate
Vagina

Fig. 7.1 Differentiation of the internal genitalia.

dysgenesis (most often associated with 45,X/46,XY mosaicism), the second most common cause of ambiguous genitalia (after virilizing congenital adrenal hyperplasia (CAH)), occupies a separate niche in both the old and the new nomenclatures.

46,XX DSDs

By far the commonest form of 46,XX DSD is CAH from 21-hydroxylase deficiency. The pathophysiology of this condition and its medical management are described in detail in chapter 8. In genetic females affected with the severe form of the disease, masculinization of the external genitalia is usually detected at birth. However, virilization can sometimes be relatively mild and may be missed in the neonatal period. At the extreme end of the spectrum, masculinization may be complete, with a penile urethra, and the neonate may be considered to be a boy with bilateral cryptorchidism. Figure 7.3 illustrates

the spectrum of virilization of the external genitalia that can be observed in girls with CAH due to 21-hydroxylase deficiency.

Much less common enzyme defects that can cause *in utero* virilization of 46,XX foetuses involve 11-β-hydroxylase and aromatase deficiencies. 3-β-ol-dehydrogenase, 17-α-hydroxylase, 17,20-lyase and the recently described deficiency in P450-oxidoreductase (an electron donor for 21-hydroxylase and 17-hydroxylase and for aromatase) do not typically induce *in utero* virilization of genetically female foetuses.

46,XY DSD

Biosynthetic defects (see Figure 7.4)

Synthetic defects in the adreno-gonadal enzyme pathways from cholesterol to testosterone (and in its reduction to DHT in genital skin) can cause ambiguous genitalia in 46,XY individuals in spite of the presence of two normally

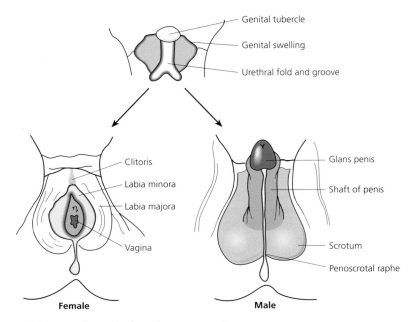

Fig. 7.2 Differentiation of the external genitalia from the common anlage.

differentiated testes. Specifically, 3-β-ol-dehydrogenase, 17,20-desmolase and 17-β-hydroxysteroid dehydrogenase deficiencies will result in reduced testosterone production during the embryonic period and therefore

Table 7.2 Previous and new classification of disorders of sex development

Previous	New
Intersex	Disorders of sex development (DSD)
• Male pseudohermaphrodite	46, XY DSD
• Undervirilization of an XY male	
• Undermasculinization of an XY male	
• Female pseudohermaphrodite	46, XX DSD
• Overvirilization of an XX female	
• Masculinization of an XX female	
True hermaphrodite	Ovotesticular DSD
XX male or XX sex reversal	46, XX testicular DSD
XY sex reversal	46, XY complete gonadal dysgenesis

ambiguous genitalia. 5-α-reductase deficiency, which results in decreased DHT production in genital skin, should also be considered in ambiguous 46,XY neonates. All of these enzyme defects are inherited in an autosomal recessive fashion and are therefore more common in consanguineous families. Lastly, a deficiency of the steroidogenic acute regulatory (StAR) protein, which transports cholesterol inside the mitochondria (see chapter), also causes an autosomal recessive form of 46,XY DSD generally with a completely female external appearance ('sex reversal') and severe adrenal insufficiency; likewise, the under-virilization of 46,XY newborns with Smith–Lemli–Opitz syndrome, an autosomal recessive multiple congenital malformation and mental retardation syndrome due to a deficiency of 7-dehydrocholesterol reductase, can be very severe.

Abnormal testicular development (testicular dysgenesis)

Leydig cell hypoplasia is suggested by severe undermasculinization, occasionally with complete 'sex reversal', in a genetic male with identifiable gonads and raised gonadotrophins. Many patients with this condition have been shown to have biallelic inactivation of the LH (luteinizing hormone)/hCG receptor. In contrast, because foetal pituitary LH only begins to control testosterone

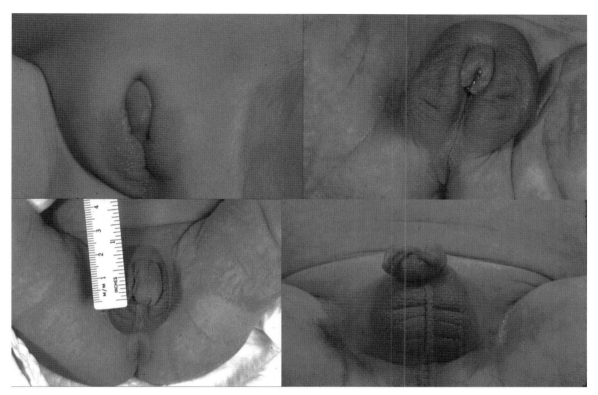

Fig. 7.3 The spectrum of virilization of the external genitalia that can be observed in girls with CAH due to 21-hydroxylase deficiency.

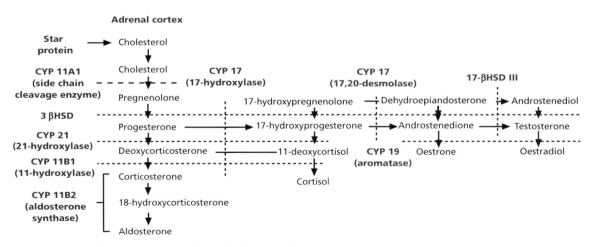

Fig. 7.4 Pathways of steroid synthesis in adrenal gland and gonads.

production by Leydig cells after 13 weeks of gestation, congenital gonadotrophin deficiency typically presents with micropenis and cryptorchidism, but not with abnormal sexual differentiation. A recently identified cause of testicular dysgenesis is inactivating mutations in steroidogenic factor 1 (SF-1), which are not always associated with adrenal insufficiency. However, a specific diagnosis remains elusive in many under-virilized males with testicular dysgenesis.

Androgen resistance

Complete androgen insensitivity syndrome (CAIS) is an X-linked disorder caused by a variety of inactivating androgen receptor (AR) mutations. These mutations can occur *de novo* or be inherited through the mother who is a healthy carrier. There may be a history of amenorrhea and infertility on the maternal side of the family. Half of the genetically male offspring of carrier mothers will be phenotypic females with absent female structures, intra-abdominal or inguinal testes and a short vagina. The diagnosis is usually made in the index case upon the discovery of gonads on palpation or at operation for an inguinal hernia in a female infant. With the increased use of amniocentesis, the diagnosis may also be suspected when a phenotypically female baby is born after a 46,XY karyotype has been found on amniocentesis. The 'classical' presentation with primary amenorrhoea in an adolescent with normal breast development but without sexual hair has become the exception.

Although completely insensitive to androgen, individuals with CAIS are normally sensitive to oestradiol which is aromatized from the high testosterone levels produced at puberty. This accounts for normal breast development and female body habitus, but there is little or no pubic and axillary hair because of the androgen resistance. AMH production by the foetal testes being normal, Müllerian structures are absent, hence the amenorrhea and the complete impossibility of fertility.

Mixed gonadal dysgenesis

Mixed gonadal dysgenesis is the term applied to 45,X/46,XY mosaicism associated with ambiguous genitalia, a streak gonad on one side and a dysgenetic testis on the other. The external and internal phenotype will depend on the degree of testicular dysgenesis. With severe androgen and AMH deficiency, the external genitalia will be under-masculinized and both vagina and uterus will be present. Regression of the uterine horn and of the Fallopian tube on the side where testicular differentiation occurred may be seen, illustrating the paracrine action

of AMH. If testicular dysgenesis is relatively mild, Müllerian regression will have occurred and the external genitalia may be male. Indeed, 45,X/46,XY mosaicism may be found in boys with unexplained short stature and features of Turner's syndrome, suggesting that in these patients the gonads are 46,XY and the growth plates 45,X.

Pure gonadal dysgenesis

In pure gonadal dysgenesis, the gonads are reduced to fibrous streaks, the external genitalia are female and Müllerian structures (i.e. female internal genitalia) are present. It can occur either sporadically or in familial form. Some 46,XY individuals have streak gonads and complete 'sex reversal'. This phenomenon has been found in some cases to be due to deletion or mutation of *SRY*. The streak gonads should be removed as soon as the diagnosis is established because of the risk of gonadoblastoma. Pure gonadal dysgenesis can also be seen in association with a 46,XX karyotype; mutations that completely inactivate the FSH receptor have been found in some cases, although these more commonly lead to premature ovarian failure.

Initial investigation of DSDs

Ambiguous genitalia are usually identified at birth and pose the dilemma of gender assignment. Both parents should be seen as soon as possible. The key points in counselling are the following:
• Initial counselling by attending staff, backed up as quickly as possible by a senior paediatrician and a paediatric endocrinologist.
• Key phrase 'there is something the matter with the way that the baby's genitals have been formed, so that we cannot at present say whether the child should be brought up as a boy or a girl'.
• Infant should be referred to as 'the baby' or 'the child' not as he, she or it!
• Mother and baby should be in a single room.
• Registration of name should be postponed.
• Urgent investigations should lead to definite gender assignment within 2 weeks.

History
• Consanguinity.
• Maternal medications.
• Maternal health including androgenic symptoms, such as an increase in body hair and acne (suggesting placental

aromatase or P450 oxidoreductase deficiency) or virilization (suggesting a tumour in the mother).

Examination

- General examination to rule out dysmorphic syndrome ± congenital anomalies.
- Palpation of the abdomen and inguinal regions for gonads.
- Meticulous description ± diagram of abnormal genitalia, using neutral words (see description of the bipotential embryo above) and including labioscrotal folds; genital tubercle; nature and size of opening below genital tubercle; identification where possible of urethral meatus and vaginal opening; and presence and site of gonad(s).
- Examination of anus.
- Measurement of blood pressure (CAH due to 11-β-hydroxylase deficiency may lead to hypertension, but this is seldom present in neonates; conversely, cortisol and aldosterone deficiency may lead to hypotension and shock).
- Medical photograph with legs spread apart and ruler next to the genital tubercle.

The degree of masculinization can be expressed as a Prader stage. Premature girls, because of the lack of subcutaneous fat, may appear to have clitoral hypertrophy. In these cases, it is useful to estimate the ratio of the distance between the anus and the posterior labial fourchette to the distance between the anus and the base of the clitoris: a ratio less than 0.5, regardless of gestational age, reasonably excludes androgenization during the first trimester.

Further investigations and management

The following professionals should be informed as soon as possible:

- Paediatric endocrinologist.
- Radiologist, surgeon and mental health professional with expertise in DSD
- Medical geneticist.

If access to the professionals listed above is difficult, then transfer to a specialist centre for specific tests or for general management may be necessary.

The following investigations should be carried out as quickly as possible:

- *Karyotype:* This takes a minimum of 3 days. In contrast, Fluorescent *in situ* hybridization (FISH) to determine the presence of a Y chromosome or DNA amplification by polymerase chain reaction (PCR) to determine the presence of SRY sequences gives a 'provisional karyotype' within hours.
- *Abdominal ultrasound to define the structures:* Uterus, intra-abdominal, inguinal or labioscrotal gonad(s) and adrenals.
- Plasma 17-hydroxyprogesterone (17-OHP).
- *Genitography:* This is usually only necessary prior to feminizing genitoplasty to define the point of confluence of the vagina and urethra.

Etiological diagnosis, sex assignment and initial management of DSDs

Figure 7.5 shows a flow diagram giving the main diagnostic possibilities. As stated above, the commonest cause of ambiguous genitalia is CAH due to 21-hydroxylase deficiency in a 46,XX baby. The diagnosis of 21-hydroxylase deficiency is based on the measurement of plasma 17-OHP, with the sample being taken on day 3 (the overlap between affected and normal being too great prior to this) and the result being requested urgently. In addition, the plasma levels of androstenedione, testosterone and dehydroepiandrosterone-sulfate (DHEAS) will be elevated in CAH. Blood glucose should be measured, although significant hypoglycaemia is seldom present. However, babies with CAH are at risk of salt wasting (an 'Addisonian crisis') and plasma electrolytes are often measured early after birth in newborns with genital ambiguity. This may give a false sense of reassurance, because plasma electrolytes are usually normal initially. Due to renal immaturity, the initial salt-wasting episode typically occurs only in the second or third week of life, so that the infant's weight should be carefully monitored even if the plasma electrolytes were normal initially. If there is significant weight loss (up to 10% weight loss is within normal limits in newborns but babies should regain their birth weight by 14 days of age) or if weight does not increase satisfactorily subsequently, plasma electrolytes should be measured again and, if hyponatraemia develops, urine sodium should be measured to document inappropriate natriuresis.

Based on their normal female internal genitalia and potential fertility, sex assignment is considered to be straightforward in virilized girls with CAH. Likewise, newborns with ambiguous genitalia due to mixed gonadal dysgenesis are usually assigned a female gender. The presence of a uterus in this condition makes assisted fertility possible. However, the gonads should be removed

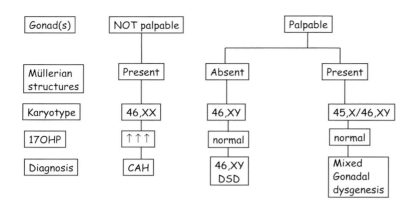

Fig. 7.5 Flowchart showing the main diagnostic possibilities in neonates with ambiguous genitalia.

as soon as the diagnosis is made because of the risk of gonadoblastoma.

Whether in CAH or in mixed gonadal dysgenesis, the psychosexual consequences of clitoral/vulvar surgery in infancy are controversial. One line of thought, with which most parents are uncomfortable, is that genital surgery should be deferred until the patient is old enough to consent.

From the points of view of diagnosis and of sex assignment, the most difficult cases are 46,XY infants with partial androgen insensitivity syndrome (PAIS) in whom the growth potential of the phallus at puberty is unpredictable. In contrast, 46,XY patients with enzyme defects have normal sensitivity to androgens and can therefore be assigned a male sex if diagnosed early enough. The diagnosis in this group of patients has classically been based on the measurement of precursor/product ratios of various plasma steroids before and after stimulation with hCG. There are many different protocols for hCG stimulation, the simplest being a single intramuscular (i.m.) injection of 3000 units/m^2 with measurement of plasma steroids 5 days later. However, several of the enzymes described above are present in various isoforms encoded by different genes (only one of which has a deleterious mutation) and expressed in different organs so that these plasma ratios may be misleading; for example, mutations inactivating *SRD5A2* will reduce 5-α reductase activity in genital skin and cause 46,XY DSD; however, *SRD5A1* is not mutated, so that the enzyme activity in the liver is intact and the plasma testosterone/DHT ratio may be normal. Molecular analysis of the relevant genes is therefore being increasingly used to establish a diagnosis based on a limited clinical and biochemical phenotype. Another example is 46,XY babies with under-virilization and salt wasting, who are likely to have 3-β-ol-dehydrogenase defi-

ciency until proven otherwise and in whom the diagnosis can be readily confirmed by analyzing the *HSD3B2* gene.

Ultimately, criteria for sex assignment include the specific diagnosis, presence of female internal genitalia (i.e. vagina, uterus), size and androgen sensitivity of the genital tubercle, parental wishes and cultural aspects. The advice given as to sex assignment should ideally result from a consensus between physicians, surgeons and psychologists of both sexes. In cases where parents and health care providers disagree and psychological support was not able to change the parents' choice, it is probably wise to let the parents' opinion prevail.

Management of CAIS should start with intensive counselling of the patients, of their parents and of all health professionals involved, to dispel any notion of 'ambiguity'. Because intra-abdominal testes have a high propensity to develop cancer, gonadectomy is recommended. The age at which gonadectomy should be performed is controversial: if the diagnosis of CAIS is certain, some argue that it is preferable for the patient to allow breast development from her endogenous estrogens. On the other hand, because testicular tumours have been reported as early as at 14 years, it seems reasonable to advise gonadectomy as soon as breast development is complete. This should, of course, be followed by hormone replacement, which is best achieved with oral contraceptives.

In contrast to CAIS, PAIS results in a wide phenotypic spectrum ranging from severely ambiguous genitalia to isolated male infertility. The management of these cases is difficult and controversial unless the degree of under-masculinization is relatively mild, in which cases they should be treated as subjects with CAIS; however, gonadectomy should be performed before puberty to avoid the risk of virilization at that time.

Psychological challenges faced by patients with DSDs and outcome

Boy or girl? This is usually the first question asked in the delivery room. It is therefore quite understandable that the birth of a child with sufficient ambiguity of the external genitalia as to make immediate gender assignment impossible is associated with great discomfort on the part of the health professionals and with great parental distress. On the other hand, the discovery, perhaps many years after birth, that the child has abnormal gonads and will be unable to have children without assistance, if at all, is also deeply wounding to many parents. Whatever the time when the DSD is discovered, it is essential for the clinician to invest as much time as possible in counselling parents. It is unrealistic to expect that all the information will be assimilated by the family at the first encounter, and several sessions will be required. It is also unrealistic to rely too much on printed information (e.g. parent booklets) in the early stages. Simple explanation, assisted by hand drawings, and tailored to the parents' psychological state, education and intellect requires time, patience and experience.

In addition to hormonal and surgical treatments as appropriate, these patients and their parents need long-term access to mental health professionals knowledgeable about DSDs. In contrast to what was often done in the past, the current thinking is to inform the parents in full, including about the karyotype, at the time of diagnosis. The anger and frustration felt by adolescents and adults in whom the diagnosis of DSD has been obscured or withheld makes a convincing case for honesty from childhood onwards. The child should therefore also be informed in a manner appropriate for his or her stage of cognitive and emotional development. Examination of the genitalia by staff and trainees at follow-up visits should be restricted to what is strictly necessary. If the child is properly counselled by the paediatrician and parents during the prepubertal years, it will be possible to give a full and honest account of the problem at adolescence. The classic difficult scenario is explaining the condition to a girl with CAIS. It may be helpful to phrase the explanation as follows: 'The great majority of girls and women have two X chromosomes and ovaries. A minority of otherwise normal women have XY chromosomes, testes in the abdomen instead of ovaries, but complete resistance to the male hormone (testosterone) made by the testes. In this situation, the body is extremely sensitive to oestrogen, which is made from the testosterone, and this results in

normal female development. However, there is no uterus and therefore you will not have menses and you will not be able to become pregnant'. Communication with women with the same condition is often helpful. Notwithstanding the use of the approach outlined above from diagnosis onwards, feelings of secrecy and shame remain common. These should be addressed so that by the time of transfer to adult care, the patient can explain his or her condition and have as little embarrassment about it as possible.

Transition to adult care

At the end of puberty and after full disclosure, patients with DSDs should be transferred to an endocrinologist or a gynaecologist with expertise in these disorders. How this is organized in practice will vary according to local circumstances, but ensuring that the transfer has actually happened is important. Especially in patients who do not need chronic medication, it is not unusual that they do not show up at the appointment made with the physician in charge of overseeing their evolution and management in adult life. Even patients on chronic replacement therapy may stop taking their glucocorticoids and present with acute adrenal insufficiency while gonadectomized or hypogonadal patients who stop their sex hormones are at risk of developing osteoporosis at an early age.

Studies of subjects with DSD in adulthood are few. The best studied, most numerous and relatively homogeneous group of patients is that of women with CAH. Some studies report no dramatic increase in psychological morbidity, good social adjustment and no deficit in self-esteem. However, the surgical techniques used in the past for feminizing genitoplasty have led to sexual difficulties in many women. It is hoped that newer techniques involving better preservation of the innervation and vascularization of the clitoris will lead to better outcomes.

Patients with 46,XY DSDs born with ambiguous genitalia are much more heterogeneous. Reports of female-to-male self-reassignment at adolescence of 46,XY subjects with 5-α reductase deficiency whose testes had not been removed in infancy are not generalizable. Importantly, almost half of 46,XY DSD subjects (mostly PAIS), reared male or female, reported that they were neither well informed about their medical and surgical history nor satisfied with their knowledge. This emphasizes the importance of the philosophy of full disclosure that is outlined above and that should now be adopted by all interdisciplinary teams that follow patients with DSD.

Common genital anomalies with no ambiguity

Fused labia

This benign problem in infant girls is likely due to their low estrogen milieu. Indeed, twice daily application of estrogen-containing creams for one to two weeks usually relieves the problem. Longer periods of application of estrogen creams may lead to breast budding. Referral to a pediatric gynecologist is only exceptionally needed. If the vaginal opening remains completely obstructed in spite of treatment with topical estrogen, a pelvic ultrasound will rule out Rokitanski syndrome (congenital absence of the vagina and uterus). However, to avoid undue anxiety, this should be performed by a radiologist with paediatric expertise, given the small size of the normal prepubertal uterus.

Isolated clitoromegaly

As described above, this is a common finding in premature infants and tends to become less obvious with the development of subcutaneous fat. On the other hand, if it is first noted after birth but is isolated (i.e. not associated with accelerated linear growth), the probability that the girl has a 'simple virilizing' form of CAH (i.e. without salt wasting) is low. A short period of watchful waiting may be in order, but it may be best to measure plasma androgens, which will also rule out the rarer but more ominous possibility of an androgen-producing tumour of the adrenals or ovaries.

Micropenis

The length of the penis should be evaluated by pressing firmly on the prepubic fat and should be compared with the existing growth curves. These show that the 10th centile for penile length in term newborns is 2.5 cm. In otherwise normal newborns with true micropenis, the presence of testes should be ascertained. If normal testes are felt with certainty, isolated gonadotrophin deficiency remains possible but can be easily ruled out by measuring plasma testosterone at about 2 months of age; indeed, the 'minipuberty of infancy' creates a critical window of opportunity to assess the integrity of the hypothalamo–pituitary–testicular axis. If no testes are felt, bilateral anorchia (which results from bilateral testicular torsion some time after sex differentiation is complete) can be ruled out by measuring plasma AMH levels as early as 3 days after birth (when FSH may still be normal due to inhibition by maternal estrogens). In infant boys with micropenis due to either gonadotrophin or anorchia, sensitivity to androgens is normal and treatment with testosterone oenanthate (25 mg i.m. monthly for 3 months) will result in a doubling of penile size.

Penile length increases until about 4 years of age and then remains stable until puberty. Therefore, by far the most common reason for referral for 'micropenis' at school age is for obese boys with a penis that is buried in prepubic fat. Anosmia may suggest an associated gonadotrophin deficiency, but in its absence these boys can be reassured by a simple physical examination as described above.

Cryptorchidism

The best time to accurately assess the presence and position of the testes is the first year of life, before the cremasteric reflex sets in. Although testicular descent may not be complete at birth in some normal term newborns (in which case one may take advantage of the 'minipuberty' to exclude gonadotrophin deficiency as outlined above), the testes should have reached a scrotal position by the end of the first year. Parents should be informed that their son has two normally descended testes and this should be noted in the health record.

If this is not done, undue concern will arise at a later age and sometimes lead to superfluous investigations and even unnecessary surgeries. Indeed, even by careful examination with warm hands, many school-age boys will have testicles that are difficult to palpate. The vast majority of these boys have retractile testes and their testes will descend permanently in the scrotum at the beginning of puberty.

If true cryptorchidism is established after repeated examinations, the extent of investigations will depend on its uni- or bilateral nature and on whether the testes are palpable or not. In the latter case, plasma AMH will establish whether there are intra-abdominal testes (in mid-childhood, plasma FSH may be normal even in the absence of functional gonads). How these intra-abdominal testes can be located by imaging is beyond the scope of this chapter; suffice is to say that ultrasound examinations are useless except if the testes are in the inguinal canal. Otherwise normal boys with incompletely descended but palpable testes, either uni- or bilaterally, can be referred for surgery without investigation.

Hypospadias

Hypospadias is defined as incomplete fusion of the urethra with the meatus on the ventral aspect of the penis – the glans, corona, shaft of penis, and (most severe) the perineum. This abnormality is commonly accompanied by chordee – curvature of the penis – caused by fibrosis of the corpus spongiosum.

Isolated hypospadias (hypospadias without micropenis and with normally descended testes in a normal scrotum) is rarely associated with an endocrine disorder. Surgeons should be asked to refer the following conditions for further investigation, including karyotype:

• Perineal hypospadias.
• Hypospadias with micropenis.
• Hypospadias with cryptorchidism ± scrotal abnormality.

However, even extensive investigation of such patients does not always lead to a specific diagnosis.

Future developments

• DSDs are relatively uncommon and affected children require help from a variety of specialized health professionals (paediatricians, endocrinologists, surgeons, gynaecologists, geneticists, psychologists, radiologists and possibly others), who are usually only available at large academic centres. Communication between these health professionals is as important as communication of each professional with the patient and with the family. Designating a primary contact person for the patient is important and this role is often assumed by the paediatric endocrinologist.
• Increased understanding of the molecular genetic basis for DSDs will clarify the aetiology in an increasing number of specific disorders.
• Long-term follow-up data are needed, in particular to help determine the optimal surgical management of the virilized genitalia in females with CAH. Multicentre studies organized jointly by paediatric endocrinologists, surgeons and psychologist are required.

• The medical, surgical and psychological management of parents, children and adolescents and adults affected by DSDs, including those born with ambiguous genitalia, has progressed greatly in part from the feedback given by affected adults but still requires considerable refinement based on continuing this dialogue.

Potential pitfalls

• Incorrect assignment of male gender to masculinized females with 21-hydroxlase deficiency. The absence of palpable gonads in an apparent male with hypospadias (or even with a penile urethra) should always arouse suspicion.
• Fusion of the labia minora, a common problem, may give the false impression of an absent vagina.
• Most school-aged boys referred for micropenis have exogenous obesity and a normal prepubertal phallus buried in surrounding fat.

Controversial points

• When should clitoroplasty and vaginoplasty be performed in girls with congenital adrenal hyperplasia?
• What are the long-term effects of exposure of the foetal brain to androgen levels that are discordant with the genetic and gonadal sex?
• When should the gonads of individuals with CAIS be removed: as soon as the diagnosis is made, or after sexual development is complete?

When to involve a specialist centre

• When a baby is born with ambiguous genitalia.
• Severe hypospadias ± cryptorchidism.
• Complete androgen insensitivity syndrome.
• Mixed or pure gonadal dysgenesis.

Case histories

Case 7.1

A 3.5 kg term newborn is of indeterminate sex, with a genital tubercle measuring 3 × 1 cm, labioscrotal folds, a single urogenital orifice and no gonad palpable. Pelvic ultrasound shows a uterus.

Question
What is the most likely diagnosis and what immediate investigations should be performed?

Answer
The most likely diagnosis is congenital adrenal hyperplasia in a genetic female. Essential investigations are the karyotype, which was 46,XX, and the 17-OHP level, which was 110 nmol/L [3663 ng/dL] on day 1 rising to above 300 nmol/L [10,000 ng/dL] on day 3. Although 17-OHP measurement should officially be deferred until day 3, a distinctly elevated level on day 1 in the context of a genital anomaly is highly suggestive.

Case 7.2

A 2.5 kg term newborn has abnormal genitalia with a gonad palpable in one labioscrotal fold and no gonad palpable on the other side. Pelvic ultrasound and genitography show a vagina and uterus. Karyotype is 45,X/46,XY. 17-OHP levels are normal.

Question
What is the diagnosis and how should the child be assigned?

Answer
The diagnosis is mixed gonadal dysgenesis with a dysgenetic testis on one side and probably a streak gonad on the other. The presence of Müllerian structures suggests that it is probably appropriate to raise this child as a female. The gonads should be removed.

Case 7.3

A 3.0 kg term newborn has a small genital tubercle (1.5 × 0.8 cm) and gonads palpable in partially fused labioscrotal folds. Pelvic ultrasound shows no uterus and genitogram shows a blind vaginal pouch. Karyotype is 46,XY; 17-OHP levels are normal.

Question
What is the most likely diagnosis and how should the child be managed?

Answer
The absence of female internal genitalia indicates that the gonads are testes which have produced AMH normally. The differential diagnosis is between a biosynthetic defect in testosterone production (rare) or, more likely, PAIS. A family history suggestive of autosomal recessive or X-linked inheritance orients to the former and latter possibility, respectively. LH, FSH and androgens should be measured in plasma before and following stimulation with hCG and, with PAIS, may show normal or high levels. In the absence of female internal genitalia, a female gender assignment would be difficult surgically. The child should be brought up as a boy unless the corpora cavernosa are inadequate.

Case 7.4

A baby is born to a 24-year-old G1P1A0 mother at 36 and 5/7 weeks of gestation, weighing 2100 g. The external genitalia are ambiguous, with a genital tubercle measuring 2 × 1 cm and partial posterior fusion of the genital folds. There are no palpable gonads. There is a posterior cleft palate, postaxial polydactyly and syndactyly of the 2nd, 3rd and 4th toes. Pelvic ultrasound shows no uterus. Karyotype is 46,XY.

Question
What is the most likely diagnosis and how should the child be managed?

Answer
The associated malformations point to a diagnosis of Smith–Lemli–Opitz syndrome. Total plasma cholesterol is low at 0.75 nmol/L and 7-dehydrocholesterol is 147 μmol/L (normally undetectable), pointing to a deficiency of 7-dehydrocholesterol reductase. This can be confirmed by DNA analysis. The prognosis should be guarded.

Useful information for patients and parents

The Androgen Insensitivity Support Group. Website: http://www.aissg.org/. It is an international consortium with good information and links to local resources.

The Accord Alliance. Website: http://www.accordalliance.org/. Provides similar services for DSDs in the broader sense.

The following professional associations of paediatric endocrinologists also have useful links for patients and parents:

- British Society for Paediatric Endocrinology and Diabetes. Website: http://www.bsped.org.uk/
- European Society for Paediatric Endocrinology. Website: www.eurospe.org/
- Pediatric Endocrine Society (North American). Website: www.lwpes.org/

Significant guidelines/consensus statement

Hughes, I.A., Houk, C., Ahmed, S.F. & Lee, P.A. (2006) Consensus statement on management of intersex disorders. *Arch Dis Child 2006 July* **91**(7), 554–63.

Further reading

Achermann, J.C. & Hughes, I.A. (2008) Disorders of sex development. In: *Williams Textbook of Endocrinology* (eds H.M. Kronenberg, S. Melmed, K.S. Polonsky & P.R. Larsen), 11th edn., pp. 783–848. Saunders Elsevier, Philadelphia.

8 Adrenal Disorders

Physiology

Adrenal anatomy and physiology

The adrenal glands are pyramidal structures which lie adjacent to the upper poles of the kidneys. The adrenal cortex is divided into three zones: the outer zona glomerulosa, middle zona fasciculata and inner zona reticularis. The main types of steroids produced by the adrenal cortex are mineralocorticoids (principally aldosterone), glucocorticoids (principally cortisol) and androgens. Steroidogenesis in the zona fasciculata (primarily cortisol) and reticularis (mainly androgen) is under hypothalamic–pituitary control; secretion of aldosterone from the zona glomerulosa is under the control of the renin–angiotensin system.

Hypothalamic–pituitary axis (Figure 8.1)

Corticotrophin-releasing hormone (CRH) is synthesized in the hypothalamus and acts on the corticotrophs of the anterior pituitary to secrete the peptide pro-opiomelanocortin (POMC). POMC is the precursor of adrenocorticotrophic hormone (ACTH). ACTH binds to its melanocortin-2 receptor (MC-2R), a cell surface receptor in the cells of the adrenal cortex. ACTH also has affinity for the melanocortin-1 receptor (MC-1R) in the skin, so that ACTH excess results in hyperpigmentation. The MC-2R is G-protein coupled, and its activation results in increased adenylate cyclase activity, which in turn increases intracellular cyclic adenosine monophosphate (cAMP). Increased cAMP activity enhances the transport of cholesterol across the mitochondrial membrane by the steroidogenic acute regulatory (StAR) protein.

Cholesterol is metabolized into three types of steroids: glucocorticoid, mineralocorticoid and androgen.

Cortisol, the principal glucocorticoid, is vital for normal health, maintaining normal glucose and blood pressure and for combating stress. It follows a circadian rhythm, with high levels on waking and a nadir at midnight. Between 80 and 90% of cortisol is bound to cortisol binding globulin (CBG), and most serum assays measure total rather than free cortisol. Cortisol exerts a negative feedback at the hypothalamic and pituitary levels. Thus, plasma ACTH concentrations will be elevated in primary adrenal insufficiency and suppressed when cortisol excess is caused by autonomous adrenal lesions or exogenous glucocorticoids. In primary adrenal insufficiency, cortisol levels will depend on the severity of the defect. In severe deficiency, cortisol is low despite massively raised ACTH, but in partial deficiency basal cortisol may be normal. However, since basal cortisol output is already maximal in this situation, there will be no further increase should a major physical stress occur and signs of acute adrenal insufficiency may then develop.

Steroid pathways

Adrenal steroidogenesis is under the control of the cytochrome P450 (CYP) and the hydroxysteroid

Practical Endocrinology and Diabetes in Children, Third Edition. Joseph E. Raine, Malcolm D.C. Donaldson, John W. Gregory, Guy Van Vliet.
© 2011 Blackwell Publishing Ltd. Published 2011 by Blackwell Publishing Ltd.

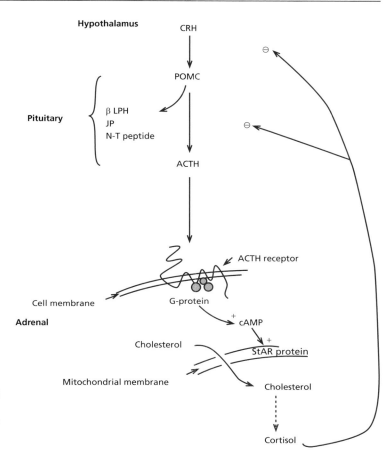

Fig. 8.1 Schematic diagram of hypothalamic–pituitary–adrenal axis. b LPH, b lipotrophic hormone; CRH, corticotrophin-releasing hormone; JP, joining peptide; N-T peptide, N-terminal peptide; POMC, pro-opiomelanocortin; StAR protein, steroidogenic acute regulatory protein; +, positive effect; –, negative effect.

dehydrogenase (HSD) enzymes. Pregnenolone may be converted along the mineralocorticoid pathway to aldosterone, along the glucocorticoid pathway to cortisol, or along the androgen pathway to testosterone (Figure 8.2). Impairment of cortisol synthesis will result from disorders affecting the StAR protein and 3-β-hydroxysteroid dehydrogenase (3-βHSD), CYP 21A2 (21-hydroxylase), CYP 11B1 (11-hydroxylase) and the CYP 17 (17-hydroxylase) enzymes. These enzyme disorders are collectively known as 'congenital adrenal hyperplasia (CAH)', as cortisol deficiency causes increased ACTH secretion and thus enlargement of the adrenal glands. Mineralocorticoid deficiency will result from StAR protein, 3-βHSD and CYP 21 deficiencies. In contrast, CYP 11B1 deficiency results in accumulation of the potent mineralocorticoid precursor deoxycorticosterone (DOC), while 17-hydroxylase deficiency also causes mineralocorticoid excess. Finally, deficiency in the enzymes proximal to testosterone – StAR protein, CYP 17 (17,20-desmolase), 17-βHSD and 3-

βHSD – results in under-masculinization of males. Lastly, 3-βHSD deficiency does not typically cause *in utero* virilization in females, because the steroid immediately above the enzyme block is dehydroepiandrosterone, a relatively weak androgen; however, mild postnatal signs of hypersecretion of this weak androgen, such as precocious pubarche, may be observed.

Mineralocorticoid synthesis

Aldosterone synthase, encoded by the *CYP 11B2* gene, converts DOC to aldosterone (Figure 8.3). Renin, secreted from the juxtaglomerular apparatus in the kidney, causes cleavage of angiotensinogen into angiotensin 1, which is in turn cleaved by angiotensin-converting enzyme (ACE) into angiotensin 2, a potent stimulator of *CYP 11B2* activity, promoting aldosterone secretion from the zona glomerulosa. Renin will therefore be elevated when aldosterone synthesis is impaired, and suppressed with aldosterone excess. Aldosterone enters the distal renal tubule

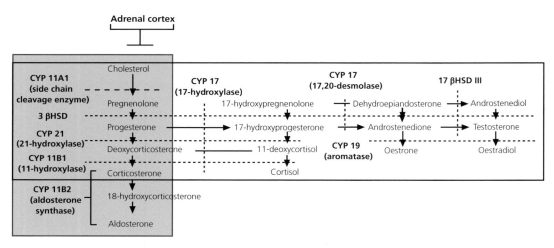

Fig. 8.2 Pathways of steroid synthesis in adrenal cortex. bHSD, b hydroxysteroid dehydrogenase. Shaded area indicates aldosterone synthesis in zona glomerulosa. Cortisol and androgen are synthesized in the zona fasciculata and zona reticularis, respectively.

cells, binds to its receptor and enters the nucleus causing transcription of messenger RNA (mRNA) and new protein synthesis. This contributes to enhanced Na^+K^+ ATPase ('the sodium pump') activity, causing sodium reabsorption in exchange for increased potassium excretion, while sodium for hydrogen ion exchange across the amiloride-sensitive epithelial sodium channel (ENaC) is also increased.

The following points should be noted:
• Cortisol has a similar affinity for the mineralocorticoid receptor as aldosterone, but is prevented from competing for this receptor by the enzyme 11-βHSD 2 which converts cortisol to cortisone. A deficiency of this enzyme causes apparent mineralocorticoid excess.
• Inactivating mutations of the ENaC or of the mineralocorticoid receptor result in failure of aldosterone action with elevated aldosterone levels – pseudohypoaldosteronism (PHA).
• Activating mutations of the ENaC result in apparent aldosterone excess despite low levels – Liddle's syndrome.
• Aldosterone excess causes sodium retention with hypernatraemia, hypokalaemia, a metabolic alkalosis and hypertension.

Investigations of adrenocortical function

Biochemical

Glucocorticoid secretion (Table 8.1)
Glucocorticoid excess and deficiency states are often difficult to diagnose because cortisol levels normally fluctuate

widely according to the time of day and degree of stress. Glucocorticoid excess results in normal or high random cortisol levels, loss of the normal circadian rhythm, an increase in urinary free cortisol and failure of plasma cortisol to suppress with low-dose dexamethasone.

Glucocorticoid deficiency is easy to diagnose if the defect is in the adrenal gland itself (primary adrenal insufficiency) because this will result in elevated ACTH levels and low cortisol levels with absent or impaired rise following synthetic ACTH (Cortrosyn® or Synacthen®) stimulation. The diagnosis is more difficult when the defect lies in the hypothalamus or pituitary gland (secondary adrenal insufficiency). In suspected secondary adrenal insufficiency, the low-dose synthetic ACTH test may be helpful. The rationale for this test is that the adrenal glands, if under-stimulated for months or years, will respond subnormally to quasi-physiological stimulation. A peak-stimulated cortisol greater than 550 nmol/L is considered normal, while a peak of less than 400 nmol/L is considered too low, and a great many patients fall in the grey zone in between. We regard a peak-stimulated cortisol level of > 500 nmol/L as 'normal' (see Table 8.1) whilst recognizing that any chosen cut-off level will be somewhat arbitrary and that the biochemical data must be interpreted in the clinical context.

Mineralocorticoid secretion (Table 8.2)
Mineralocorticoid deficiency is assessed by measurement of plasma and urinary electrolytes, and of plasma renin and aldosterone.

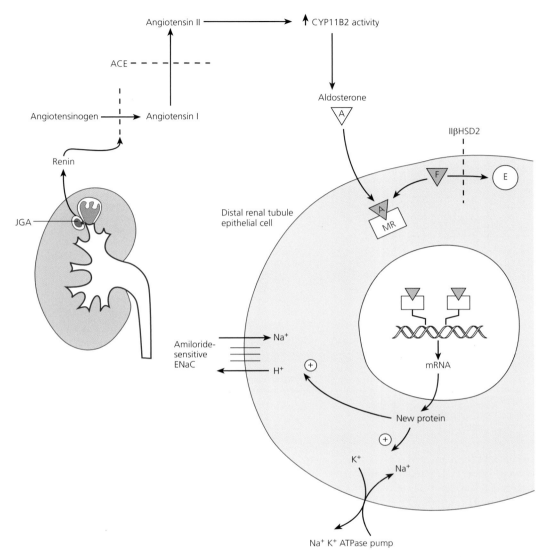

Fig. 8.3 Schematic diagram of aldosterone stimulation and action. A, aldosterone; ACE, angiotensin converting enzyme; E, cortisone; ENaC, epithelial sodium channel; F, cortisol; JGA, juxtaglomerular apparatus; MR, mineralocorticoid receptor; 11βHSD2, 11-beta-hydroxysteroid dehydrogenase 2.

Adrenal androgen secretion (Table 8.3)

Adrenal androgen status is assessed by plasma steroid analysis under basal and stimulated conditions. Salivary or capillary profiles collected at home for 17-hydroxyprogesterone (17-OHP) and androstenedione measurement are valuable in the monitoring of adrenal enzyme disorders, notably CAH resulting from 21-hydroxylase deficiency.

Glucocorticoid excess

Cushing's syndrome

Cushing's syndrome, unless iatrogenic, is very rare in childhood (Figure 8.4). However, its principal feature, obesity, is extremely common, so that the possibility of Cushing's syndrome is often raised.

Table 8.1 Investigation of glucocorticoid secretion.

Basal samples	Reference values
Plasma	
Fasting glucose	4–7 mmol/L
08.00 h ACTH	<20 mU/L
24.00 h (sleeping) cortisol	<50 nmol/L
08.00 h cortisol	200–700 nmol/L
Saliva	
08.00 h cortisol	6.5–28 nmol/L (usually 9–16) median 14.5
18.00 h cortisol	≤10 (mean 1.4)
Urine	
Urinary-free cortisol (random)	<25 μmol/mmol creatinine
Suppression tests	
Low-dose dexamethasone (0.5 mg 6-hourly × 8)	<50 nmol/L at 09.00 h 48 h after first dose
High-dose dexamethasone (2 mg 6-hourly × 8)	<50% basal value 48 h after first dose
Stimulation tests	
CRH (1 μg/kg IV)	Doubling of ACTH (usually to 8–25 mU/L)
	Cortisol peak ≥600 nmol/L with >20% increase over basal value
Standard short Synacthen (250 μg/m² IV)	Peak value >500 nmol/L ± doubling of basal value
Low-dose short Synacthen (500 ng/m² IV)	Peak value >500 nmol/L ± doubling of basal value
Insulin hypoglycaemia (min blood glucose <2.2 mmol/L)	Peak value >500 nmol/L
Metyrapone test	Doubling of plasma 11 deoxycortisol and urinary tetrahydrodeoxycortisol

Reference values are taken from the Institute of Biochemistry, Glasgow Royal Infirmary. Salivary cortisol data kindly provided by Dr J. Schulga are derived from 147 healthy children aged 5–15 years. Abbreviations: ACTH, adrencocorticotrophic hormone; CRH, corticotrophin-releasing hormone.

Imaging

If a central cause for glucocorticoid excess or deficiency is discovered, imaging of the hypothalamic–pituitary axis by magnetic resonance imaging (MRI) will be required. Adrenal ultrasound is a useful screening test for adrenal enlargement, but computed tomography (CT) or MRI will be needed to identify small lesions.

Causes

The causes of Cushing's syndrome in childhood are the following:

• *Iatrogenic:* Oral steroids, inhaled steroids, skin preparations containing steroids and steroid nose drops
• Cushing's disease (ACTH-secreting pituitary tumour)
• Adrenal tumour (cortical adenoma or carcinoma)

• *Primary adrenal hyperplasia:* Bilateral micronodular dysplasia (+/– Carney complex) and McCune–Albright syndrome
• Ectopic ACTH syndrome

Clinical diagnosis

Symptoms
• Obesity
• Slow growth (overtaken by siblings and peers)
• Fatigue
• Emotional lability

Signs
• Cushingoid habitus with moon face, central obesity and buffalo hump
• Facial plethora
• Acne
• Hirsutism

Table 8.2 Investigation of mineralocorticoid secretion.

Electrolytes	Normal values	Mineralocorticoid excess	Mineralocorticoid deficiency
Sodium	Na 135–145 mmol/L	Normal or ↑	↓
Potassium	K 3.5–4.5 mmol/L	Normal or ↓	↑
Aldosterone (ρ mol/L)*			
Infants <1 month	1000–5500	↑ in hyperaldosteronism	↓ in hypoaldosteronism
Infants 1–6 months	500–4500	↓ in AME and Liddle's syndrome	↑↑ in PHA
Infants 6–12 months	160–3000		
Children 1–4 years	70–1000		
Children 5–15 years	30–600		
Adults	30–420		
Plasma renin activity (ng/ml/h)† (supine for 30 min)			
Infants (<1 year)	<31	Suppressed	↑
Children 1–4 years	<26		
Children 5–15 years	<9		
Adults	<2.6		

*Aldosterone data obtained using Diagnostic Products Corporation Coat-A-Count Aldosterone Kit. †Plasma renin activity data obtained using BioChem ImmunoSystems Renin Maia Kit (Code 129640). Abbreviations: AME, apparent mineralocorticoid excess; PHA, pseudohypoaldosteronism.

- Striae
- Hypertension

Auxology
- Height below mid-parental centile.
- Height velocity subnormal
- Bone age usually delayed

The crucial difference between obesity, as a result of Cushing's syndrome/disease, and exogenous obesity is in the growth pattern. Cushing's syndrome/disease is almost always associated with a slower, and exogenous obesity with a faster, rate of linear growth. Appreciation of this difference in auxology will largely protect children with simple obesity from being investigated for Cushing's syndrome, although the occasional child with familial short stature and exogenous obesity may cause confusion. It is important not to subject children with simple obesity to investigation of Cushing's syndrome since serum and urine cortisol levels are often elevated in these subjects. Steroid biochemistry should also be interpreted with care in adolescent girls who may be on the oral contraceptive pill since this treatment increases CBG levels and hence plasma cortisol.

Investigations
Where exogenous steroid excess (by a steroid other than cortisol) is suspected, a low or undetectable 8.00 a.m.

plasma cortisol will usually confirm suppression of the pituitary–adrenal axis (Table 8.1) and a low-dose ACTH test is seldom necessary. If the features of Cushing's syndrome are accompanied by virilization, then an adrenal tumour is likely and an adrenal MRI (or CT) scan should be performed. If neither of the above applies and Cushing's syndrome or disease is seriously suspected, then careful evaluation is required.

Diagnosis of Cushing's syndrome or disease
The following sequence can be carried out in a non-specialist centre:
- Measurement of plasma cortisol levels at 8.00 a.m. and 4.00 p.m., looking for loss of the normal circadian rhythm.
- Measurement of plasma or salivary cortisol at midnight (value < 50 nmol/L).
- Measurement of plasma cortisol levels at 8.00 a.m. after taking dexamethasone 1 mg *per os* (orally) (p.o.) at 11.00 p.m. the night before (if cortisol < 50 nmol/L, Cushing's syndrome or disease is reasonably excluded). If the patient is very obese (> 100 kg), use 2 mg of dexamethasone.
- Measurement of three consecutive 24-hour urinary free cortisol estimations, looking for elevated cortisol excretion.

Aetiological diagnosis of hypercortisolism
This can be difficult. Referral to a specialist centre is recommended.

Table 8.3 Investigation of adrenal steroid precursors and androgens.

17-hydroxyprogesterone

Plasma (nmol/L) of plasma

Normal neonates	<13	
Stressed/preterm neonates	<40	
Neonates with CAH	>100	
Adults		
Basal	<13	
60 min after 250 μm i.v. Synacthen	<20	

Blood spot (nmol/L of blood)	**Extraction assay**	**Direct assay**
Stressed/preterm neonates	<70	<140
Neonates with CAH	>180	>350

Saliva (nmol/L of saliva)

Children 5–15 years 09.00 h	0.16–0.66 (median range 0.22–0.4)	

Androstenedione (mean ± SD)	Male	Female
Plasma (nmol/L)		
1–2 months	1.5 ± 0.45	0.66 ± 0.24
>6 months–adrenarche	<0.4	<0.4
Adult male	3.7 ± 0.9	
Adult female		
follicular phase		2.7 ± 1.0
luteal phase		5.2 ± 1.5
Saliva		
5–15 years 09.00 h	0.04–0.96 (median range 0.2–0.7)	

Testosterone (mean ± SD)	Male	Female
Plasma (nmol/L)		
First week	1.15 ± 0.15	0.45 ± 0.3
1–2 months	8.8 ± 2.7	0.28 ± 0.13
>6 months–prepubertal	<0.3	<0.3
Adult male	19.8 ± 4.7	
Adult female		
follicular phase		0.75 ± 0.2
luteal phase		1.28 ± 0.3

Dehydroepiandrosterone sulphate (μmol/L)	Male	Female
Infancy, pre-adrenarche	<2	<2
Adult	2–9	2–11

Blood spot 17-hydroxyprogesterone data are from A. M. Wallace *et al.* (1986). Salivary data are from Dr Schulga (see Table 8.1). Plasma androstenedione and testosterone data are from M. G. Forest (1993).

- *ACTH measurement at 8.00 a.m.:* Undetectable values suggest a primary adrenal lesion, detectable levels pituitary Cushing's and elevated levels ectopic ACTH syndrome (very rare in children).
- **High-dose dexamethasone suppression test**, measuring 9.00 a.m. plasma cortisol, then giving dexamethasone 2 mg at 9.00 a.m., 3.00 p.m., 9.00 p.m. and 3.00 a.m. × 2, i.e. eight doses over 48 hours, then re-measuring 9.00 a.m. plasma cortisol. A fall in cortisol to below more than 50% of the basal value is suggestive of pituitary Cushing's (Cushing's disease), while failure to suppress suggests a primary cause or ectopic ACTH syndrome.
- *CRH test:* Giving CRH 1 μg/kg intravenously after overnight fast and measuring cortisol and ACTH at −15, 0, 15, 30, 45, 60, 90 and 120 minutes. A rise in plasma cortisol to > 600 nmol/L suggests pituitary Cushing's, no rise in plasma cortisol and undetectable ACTH suggests a primary lesion, and no rise in cortisol with elevated ACTH suggests ectopic ACTH secretion.

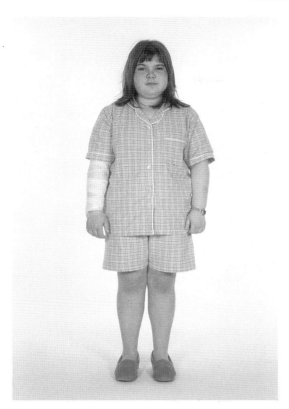

Fig. 8.4 A 10-year-old girl with Cushing's disease causing obesity and growth failure.

- According to the ACTH level, imaging of either adrenal (CT or MRI) or pituitary (high-resolution MRI) should be carried out.
- The final step in the investigation of Cushing's disease is bilateral inferior petrosal sinus sampling via femoral vein catheters. This technique, which should only be carried out in a specialist centre, is helpful in confirming that the ACTH secretion is of pituitary origin and not from an ectopic lesion. It may also identify on which side of the pituitary gland the adenoma is located.

Treatment

Iatrogenic Cushing's syndrome must be managed by withdrawal of the glucocorticoid preparation or, if this is not possible, by minimizing the dosage given, or converting to an alternate day regimen. If severe adrenal suppression has occurred, hydrocortisone replacement may be required for months, or even years, following treatment. Treatment of an adrenal or pituitary tumour is by surgical resec-

tion, followed by hydrocortisone replacement if the other adrenal gland is suppressed. After bilateral adrenalectomy, mineralocorticoids should be given as well.

Cushing's disease is treated by trans-sphenoidal surgical exploration with removal of the microadenoma. If none is identified, but petrosal sinus sampling has suggested lateralization of ACTH secretion, then a hemi-hypophysectomy can be carried out. A postoperative cortisol level of <50 nmol/L [<1.4 µg/dL] indicates that the adenoma has been completely removed and the patient is cured. The treatment of choice for Cushing's disease following failed pituitary exploration is direct pituitary irradiation. The alternative, bilateral adrenalectomy, carries a risk of pituitary tumour development with hyperpigmentation (Nelson's syndrome).

The ectopic ACTH syndrome may be seen as part of an established malignancy. Occasionally, small carcinoid lesions (e.g. lungs, pancreas) may be responsible, requiring location by CT scanning with selective venous sampling where necessary, and surgical removal.

Cushing's syndrome caused by bilateral micronodular dysplasia with or without primary pigmentation (Carney's syndrome), or the McCune–Albright syndrome, should be treated medically if features are mild to moderate, otherwise by bilateral adrenalectomy. When surgical resection is impossible (e.g. with infiltrating carcinoma), or in pituitary Cushing's disease when there may be a delay of several months before remission occurs (e.g. following radiotherapy), then medical therapy must be given. Useful agents include metyrapone and ketoconazole. In adrenal carcinoma, the adrenal cytotoxic o,p'-dichlorodiphenyl-dichloroethane (o,p'-DDD) (mitotane) is of temporary benefit.

Follow-up

After definitive treatment of Cushing's syndrome, patients should be seen 3-monthly to monitor growth rate, body composition and signs of recurrence.

Glucocorticoid deficiency

Adrenal insufficiency caused by hypothalamic–pituitary disease—secondary adrenal insufficiency (SAI)

Causes
The causes of SAI are as follows:
- Congenital:

- idiopathic congenital hypopituitarism;
- septo-optic dysplasia;
- other mid-line central nervous system (CNS) disorders; or
- isolated ACTH deficiency.
- *Acquired:*
  - craniopharyngioma;
  - cranial irradiation (e.g. for head and neck tumours);
  - surgery to hypothalamic–pituitary area;
  - steroid therapy; or
  - rare causes of hypopituitarism (e.g. vascular insult, trauma, meningitis).

Clinical features

ACTH deficiency is usually seen in association with several other anterior pituitary hormone deficiencies. Severe ACTH deficiency at birth causes hypoglycaemia, poor feeding, convulsions and jaundice. The jaundice is of the cholestatic type and resolves once hydrocortisone is started.

In older children, the symptoms of SAI are non-specific. Cortisol deficiency is responsible for tiredness and lack of energy, with increased susceptibility to and a longer recovery period from minor illnesses.

Investigations

In the newborn infant, dynamic studies are difficult to perform. If congenital hypopituitarism is strongly suspected (hypoglycaemia, jaundice, micropenis, low plasma thyroxine (T4) and random plasma cortisol levels less than 50 nmol/L [1.4 μg/dL]), then replacement should be instituted without delay. In more doubtful cases where the child is reasonably stable, 1 μg ACTH can be given intravenously and the cortisol response assessed at 30 minutes. Peak values of <550 nmol/L [<19 μg/dL] are suggestive of prenatal hypostimulation of the adrenal glands.

In children with suspected SAI, especially survivors of cancer, investigation depends on the severity of symptoms and the clinical context. Children who have received doses of >3000 cGy are particularly at risk. Cortisol secretion can be assessed by carrying out a low-dose ACTH test, or a salivary cortisol profile. An undetectable plasma dehydroepiandrosterone sulfate (DHEAS) level at an age when adrenarche should have occurred (> 8 years) is indirect evidence of at least partial ACTH deficiency.

Treatment

Hydrocortisone, 10 mg/m^2 per day should be given either in morning and evening or three times a day. Treatment during an intercurrent illness or during surgery is as for 21-hydroxylase deficiency (see below). Once the child is on glucocorticoid replacement, biochemical monitoring is not usually necessary.

Primary adrenal insufficiency

Causes

- *Congenital:*
  - Adrenal hypoplasia – X-linked (including **D**osage-sensitive sex reversal, **A**drenal hypoplasia critical region, on chromosome **X**, gene **1**(DAX-1 mutation)), or autosomal recessive
  - Congenital adrenal hyperplasia
  - Familial glucocorticoid deficiency (autosomal recessive)
- *Acquired:*
  - Isolated autoimmune adrenalitis (Addison's disease)
  - Adrenalitis associated with other autoimmune endocrinopathies
  - Adrenoleukodystrophy (ALD)
  - Tuberculosis
  - Bilateral adrenalectomy
  - Drugs (e.g. cyproterone)

Congenital adrenal hypoplasia

In the newborn period, cortisol deficiency will cause hypoglycaemia and jaundice, while aldosterone deficiency will result in hyponatraemia, hyperkalaemia, poor feeding, vomiting and failure to thrive. Investigations will show elevated renin and ACTH, but low or normal 17-OHP. Symptoms usually start from day 10 onwards. Boys with the DAX-1 mutation may have bilateral cryptorchidism in infancy and gonadotrophin deficiency in adolescence.

Familial glucocorticoid deficiency

Familial glucocorticoid deficiency (FGD, also known as 'hereditary unresponsiveness to ACTH') is an autosomal recessive disorder in which the adrenal cortex is unable to respond to ACTH. In about 25% of cases, a mutation on the ACTH receptor MC2-R can be identified. These children, who tend to be tall, are classified as having FGD type 1. FGD without an MC2-R mutation is termed FGD type 2. Recently, mutations in a new gene encoding a protein called melanocortin 2 receptor accessory protein (MRAP) have been identified in some cases of FGD type 2. It is thought that MRAP may play a role in the processing, trafficking or function of the MC2-R. In a number of children with FGD, the genetic mechanism is still unknown (FGD type 3).

FGD causes severe cortisol deficiency, presenting with jaundice, poor feeding, failure to thrive and hypoglycaemia in infancy. Older children may present with collapse and coma, sometimes with fatal consequences so that the diagnosis is only made post mortem. Investigations show elevated ACTH, low cortisol with poor or no response to ACTH and normal renin levels. Plasma potassium is usually normal but a degree of hyponatraemia may be present. This is attributable to cortisol deficiency causing impaired water secretion at the renal tubule.

Treatment

Congenital adrenal hypoplasia should be treated similarly to 21-hydroxylase deficiency (see below), although the dose of hydrocortisone used can be somewhat lower (as there is no need to suppress ACTH to prevent hyperandrogenism). FGD should be treated with hydrocortisone but not fludrocortisone or salt.

Acquired adrenal insufficiency

Causes

Autoimmune adrenalitis (Addison's disease) is the most common cause of acquired primary adrenal deficiency. Although seen in isolation, it may also be associated with other autoimmune disorders, such as diabetes mellitus and Hashimoto's thyroiditis, and with the polyglandular autoimmune (PGA) syndromes. PGA 1, also known as autoimmune polyendocrinopathy with endocrinopathy and cutaneous ectodermal dystrophy (APECED), is a generally recessive condition caused by mutations of the *AIRE* gene on chromosome 21 and has its onset in childhood and adolescence. Components of APECED syndrome include the following:

- *Endocrine disorders:*
  - Addison's disease;
  - hypoparathyroidism;
  - primary ovarian failure;
  - diabetes mellitus; and
  - hypophysitis.
- *Non-endocrine disorders:*
  - vitiligo;
  - alopaecia;
  - malabsorption;
  - hepatitis;
  - keratitis; and
  - immune deficiency – increased prevalence of infections, particularly mucocutaneous candidiasis.

ALD is an X-linked disorder affecting both the CNS and the adrenal cortex. Onset may be in childhood or early adulthood. The phenotype is highly variable,

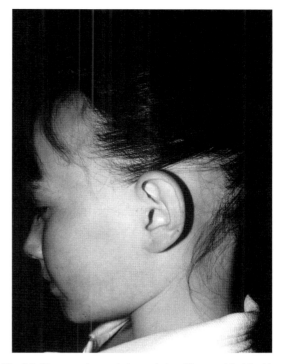

Fig. 8.5 Pigmentation and alopaecia in a 10 year-old-girl with nail dystrophy caused by *Candida*. Investigations showed both Addison's disease and hypoparathyroidism. Genetic studies showed a homozygous 13-bp deletion in exon 8 of the autoimmune regulator gene on chromosome 21q22.3.

even within families, so that the presence and severity of neurological impairment and adrenal failure varies from case to case. Severely affected individuals suffer progressive neurological disability, and ultimately death. The neurological symptoms may precede those of adrenal insufficiency, or vice versa. Therefore, all males presenting with primary adrenal insufficiency other than CAH must be investigated for ALD.

Clinical features of primary adrenal insufficiency

Symptoms include tiredness, weight loss, polyuria, increasing pigmentation (Figure 8.5) and, in the final stages, vomiting, drowsiness and coma. Examination shows increased pigmentation, especially in the skin creases, old scars and buccal mucosa, with signs of recent weight loss, and low or normal blood pressure.

Investigations

ACTH is elevated (often >1000 mU/L) and plasma renin activity is high. Fasting glucose is normal or low. Basal

Table 8.4 Dosage schedules for mineralocorticoid, glucocorticoid and salt therapy in adrenal disorders.

Disorder	Mineralocorticoid	Glucocorticoid	Salt
Hypothalamo–pituitary-adrenal insufficiency	Not required	Hydrocortisone 8–10 mg/m^2/day	
Primary adrenal insufficiency (Addison's disease)	Fludrocortisone 100 μg/day from birth to adolescence, then 150 μg/day	Hydrocortisone 10–12 mg/m^2/day	
Congenital adrenal hypoplasia	As for primary adrenal insufficiency	For first 6 months consider treatments as for CAH. (see pp. 140–1), then hydrocortisone 10–12 mg/m^2/day	
FGD	Not required	As for Primary adrenal insufficiency (Addison's disease)	
CAH (21-hydroxylase deficiency)			
Salt-wasting	Fludrocortisone 100 μg/day from birth or 150 μg/m^2/day, whichever is greater	For first 6 months of life see pp. 140–1 Oral hydrocortisone 10–15 mg/m^2/day thereafter. Prednisolone 3–5 mg/m^2/day in late pubertal girls	5 mmol/L/kg/day in three divided doses for first year
Simple virilizing	As above if plasma renin activity ↑ at diagnosis	As above	Not required
Pseudohypoaldosteronism	Not usually effective		Sodium chloride 10–40 mmol/kg/day + calcium resonium

Abbreviations: ACTH, adrenocorticotrophic hormone; CAH, congenital adrenal hyperplasia; FGD, familial glucocorticoid deficiency.

cortisol is low or normal with no rise following ACTH administration. In acute adrenal insufficiency, sodium is low, potassium is high and there may be severe hypoglycaemia. In ALD, the diagnosis is established by measuring very long chain fatty acids (VLCFA) in plasma. Given the association between Addison's disease, other endocrinopathies and ALD, the following further investigations are recommended:

• VLCFA in males
• Autoantibody screen (adrenal, thyroid, islet cell, parietal cell)
• Calcium and phosphate
• Thyroid function
• Full blood count (FBC), vitamin B$_{12}$ and folate
• Liver function tests

Thyroid function, FBC, calcium and phosphate and liver function tests should be repeated annually to detect the development of other autoimmune diseases.

Treatment

Acute adrenal insufficiency is managed by intravenous (IV) fluids with 0.9% saline and added 5% glucose, IV hydrocortisone (see p. 167) and conversion to oral hydrocortisone and fludrocortisone once recovery has occurred (Table 8.4).

Follow-up

Once a patient is on established treatment with hydrocortisone and fludrocortisone, clinical monitoring and adjusting the dosage as body surface area increases is usually sufficient and there is no need for laboratory investigations.

Mineralocorticoid excess

Apart from the secondary hyperaldosteronism seen in cardiac and renal patients and in chronic volume depletion (leading to activation of the renin–angiotensin system), mineralocorticoid excess is very rare.

Causes

- Secondary hyperaldosteronism.
- *Iatrogenic:*
  - fludrocortisone overdosage; and
  - carbenoxolone therapy or liquorice ingestion.
- Aldosterone-secreting adrenal adenoma/hyperplasia (Conn's syndrome).
- *Enzyme gene mutations:*
  - CYP 11B1 (11-hydroxylase) deficiency;
  - CYP 17 (17-hydroxylase) deficiency;
  - 11-βHSD 2 deficiency; and
  - CYP 11B2 mutation.
- Activating mutation of amiloride-sensitive epithelial sodium channel (Liddle's syndrome).

Secondary hyperaldosteronism does not normally present to the endocrinologist. Fludrocortisone overdosage may result in hypertension with or without hypokalaemia. Carbenoxolone is rarely used, but liquorice addiction can cause the syndrome of apparent mineralocorticoid excess (AME), brought about by 11-βHSD 2 inhibition (see below). Aldosterone-secreting adrenal adenomas are rare in childhood, and other causes of hyperaldosteronism must be ruled out before invasive procedures, such as selective adrenal vein sampling, are performed.

Two of the enzyme disorders causing CAH, CYP 11B1 (11-hydroxylase) and CYP 17 (17-hydroxylase) deficiencies, cause hypertension with hypokalaemia. 11-hydroxylase deficiency causes virilization in girls and sexual precocity in boys from infancy, but affected children are hypertensive because of the high levels of DOC, rather than salt-losing as in 21-hydroxylase deficiency. 17-hydroxylase deficiency causes cortisol and androgen deficiency but mineralocorticoid excess, so that affected 46,XY individuals are phenotypically female and may present with pubertal failure in association with hypertension and hypokalaemia. Deficiency of the enzyme 11-βHSD 2 results in failure to metabolize cortisol to cortisone, with consequent occupation of mineralocorticoid receptors by cortisol (Figure 8.3). The clinical features are those of mineralocorticoid excess but aldosterone levels are suppressed, hence the term **apparent** mineralocorticoid excess (AME).

Mutations of the *CYP 11B2* gene may lead to a chimeric enzyme which is under ACTH control, resulting in glucocorticoid-suppressible hyperaldosteronism. This condition should be suspected in the hypertensive adolescent, with or without hypokalaemia, in whom there is a family history of hypertension and cerebral haemorrhage. Treatment is with dexamethasone or amiloride.

Liddle's syndrome is autosomal dominant and caused by an activating mutation of the ENaC, leading to increased sodium absorption with aldosterone and renin suppression. Treatment is with amiloride.

Mineralocorticoid deficiency

Causes

Aldosterone deficiency
- Congenital adrenal hypoplasia.
- Addison's disease.
- *Enzyme disorders:*
  - StAR protein deficiency;
  - 3-βHSD deficiency;
  - CYP 21 (21-hydroxylase) deficiency; or
  - CYP 11B2 (aldosterone synthase) deficiency.

Aldosterone resistance (pseudohypoaldosteronism)
- Autosomal dominant or sporadic – affects renal tubule.
- Recessive – affects kidneys, colon, and sweat and salivary glands.

Clinical features and investigation

Mineralocorticoid deficiency causes salt-wasting with polyuria, vomiting, dehydration and hyperkalaemia which, if severe and untreated, leads to cardiac arrest. In older children, the salt-wasting tendency is partially offset by an instinctive increase in salt intake. Congenital adrenal hypoplasia and Addison's disease are discussed above; the three types of CAH causing salt-wasting are discussed below.

Pseudohypoaldosteronism may be associated with salt-wasting and dangerous hyperkalaemia in the newborn period. Affected infants do not respond to large doses of fludrocortisone, and treatment consists of generous sodium replacement (Table 8.4) and resins to combat hyperkalaemia. The dominant and sporadic forms are milder and resolve with age. The autosomal recessive variety, caused by inactivating mutations in the ENaC, is severe and runs a protracted course.

Sex steroid excess

Androgen excess

Adrenal causes of androgen excess
- Exaggerated adrenarche
- Adrenocortical adenoma and carcinoma
- *Congenital adrenal hyperplasia:*
  - CYP 21 (21-hydroxylase) deficiency and CYP 11β1 (11-hydroxylase) deficiency
  - 3-βHSD deficiency in females
  - 11-βHSD 1 deficiency

The most common cause of mild androgenicity, observed most often in girls, is an exaggerated form of the adrenal puberty (adrenarche) that occurs between the ages of 6 and 8 years (see Chapter 5). However, signs of severe androgenicity — with clitoral or phallic enlargement — in girls or prepubertal boys suggest an androgen-secreting tumour or an enzyme defect.

Adrenocortical tumour

Clinical features
Significant androgenic features develop over a period of weeks or months in a child of previously normal stature. In boys, the testes are prepubertal (Figure 8.6). Height status, growth rate and bone age may be increased or normal, depending on the duration of the illness.

Investigations
These show a marked elevation of one or more of the adrenal androgens, androstenedione and dehydroepiandrosterone-sulfate (DHEAS). Ultrasound, followed by CT or MRI scanning, should be obtained without delay.

Treatment
Treatment is by surgical removal wherever possible. If the tumour is well circumscribed and <5 cm in diameter, the prognosis is good. Pathological features are usually not helpful in predicting the risk of recurrence or of metastases.

Adrenal enzyme defects

21-hydroxylase deficiency is by far the most common adrenal enzyme disorder and will be discussed in detail. 11- and 17-hydroxylase deficiencies are discussed above (see p. 163). 3-βHSD deficiency in females causes mild

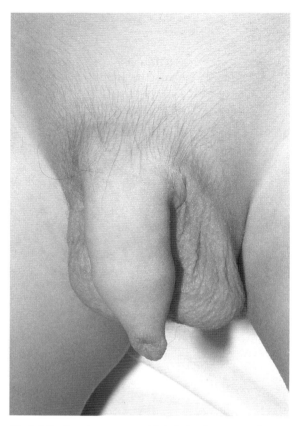

Fig. 8.6 Penile enlargement, pubic hair development and scrotal laxity with prepubertal (2 mL) testes in a 2-year-old boy. Investigation showed a small tumour in the right adrenal cortex.

postnatal androgenization because of high DHEAS levels. A relatively newly discovered cause of congenital adrenal hyperplasia, associated with a spectrum of bone abnormalities called the Antley–Bixler syndrome, is due to inactivating mutations in the gene encoding P450 oxidoreductase, the electron donor for 21- and 17-hydroxylases and for aromatase; this condition may be more common than previously thought, especially in Japan. The very rare 11-βHSD 1 deficiency has been reported as causing virilization in adult females because of cortisol deficiency and increased ACTH drive.

21-hydroxylase deficiency

Incidence
The incidence varies from 1 in 2500 births in Yupik Eskimos to 1 in 30,000 in some countries; the overall

incidence (including the United Kingdom) is approximately 1 in 15,000 births.

Pathogenesis and classification

21-hydroxylase deficiency results from mutations in the *CYP21B* gene, which is situated on chromosome 6. The phenotype of 21-hydroxylase deficiency correlates reasonably well with the following genotype:
• Salt-wasting 21-hydroxylase deficiency (SW 21-OHD) results from a child inheriting two severe mutations, leading to complete or near-complete loss of 21-B function, with <1% of normal 21-hydroxylase activity.
• Simple virilizing 21-hydroxylase deficiency (SV 21-OHD) occurs if one of the two mutations (e.g. point mutation Ile172Asn) is relatively mild with 1–5% preservation of 21-hydroxylase activity. Significant salt loss does not occur, although plasma renin activity is often elevated.
• Non-classical or late onset 21-hydroxylase deficiency (NC 21-OHD) results if one mutation is mild (e.g. Val 281Leu). The condition is seen in females from adolescence onwards and causes androgenicity with or without the polycystic ovary syndrome.

Clinical features

SW 21-OHD in females presents with virilization at birth. The clitoris is enlarged and there generally is posterior fusion of the labia majora (Figure 8.7). The vagina and urethra usually enter a common urogenital sinus, with the distal end of the vagina becoming increasingly more distant from the pelvic floor with the severity of virilization. Virilization can be graded in severity according to the Prader classification (Figure 8.8).

Males with SW 21-OHD usually present in the second week of life, with a salt-losing crisis heralded by poor feeding, vomiting, poor weight gain and listlessness. Examination shows dehydration with pigmentation of the scrotum. Biochemistry reveals hyponatraemia, hyperkalaemia and, occasionally, hypoglycaemia. Death may occur before the diagnosis is considered. For this reason, neonatal screening for SW 21-OHD is being implemented in an increasing number of countries. However, this is not yet universal because the positive predictive value of a high 17-OHP is very low, especially in premature or stressed neonates.

Boys with SV 21-OHD, and girls with SV 21-OHD in whom virilization at birth has been mild and/or missed, will present later in childhood (usually 2–4 years) with signs of androgen excess – enlarged penis or clitoris, pubic hair, greasy skin, long-standing growth acceleration and advanced bone age. Both girls and boys with SV 21-OHD tend to develop true puberty early because of the early

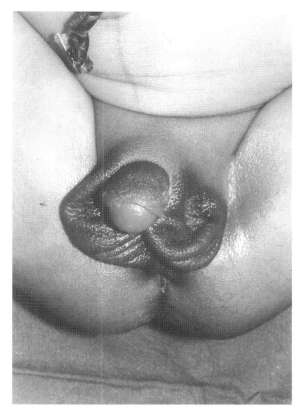

Fig. 8.7 Severe virilization with fusion and scrotalization of labia majora and gross clitoral enlargement in female infant with 21-hydroxylase deficiency.

exposure of the hypothalamic–pituitary axis to sex hormones ('priming'). The combination of advanced bone age because of androgen excess, compounded by true puberty, leads to premature closure of the epiphyses and an adult height below the mid-parental centile.

NC 21-OHD is a rare cause of hyperandrogenism in adolescent and adult females and should be considered in the differential diagnosis of the polycystic ovary syndrome.

Diagnosis

SW 21-OHD is diagnosed in females with ambiguous genitalia, no palpable gonads, hyperpigmentation of the labia majora and a uterus on ultrasound, and in boys with a salt-wasting crisis. Biochemical confirmation is based on high plasma androgens and 17-OHP (values usually >100 nmol/L [>3300 ng/dL]).

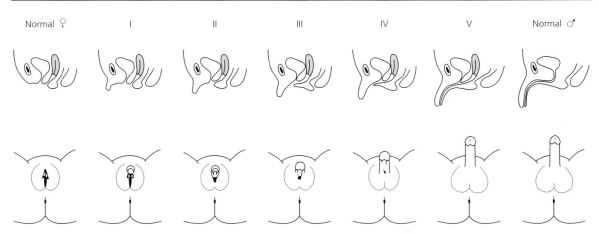

Fig. 8.8 Prader classification of five stages of virilization in the female infant.

In SV and NC 21-OHD, 17-OHP elevation is milder. Levels are best measured between 8.00 a.m. and 9.00 a.m. to capture the morning 17-OHP peak. ACTH stimulation will demonstrate raised levels of 17-OHP. In this context, the standard dose of ACTH is used (250 μg), 17-OHP is measured at 0 and 60 minutes and the values compared to the nomogram published by New *et al.* in 1983.

Prenatal management

After the birth of a child affected with 21-OHD, the genotype of parents, affected child and healthy siblings can be determined. In future pregnancies, chorionic villus sampling at 9–10 weeks' gestation or amniocentesis at 14–16 weeks enables the sex and genotype of the foetus to be determined.

The main purpose of prenatal testing is to assist with maternal dexamethasone treatment. Pre-pregnancy counselling as to the pros and cons of this intervention is important. If prenatal treatment is to be given, it should be started at a dosage of 20 μg/kg per day as early as possible (preferably by 4–6 weeks' gestation). This high dose is required to suppress embryonic/foetal ACTH secretion and should be continued throughout pregnancy if the foetus is an affected female, but stopped if the foetus is male or an unaffected female. In some centres, examination of maternal venous blood for male foetal cells by *in situ* hybridization techniques can be performed as soon as pregnancy is confirmed so that dexamethasone treatment can be stopped immediately if the foetus is male. The demonstrated benefit of reducing or preventing virilization in girls must be offset against the unknown long-term effects of prenatal dexamethasone treatment on the

exposed children and, to a lesser extent, the side effects of hypertension, weight gain, striae and mood changes in the mother. Prenatal treatment for 21-OHD should only be undertaken according to a strictly audited national protocol.

Neonatal management

Diagnosis and management of 21-OHD in newborn females is part of disorder of sex development (DSD) management (see Chapter 7). The following protocol is recommended:

1 Inform parents that there is doubt as to the gender of the child but that steps will be taken to make the decision within 4 days if at all possible.

2 Urgent polymerase chain reaction (PCR) analysis for sex determining region of the Y chromosome (SRY) sequences, fluorescent *in situ* hybridization (FISH) analysis for SRY and standard karyotyping.

3 Pelvic ultrasound to document the presence of a uterus.

4 Surgical evaluation.

5 Plasma electrolyte and glucose measurement.

6 2 mL heparinized blood for 17-OHP, ideally obtaining result on the same day.

N.B.: Normal newborns may have high 17-OHP levels before 72 hours of age, so that blood should only be taken on the third day. Plasma androgens should also be measured.

Once the diagnosis has been confirmed, treatment must be started immediately with the following protocol:

1 Fludrocortisone 0.05 to 0.100 mg per day.

2 Sodium chloride 5 mmol/kg per day in three divided doses given as either 6% (1 mmol/mL), 15%

(2.5 mmol/mL), or 30% (5 mmol/mL) solution. The solution may be added to milk feeds or given separately (e.g. if mother is breast-feeding).

3 Hydrocortisone 20 mg/m^2 per day in three divided doses.

In males presenting with a salt-losing crisis and in missed/incorrectly assigned females, the following is recommended:

1 Measurement of electrolytes, glucose and 17-OHP.

2 Give 10–30 mL/kg of 0.9% saline over 1–3 hours depending on the degree of dehydration, then 0.9% saline at a rate sufficient to provide maintenance, and correct any deficit over 24 hours. Add potassium when plasma potassium <4 mmol/L and give 10% dextrose 2–4 mL/kg if capillary glucose < 3 mmol/L.

3 Hydrocortisone 25 mg intravenously immediately and 12.5 mg subsequently 6 hourly until enteral administration can be started.

4 When plasma sodium is normal and the infant is stable, start fludrocortisone, sodium chloride and hydrocortisone as above.

Management in infancy

Glucocorticoid therapy

Treatment consists of oral hydrocortisone, approximately 15 mg/m^2 per day in three divided doses. Suspensions are unreliable and 10 mg hydrocortisone tablets should be given halved or quartered, asking the pharmacy to prepare sachets if smaller doses are needed.

Fludrocortisone therapy

Fludrocortisone 0.05 to 0.100 mg per day, provided that this is not associated with hypertension.

Salt therapy

The dosage of 5 mmol/kg per day should be maintained for the first 12 months of life and is usually discontinued at, or shortly before, the first birthday.

Education and surveillance

A great deal of time must be invested in counselling the parents at diagnosis. Parent information leaflets are very useful. Contact with a family with an affected child of similar sex can also be very helpful. Management of acute illness should be carefully discussed, and the parents instructed in capillary glucose measurement as well as in the giving of intramuscular hydrocortisone in emergency. Detection of hypoglycaemia is important, because it is now recognized that the adrenal medullary output

Table 8.5 Preoperative and emergency intramuscular (I.M.), bolus, and infusion rate for hydrocortisone dosage (mg) according to body weight and age in months (m) and years (yr) in infants and children with adrenal insufficiency including congenital adrenal hyperplasia.

Age	Weight (kg)	I.M. dose	bolus dose	mg/hr
				Subsequent 6-hrly infusion rate
<6 m	3–7	12.5	6.25	0.5
6 m–5 yr	7–20	25	12.5	1
5–10 yr	20–30	50	25	2
10 yr	30	100	50	3

12.5 mg for infants up to 6 months, 25 mg from 6 months to 5 years, 50 mg from 5 to 10 years, and 100 mg thereafter

of epinephrine is adversely affected in cortisol deficiency leading to impaired gluconeogenesis and hepatic glucose output (Weise *et al.* 2004).

The infant should be reviewed weekly until the parents are comfortable with management, thereafter 1- to 3-monthly during infancy. Weight and length are measured on each occasion with blood pressure, plasma steroids and renin at least 3-monthly. Routine measurement of electrolytes is not indicated if the child is thriving.

Management of acute illness (see Table 8.5)

Infancy is a prime time for acute illness, including gastroenteritis. The key to successful management is correct parental instruction facilitated by provision of a CAH therapy card (similar to the asthma card). A CAH therapy card is shown in Appendix 2. In North America, it is common practice to prescribe a Medic-Alert® bracelet to all patients who are glucocorticoid-dependent. If the following procedure is followed, children with CAH rarely need admission to hospital and duration of hospital stay will be minimized:

1 If the child has an intercurrent illness but is well, feeding and playing normally, and is not febrile, then no change in dosage is required.

2 If the child is unwell with fever, reduced activity, etc., then the oral total daily dosage of hydrocortisone is doubled and given in three divided doses.

3 If the child is particularly unwell, especially if there is vomiting, drowsiness or diarrhoea – in which case oral hydrocortisone will not be reliably absorbed – give hydrocortisone intramuscularly in a dose of 12.5 mg for infants up to 6 months, 25 mg from 6 months to 5 years, 50 mg from 5 to 10 years, and 100 mg thereafter (see Table 8.5). If the parents are unable or unwilling to give intramuscular hydrocortisone, then the child should be taken to hospital immediately.

4 If the child does not respond to the intramuscular injection, parents should bring the child immediately to hospital. Under these circumstances:

- Take blood for glucose (for bedside and laboratory assays), electrolytes and FBC.
- Give a bolus of glucose if glucose <3 mmol/L (54 mg/dL) as with neonatal management.
- Give hydrocortisone intravenously if not given intramuscularly by parents (dosage as above).
- Give 10–30 mL/kg 0.9% saline over 1–3 hours depending on the degree of dehydration, followed by 0.9% saline and 5% dextrose to provide maintenance and correct any deficit. Add potassium as indicated by electrolytes.
- Give hydrocortisone injections 6 hourly (dosage given in Table 8.5) until the child is able to tolerate oral medications. An alternative is to give the hydrocortisone in the form of a 50 mg/50 mL 0.9% saline (1 mg/mL) solution as an infusion at 0.5, 1, 2 or 3 mL/h depending on the child's age and weight (see Table 8.5).

Genital surgery

Current practice is to perform clitoral recession by excising the shaft, carefully preserving the neurovascular supply to the tip. Surgery is usually between 6 and 12 months of age. Vaginoplasty may be performed at the same time but there is an argument in favour of leaving this procedure until much later in childhood to prevent stenosis (see Chapter 7).

Medical management of children undergoing surgery

On the day of surgery, hydrocortisone should be given intravenously at the doses stated in Table 8.5 as soon as an IV line is established. Thereafter, half of this initial dose should be given 6 hourly or a hydrocortisone infusion given until the child is able to tolerate oral medications (see Table 8.5). This high dose hydrocortisone treatment also covers the mineralocorticoid needs of these patients.

Management of linear growth

Chronic treatment consists of daily or twice daily fludrocortisone therapy to replace aldosterone, and twice or thrice daily hydrocortisone to suppress ACTH secre-

tion and thus prevent virilization. The limitation of this approach is that the glucocorticoid regimen fails to mimic normal cortisol secretion. Moreover, even if ACTH secretion is normalized, the presence of the enzyme block will still cause androgen excess. Therefore, to achieve satisfactory adrenal suppression, a slightly supraphysiological dose of glucocorticoid is needed. Conversely, insufficient glucocorticoid dosage will result in androgen excess, early epiphyseal fusion and decreased adult height.

It is also evident that frankly excessive glucocorticoid administration will result in Cushingoid features, obesity and slow growth with decreased adult height. What is less obvious is that lesser degrees of glucocorticoid overdosage will cause hyperphagia resulting in obesity with normal or increased height velocity and advancing bone age, tempting the clinician to make a further increase in hydrocortisone dosage.

With these considerations in mind, the clinician needs to make a careful judgment as to the optimal glucocorticoid dose, taking the clinical assessment, height velocity, bone age and biochemical profile into account, and being mindful that compliance problems are common, especially during adolescence.

Hydrocortisone – 10–15 mg/m^2 per day – is usually given in two to three doses, titrating the dosage so that the height velocity is 4–7 cm per year. The manner in which the daily glucocorticoid dose should be administered is controversial. Some favour giving a thrice-daily dose, equally divided, in pre-school children, then a twice-daily dose from school age (when compliance with a thrice-daily regime becomes problematic), giving a third of the dose in the morning and two-third in the evening (to suppress the morning 17-OHP surge). Fludrocortisone should be given at 0.150 mg/m^2 per day to bring plasma renin into the reference range.

At clinic visits (no less than every 6 months), the following should be done:

- Measurement of height, weight, height velocity and body mass index (BMI) and (in older children) pubertal stage.
- Examination for features of over-treatment (Cushing's syndrome) and under-treatment (including pigmentation and signs of androgen excess).
- Measurement of blood pressure (to monitor fludrocortisone dosage).
- Bone age should be evaluated yearly.
- Most practitioners also measure plasma 17-OHP, androgens and renin activity biannually; this should ideally be done in the morning before taking the tablets. Some centres also measure 17-OHP and androstenedione

on capillary samples taken by the patient throughout the day. Normalization of 17-OHP and androstenedione may reflect over-treatment with glucocorticoid and suppression of renin may reflect over-treatment with mineralocorticoid. However, there is great individual variation in biochemical profiles, and surveillance is based primarily on clinical parameters (growth in height and weight, bone age, pubertal progression and blood pressure).

Morbidity

The sources of morbidity for parents and individuals with CAH are as follows:

A. *Parents:*

    1 Shock of initial diagnosis.

    2 In female infants, distress at the genital anomaly and uncertainty about gender at birth.

    3 Anxiety over genital surgery and sequellae.

B. *Patients:*

    1 Acute illness.

    2 Learning disability in some salt-wasting patients.

    3 *Growth:*
- poor growth 0–2 years;
- overgrowth 2–10 years;
- early puberty;
- decreased adult height; and
- obesity.

    4 *Urogenital problems:*
- urinary tract infection;
- incontinence; and
- vaginal stenosis (haematocolpos, difficulty with tampon insertion and later with sexual intercourse).

    5 *Psychosexual:*
- self-esteem/confidence;
- sexual activity;
- sexual orientation; and
- fertility.

The principal causes of morbidity are the complications of surgery in girls, and of obesity in both sexes, particularly girls. Possible future strategies to minimize these problems include the use of prenatal dexamethasone, bilateral adrenalectomy during infancy in those with SW 21-OHD associated with severe genotype, and ther-

apy with anti-androgens and aromatase inhibitors, such as testolactone and anastrozole. However, none of these therapeutic options have become standard, despite having been under discussion for some years.

Oestrogen excess

Feminizing adrenal adenomas are exceedingly rare, but difficult to diagnose in that they mimic true precocious puberty in girls. The clue that the source of sexual precocity lies outside the hypothalamic–pituitary axis is the luteinizing hormone-releasing hormone (LHRH) test which shows suppression of luteinizing hormone (LH) and follicle stimulating hormone (FSH) levels.

Sex steroid deficiency

Adrenal androgen deficiency

Causes
- Adrenal hypoplasia.
- *Enzyme disorders:*
  - StAR protein deficiency;
  - 3-βHSD deficiency;
  - 17-hydroxylase deficiency;
  - 17,20-desmolase deficiency;
  - 17-βHSD deficiency.

The androgen deficiency in boys with adrenal hypoplasia is insignificant because gonadal androgen synthesis is intact. However, severe enzyme deficiency affecting both adrenal and gonadal androgen synthesis results in undermasculinization with complete sex reversal in the more severe cases, and ambiguous genitalia in less severe cases. Management is discussed in Chapter 7.

Oestrogen deficiency

Oestrogens are responsible for closure of the epiphyses at adolescence. Gene mutations inactivating the aromatase enzyme and the oestrogen receptor are associated with tall stature.

Adrenal medullary disorder

Phaeochromocytoma

Phaeochromocytoma is a chromaffin cell tumour which usually occurs as a single adrenal tumour, but can be bilateral or extra-adrenal. It may be seen in isolation, either as a familial or sporadic disorder. Phaeochromocytoma may also occur in association with neurofibromatosis type 1 as part of the multiple endocrine neoplasia (MEN) syndromes: MEN type 2A (hyperparathyroidism, phaeochromocytoma, medullary thyroid carcinoma), MEN type 2B (phaeochromocytoma, medullary thyroid carcinoma, and tongue neuromas) and in von Hippel–Lindau syndrome, all of which are dominant in inheritance.

Although extremely uncommon in childhood, phaeochromocytoma is an important cause of hypertension. It is suggested by the combination of episodic pallor, sweating and headaches, with either sustained hypertension or raised blood pressure during a symptomatic episode. The diagnosis is made by examining urine catecholamine metabolites in children with hypertension and in children with symptoms suggestive of a phaeochromocytoma, even in the absence of hypertension.

Neuroblastoma

Neuroblastoma usually presents to the general paediatrician or oncologist. The diagnosis is suggested by hypertension in the context of malaise, sweating, pallor and an abdominal mass. There is an increase in catecholamine metabolites in the urine.

Future developments

• The molecular genetic basis for rare adrenal disorders is becoming more clear as progress continues in the field.
• Conventional therapy for 21-hydroxylase deficiency may be overtaken by new strategies to reduce adrenal androgen production.
• Multicentre studies are needed in order to evaluate optimal surgical approach to female masculinization.
• The potential long-term risks of prenatal dexamethasone will be demonstrated or disproved through long-term surveillance of all exposed children.

Potential pitfalls

• Gender mis-assignment as male of a fully masculinized female infant affected by 21-hydroxylase deficiency.
• Incorrect diagnosis of salt-losing crisis in a male with hyponatraemia, caused by obstructive uropathy from urethral valves (elevation of 17-hydroxyprogesterone may occur in this situation because of acute stress, but androgens will be normal).
• Incorrect diagnosis of congenital adrenal hyperplasia in child with adrenal tumour.

• Non-specific symptoms, such as vomiting and hypoglycaemia, in a patient with one endocrine disorder (such as diabetes) should alert the clinician to the possibility of a different endocrine problem (such as Addison's disease).

Controversial points

• Should pituitary surgery for Cushing's disease be performed in one or two designated national centres?
• What is the optimal treatment regimen for infants with 21-hydroxylase deficiency?
• Is antenatal dexamethasone given to prevent virilization in foetuses at risk of 21-hydroxylase deficiency standard of care or investigational?

When to involve a specialist centre

• When Cushing's syndrome is either seriously suspected or confirmed.
• Endogenous primary and secondary adrenal insufficiency states.
• Conditions causing mineralocorticoid excess.
• Congenital adrenal hyperplasia.
   N.B.: Involvement of a specialist centre does not preclude a shared care arrangement.

Transition

• The care of adolescents and young adults with congenital adrenal hyperplasia is greatly facilitated by their being seen jointly by their paediatrician and an adult physician in a transition clinic setting. While a single visit may suffice, some patients benefit from being seen several times in the transition clinic prior to adult transfer.
• Adolescent females with genitourinary problems related to CAH and its surgery may need joint assessment, sometimes involving joint examination under anaesthesia by a paediatric surgeon, plastic surgeon and gynaecologist with an interest in feminizing genitoplasty.

Emergency management

Correct emergency management depends on: (1) recognizing adrenal insufficiency in an acute situation; and (2) giving appropriate glucocorticoid, glucose, electrolyte and fluid treatment to known or suspected cases.

Recognizing adrenal insufficiency

The cardinal symptoms include vomiting, diarrhoea (often mistakenly thought to be infectious in nature) and altered consciousness, and with/without a background history of poor feeding, poor weight gain/weight loss.

Signs of adrenal insufficiency include dehydration, shock, hyperpigmentation (in primary adrenal insufficiency) and genital anomaly (in genetic females with 21-hydroxylase deficiency).

Investigation suggesting adrenal insufficiency includes hypoglycaemia, hyponatraemia (due to salt-wasting from aldosterone deficiency, and with/without water retention due to cortisol deficiency), hyperkalaemia and acidosis.

In the newborn, adrenal insufficiency causes hypoglycaemia, prolonged jaundice and, sometimes, a neonatal hepatitis-like syndrome with conjugated bilirubinaemia and raised liver transaminases. There may be associated features such as roving nystagmus (in septo-optic dysplasia) and low T4 with low/normal thyroid stimulating hormone (TSH) in hypopituitary states.

It is particularly important to consider adrenal insufficiency in a newborn infant with unexpected hypoglycaemia, for example when neither the gestation nor birth weight explains this problem, and especially if there is concurrent jaundice.

Appropriate management of adrenal insufficiency (see Table 8.1)

Hospital admission is almost always required in a patient with known adrenal insufficiency who develops vomiting. Such patients should always be seen at the hospital, and only allowed to leave the emergency department after a senior member of staff has been consulted.

- Families should be encouraged to show their adrenal insufficiency or CAH card to the emergency staff.
- Capillary glucose and vital signs should be recorded on arrival by the nursing staff. After the medical history and examination has been completed, a cannula should be inserted and blood taken for glucose, electrolytes and (if intercurrent infection is a possibility) FBC and inflammatory markers. Blood, urine and stool cultures may also be indicated.
- A bolus injection of hydrocortisone should be given (unless intramuscular injection has already been given recently), and fluid management should be as set out in the section on emergency management of 21-hydroxylase. Hydrocortisone may be given either as 6-hourly injections or as a continuous infusion (see Table 8.5).
- Before discharge, the glucocorticoid and mineralocorticoid dosages, together with the family situation regarding education and compliance, should be reviewed.

Case histories

Case 8.1

A 4-year-old boy with known asthma is admitted acutely with a convulsion, and is found to be hypoglycaemic (blood glucose 0.8 mmol/L [14 mg/dL]). For the past year his asthma has been well controlled on fluticasone propionate 500 µg twice daily, but recently he has been lethargic and has had more than his fair share of intercurrent illnesses. On examination (after glucose administration), his consciousness level is normal. He looks slightly Cushingoid with some increase in body hair, especially over the back. Height is on the 3rd centile (mid-parental height 25th centile), weight on the 50th centile, and blood pressure is 120/50. Random plasma cortisol <24 nmol/L [<1 mg/dL].

Question

How can this boy's Cushingoid features be reconciled with his gross adrenal impairment?

Answer

This boy has an iatrogenic combination of Cushing's syndrome (causing the facial appearance, increase in body hair, a degree of growth failure and an increased tendency to infections), together with adrenal suppression (lethargy, hypoglycaemia). He is receiving over twice the licensed paediatric dose of fluticasone (400 µg daily). He will require hydrocortisone replacement while the respiratory team modifies his therapy, and his adrenal status should be re-evaluated if and when the dose of inhaled steroid is reduced.

Case 8.2

Four hours after delivery at 41 weeks' gestation with birth weight 3740 g, a baby boy becomes dusky while breastfeeding. True blood glucose is 1.1 mmol/L [<20 mg/dL]. On examination, the baby is noted to have a very small penis. He is started on a glucose infusion. Plasma cortisol is < 30 nmol/L and LH and FSH are unmeasurable (<0.5 units/L).

Question

What is the diagnosis, and what other system should be examined in detail?

Answer
This baby has hypopituitarism with complete gonadotrophin deficiency leading to micropenis and ACTH deficiency resulting in hypoglycaemia. Associated central hypothyroidism is documented by a very low plasma free T4 level (2.9 pmol/L), contrasting with an inappropriately normal plasma TSH (3.5 mU/L). On day 6, the baby is seen by an ophthalmologist who confirms that the optic discs are small with a 'double ring' sign, consistent with a diagnosis of septo-optic dysplasia.

Case 8.3
A 14-year-old boy is found to be hypertensive (blood pressure 170/130) when he consults his family practitioner with headache. Investigations show normal electrolytes and renal imaging, but plasma aldosterone is elevated at 990 pmol/L [36 ng/dL] and renin completely suppressed. There is a family history of hypertension, with maternal uncle and grandmother dying young of stroke and the mother being hypertensive during pregnancy.

Question
What diagnostic possibilities should be considered and what further investigations should be performed?

Answer
The family history of hypertension in a boy with high aldosterone levels strongly suggests glucocorticoid-suppressible hyperaldosteronism. Molecular genetic studies confirmed a chimeric *CYP 11B1/2* gene in both mother and son, and the boy's aldosterone suppressed quickly with dexamethasone. Detailed adrenal imaging in search of adenoma or hyperplasia was unnecessary in this case.

Case 8.4
A boy was admitted, aged 4.7 years, with a short history of vomiting and acidosis. On arrival at the hospital he was comatose; investigations showed plasma sodium 132 mmol/L, cortisol 228 nmol/L (inappropriately low for such a sick child) and ACTH 41 mU/L (normal <20 mU/L). Despite intensive care he died of cerebral oedema. He was found at post mortem examination to be hyperpigmented with small adrenal glands. Nasopharyngeal aspirate was positive for influenza A.

His two surviving brothers underwent stimulation testing with synthetic ACTH (Synacthen). Aged 1.6 years, the second brother showed adrenal insufficiency with no response to Synacthen, basal/peak cortisol 321/343 nmol/L, but ACTH (7 mU/L), renin and electrolytes normal. He was treated with hydrocortisone but not fludrocortisone. The youngest brother showed a normal peak cortisol of 680 nmol/L aged 3 months and was not treated.

Aged 1.9 years, the second brother became drowsy and began vomiting after his oral hydrocortisone at 8 a.m. His mother gave him intramuscular hydrocortisone and brought him to hospital where biochemistry showed true blood glucose 1.8 mmol/L, sodium low at 127 mmol/L, but potassium normal at 4.3 mmol/L. He was given a 2-mg/h hydrocortisone infusion, together with IV 0.45% saline, 5% dextrose and 10 mmol of KCl per 500 mL, and he made a good recovery.

Questions
1 What is the differential diagnosis of this family's adrenal disorder?
2 What investigations should be carried out to try and ascertain the diagnosis?
3 How can the low sodium on admission be explained, given that recent renin measurement was normal?

Answers
1 Congenital adrenal hyperplasia is unlikely, given the small adrenal glands in the oldest brother at post mortem. By contrast, X-linked congenital adrenal hypoplasia is a possibility, although these children commonly present in infancy with salt wasting. Familial glucocorticoid deficiency, inherited as an autosomal recessive, is another possibility and would be in keeping with intact mineralocorticoid function. Triple A (or Allgrove) syndrome, another autosomal recessive disorder, can present with adrenal insufficiency prior to the development of alacrima and achalasia. Finally, X-linked ALD can present with adrenal insufficiency rather than neurological signs.
2 Molecular genetic analysis was negative for DAX-1 and ACTH-receptor mutations, but very long-chain fatty acids were elevated in both surviving siblings and mutational analysis indicated that all three brothers shared the common mutation for ALD (*c.1415_1416delAG*). MRI scan of brain was normal in both surviving brothers initially but when subtle

white matter changes were found on surveillance scanning in the second brother at 10 years of age he underwent a successful pre-emptive bone marrow transplant.

3 The low plasma sodium on admission at 1.9 years is attributable to impaired water excretion secondary to cortisol deficiency. Cortisol deficiency could partly explain the development of cerebral oedema seen in the deceased brother.

Comment

This family's case history shows the potentially rapid and devastating nature of acute adrenal decompensation, especially in infants and preschool children. Meticulous education of the parents, best given by the endocrine specialist nurse, is the cornerstone of management.

Useful information for patients and parents

The Congenital Adrenal Hyperplasia Support Group: This group, which was formed in 1991 to assist families affected by congenital adrenal hyperplasia, offers support to families and patients, aims to increase awareness of the condition to the public and to the medical profession, and to raise funds to support research. Website: www.livingwithcah.com

Child Growth Foundation: CGF offers support to patients and families with CAH; CGH and & Serono publish 'Congenital Adrenal Hyperplasia; Series No: 6. Website: http://www.childgrowthfoundation.org

Warne, G.L. (2009) *Your Child With Congenital Adrenal Hyperplasia*. Royal Children's Hospital, Victoria ISBN 0-7316-5816-7

Kelton Sheila (2009) *Congenital Adrenal Hyperplasia (CAH)*. Family Researched Library. British Columbia's Children's Hospital, Vancouver. email: famreslib@cw.bc.ca

CARES Foundation: *This USA-based organisation offers support to families and individuals with CAH. Website: www.caresfoundation.org*

Significant guidelines/consensus statements

Nieman, L.K., Biller, B.M.K., Findling, J.W. *et al.* (2008) The diagnosis of Cushing's syndrome: an endocrine society clinical practice guideline. *JCEM* **93**(5), 1526–1540.
Joint LWPES/ESPE CAH Working Group (2002) Consensus statement on management of 21-hydroxylase deficiency from the Lawson Wilkins Pediatric Endocrine Society and The European Society for Paediatric Endocrinology. *J Clin Endocrinol Metab* **97**(9), 4048–4053.

Further reading

New, M.I., Lorenzev, F., Lerner A.J. *et al.* (1983). Genotyping eteroid 21-hydroxylase deficiency hormonal reference data. *Journal of Clinical Endocrinology and Metabolism.* **57**(2):320–326.

Perry, R., Kecha, O., Paquette, J. *et al.* (2005) Primary adrenal insufficiency in children: twenty years experience at the Sainte-Justine Hospital, Montreal. *Journal of Clinical Endocrinology and Metabolism* **90**(6), 3243–3250.

Savage, M.O., Chan, L.F., Afshar, F. *et al.* (2008) Advances in the management of paediatric Cushing's disease. *Horm Res* **69**(6), 327–333.

Stratakis, C.A. (2008) Cushing syndrome caused by adrenocortical tumors and hyperplasias (corticotropin- independent Cushing syndrome). *Endocr Dev* **13**, 117–132.

Weise, M., Mehlinger, S.L., Drinkard, B. *et al.* (2004). Patients with classic congenital adrenal hyperplasia have decreased epinephrine reserve and defective glucose elevation in response to high-intensity exercise. *J Clin Endocrinol Metab* **89**, 591–597.

9 Salt and Water Balance

Physiology and pathophysiology

Control of salt balance

Regulation of salt balance is achieved primarily through activation of the renin–angiotensin–aldosterone system and the release of atrial natriuretic peptide. Renin is secreted by the juxtaglomerular cells of the kidney in response to sodium depletion or extracellular fluid volume restriction. Renin converts angiotensinogen to angiotensin I which, in turn, is metabolized by angiotensin-converting enzyme to angiotensin II. Angiotensin II stimulates the production of aldosterone from the zona glomerulosa of the adrenal cortex. Aldosterone secretion can also be stimulated directly by adrenocorticotrophic hormone (ACTH) although the physiological importance of this mechanism is unclear. Potassium ions also facilitate the secretion of aldosterone. By contrast, the secretion of both renin and aldosterone may be inhibited by atrial natriuretic peptide.

Aldosterone binds to the mineralocorticoid receptor which increases the reabsorption of sodium in the kidney, sweat and salivary glands. Sodium ions are exchanged for potassium and hydrogen ions in the distal tubule. Cortisol also has a strong binding affinity for the mineralocorticoid receptor but is prevented from doing so as a result of metabolism to inactive cortisone by 11-β-hydroxysteroid dehydrogenase-2 in aldosterone-selective tissues.

Control of water balance

Water balance is maintained as a result of the inter-relation between thirst, renal function and the antidiuretic hormone arginine vasopressin (AVP). Vasopressin is synthesized in the supraoptic and paraventricular nuclei of the hypothalamus and transported along the supraoptic–hypophyseal tract to be stored in the posterior pituitary. Vasopressin release is regulated by osmoreceptors in the hypothalamus which detect changes in plasma osmolality from 280 to 295 mOsm/kg as may occur with loss of extracellular water. High concentrations of vasopressin may also be secreted following baroreceptor-detected reductions in blood volume or blood pressure of 5–10%. Baroreceptors are located in the carotid arch, aortic sinus and left atrium and modulate vasopressinergic neuronal function via vagal and glossopharyngeal stimulation of the brainstem.

Vasopressin binds to a V2 receptor in the renal collecting tubule which regulates the insertion of water channel proteins (aquaporin 2) into the cell membrane. These allow water to flow along an osmotic gradient into the cells lining the collecting duct. Further aquaporins (aquaporin 4) allow this water to pass to the renal interstitium and circulation. This regulatory mechanism maintains plasma osmolality between 282 and 295 mOsm/kg. When the plasma osmolality exceeds 295 mOsm/kg, vasopressin secretion cannot be increased further and fluid balance is maintained by increased thirst leading to increased fluid intake. The vasopressin effect is under negative feedback modulation by locally generated prostaglandins

Practical Endocrinology and Diabetes in Children, Third Edition. Joseph E. Raine, Malcolm D.C. Donaldson, John W. Gregory, Guy Van Vliet.
© 2011 Blackwell Publishing Ltd. Published 2011 by Blackwell Publishing Ltd.

in the medullary collecting duct cells. Glucocorticoids are also required for free water excretion so that inadequate replacement in hypopituitary patients with diabetes insipidus (DI) will adversely affect DI control.

Hyponatraemia

Aetiology

Hyponatraemia may occur either as a result of salt and water depletion in which salt loss exceeds water loss or following fluid overload with relatively more water than salt. The general mechanisms for the development of hyponatraemia are shown in Table 9.1.

Hyponatraemia associated with extracellular fluid loss is not always a direct consequence of the fluid loss, which is frequently hypotonic or isotonic by comparison with plasma, but may be caused by replacement of these fluid losses with hypotonic fluid (e.g. drinking of water alone or use of hypotonic intravenous (IV) fluids).

History and examination

When a child presents with hyponatraemia for which the cause is not immediately apparent, the following points should be highlighted in the history:

1 *Features suggestive of salt loss:*
   - The presence of symptoms causing excess fluid and sodium loss (e.g. vomiting, diarrhoea, polyuria) or a compensatory decrease in urine production which may occur when sodium loss has occurred from the skin or gut.
   - Evidence that hyponatraemia is precipitated by intercurrent illness and associated with hyperkalaemia and hypoglycaemia which might suggest adrenal failure.
   - Symptoms of malabsorption or recurrent chest infections or a tendency for hyponatraemia to develop during hot weather which may be indicative of cystic fibrosis.
   - The use of medication (e.g. diuretics) which predispose to hyponatraemia.
   - Family history of consanguinity and of specific disorders such as cystic fibrosis, congenital adrenal hyperplasia or hypoplasia, and pseudohypoaldosteronism.

Table 9.1 Causes of hyponatraemia.

Mechanism	Examples
Salt loss	
Renal disease	Renal tubular defects (e.g. Fanconi, Barrter syndromes)
	Chronic renal failure
	Interstitial nephritis
	Renovascular hypertension
	Diuretic treatment
	Cisplatin toxicity
Aldosterone deficiency	Inherited enzyme disorders (e.g. 21-hydroxylase deficiency), Addison's disease
Aldosterone resistance	Pseudohypoaldosteronism
Cutaneous loss	Excess sweat sodium loss in cystic fibrosis, fluid loss in burns
Gastrointestinal	Vomiting and diarrhoea (e.g. in gastroenteritis)
	Intestinal obstruction (e.g. intussusception)
Water excess	
Renal disease	Acute nephritic syndrome, acute and chronic renal failure
Hypovolaemia causing increased proximal renal tubular reabsorption	Cirrhosis, congestive heart failure, nephrotic syndrome
Excessive water intake	Iatrogenic – excessive intravenous fluid replacement
	Primary polydipsia
ADH excess	Syndrome of inappropriate ADH secretion (e.g. in meningitis, pneumonia)
	Overtreatment with DDAVP

Table 9.2 Clinical signs of volume depletion and overload.

Volume depletion	Volume overload

1 Weight loss
2 Intravenous compartment depletion with
  • ↓ tissue perfusion
  • fast, low volume pulse
  • blood pressure typically low (but may be normal/high due to vasoconstriction)
  • slow capillary refill (> 2 secs)
  • impaired consciousness
  • pallor due to vasoconstriction
3 Interstitial compartment depletion
  • ↓ skin turgor
  • sunken eyes
  • dry mucous membranes
4 Increased urine osmolality
Urine sodium low or high depending on aetiology
	1 Weight gain
	2 Intravenous compartment expansion
	  • fast, high volume (bounding) pulse
	  • high blood pressure
	  • raised jugular venous pressure
	  • gallop rhythm
	  • liver engorgement
	3 Interstitial compartment expansion
	  • peripheral oedema with puffy eyes, ankle and sacral oedema, ascites
	4 Urine osmolality increased or decreased depending on aetiology

2 *Features suggestive of water retention:*
   • Excess daily fluid intake.
   • Symptoms suggestive of an underlying central nervous system or respiratory disorder (e.g. meningitis, raised intracranial pressure, pneumonia) associated with the syndrome of inappropriate antidiuretic hormone secretion (SIADH).
   • Symptoms suggestive of heart failure, renal, liver or thyroid disease.

The following points should be highlighted in the clinical examination:

1 The patient should always be weighed.

2 If sodium loss has occurred, clinical signs of volume depletion may be present as shown in Table 9.2.

Evidence of growth impairment may suggest a longstanding cause of hyponatraemia resulting from sodium loss. Careful clinical examination should be undertaken of all systems for signs suggestive of intracranial or respiratory disease, cardiac, hepatic, renal or adrenal failure or hypothyroidism.

3 If signs of volume depletion are absent, this may imply either previous fluid replacement with hypotonic fluids or the presence of water retention. In the latter circumstances, there may be evidence of oedema or rapid recent weight gain. The clinical signs of volume overload are shown in Table 9.2. The rapid onset of a hypo-osmolar state may be associated with neurological manifestations including anorexia, apathy, confusion, headaches, weakness and muscle cramps. More severe symptoms may include vomiting, depressed deep tendon reflexes, bulbar or pseudobulbar palsy, Cheyne–Stokes breathing, psychotic behaviour, seizures, coma and death.

Investigations

• Serum and urine electrolytes and creatinine to calculate urinary sodium losses.
• Serum and urinary osmolalities.
• Plasma renin activity, aldosterone, 17-hydroxy progesterone and cortisol.
• Thyroid function tests (TFT).
• Other investigations as indicated for cardiac, respiratory, hepatic, renal or intracranial disease.
• If the patient is normo-osmolar, plasma proteins, lipids and glucose.

Differential diagnosis

Hyponatraemia can be spurious either as a result of contamination of the blood sample taken from an IV cannula with hypotonic IV fluids or because of interference with the flame photometer assay by excess serum lipids or proteins.

The key requirement in the assessment of a patient with hyponatraemia is to distinguish between causes associated with excess sodium loss and those associated with water retention, for example in SIADH. The clinical distinction between these two states is summarized in Table 9.2.

If the cause of the hypo-osmolar state is not clear at presentation, urine osmolalities >100 mOsm/kg associated with urinary sodium concentrations >20 mmol/L suggest acute SIADH or renal, adrenal or cerebral salt

Table 9.3 Causes of syndrome of inappropriate antidiuretic hormone secretion (SIADH).

Cause	Examples
Central nervous system disorders	Meningitis, encephalitis, trauma (including surgery), hypoxia, haemorrhage, ventriculo-peritoneal shunt obstruction, Guillain–Barré syndrome
Respiratory disorders	Pneumonia, tuberculosis
Tumours	Thymoma, lymphoma, Ewing's sarcoma
Drugs	
• AVP stimulants	Phenothiazines, tricyclic antidepressants, vincristine,
• AVP potentiators	narcotics DDAVP, prostaglandin synthetase inhibitors
• Other	Chlorpropamide, cyclophosphamide, Carbamazepine

wasting. Urine osmolalities >100 mOsm/kg associated with urinary sodium concentrations <20 mmol/L suggest hypovolaemia or longer standing SIADH. Plasma renin is usually suppressed in SIADH but elevated in hypovolaemia. When it is uncertain whether SIADH is the cause of the hyponatraemia, a hypertonic saline infusion test (see below) may confirm SIADH by the demonstration of an exaggerated AVP response to the osmotic challenge.

Diagnosis

The causes of hyponatraemia are summarized in Table 9.1. Mineralocorticoid deficiency may be a consequence of idiopathic congenital adrenal hypoplasia or aplasia, biosynthetic defects of aldosterone synthesis (e.g. congenital adrenal hyperplasia) or acquired primary adrenal failure (e.g. Waterhouse–Friderichsen syndrome, autoimmune disease or following surgical removal). While combined mineralocorticoid and glucocorticoid deficiency will cause hyponatraemia through salt loss, glucocorticoid deficiency (e.g. in hypopituitarism) will cause hyponatraemia due to impaired water excretion. Resistance to aldosterone may occur as a result of absence or abnormal function of the mineralocorticoid receptor. Abnormalities of mineralocorticoid physiology are discussed in more detail in Chapter 8.

The various causes of SIADH are summarized in Table 9.3.

Treatment

Where hyponatraemia is a consequence of sodium loss and in the context of clinical signs of significant hypovolaemia, IV colloid or 0.9% saline should be given until there is clinical evidence of circulatory improvement.

Adrenal insufficiency should be treated with fludrocortisone and glucocorticoids (see Chapter 8).

SIADH should be anticipated in individuals who have experienced significant head trauma or intracranial surgery and careful postoperative supervision of fluid balance is required. SIADH should be treated by fluid restriction which may, on occasions, amount to only 40% of normal intake. Where severe or symptomatic hyponatraemia or excessive thirst makes this approach impractical, then treatment to either increase water excretion or to raise the plasma sodium should be used. Water excretion will be enhanced by the tetracycline antibiotic demeclocycline which impairs the renal response to vasopressin and has been used in adults, giving 3–5 mg/kg 8-hourly. An alternative is the newly licensed V2 receptor antagonist Tolvaptan. Plasma sodium can be raised using hypertonic (3%) saline (0.1 mL/kg/min for 2 hours), aiming to increase plasma sodium concentration by about 10 mmol/L. In this context, it may be necessary to give furosemide with replacement of excreted urinary electrolytes to prevent hypervolaemia. This treatment should be reserved for those with significant neurological symptoms following the relatively acute onset of SIADH, as there is a risk of lethal pontine myelinosis if serum sodium concentrations rise too rapidly (>10 mmol/L per day).

Endocrine hypertension

Aetiology

Hypertension in childhood as a result of endocrine pathology is usually a consequence of either glucocorticoid or catecholamine excess as shown in Table 9.4.

Table 9.4 Causes of endocrine hypertension.

Mechanism	Examples
Steroid-mediated	
Glucocorticoid excess	Iatrogenic (pharmacological doses, or over-replacement in deficiency states)
	Cushing's syndrome
	Apparent mineralocorticoid excess (AME)
Mineralocorticoid excess	11β-hydroxylase deficiency 17α-hydroxylase deficiency
	Liddle's syndrome
	Dexamethasone-suppressible hyperaldosteronism
Catecholamine-mediated	Phaeochromocytoma, ganglioma, neuroblastoma

History and examination

Key points to highlight in the history and on clinical examination include the following:

• A history of intermittent headaches, sweating, flushes, nausea or vomiting is suggestive of a phaeochromocytoma.

• *Other affected family members*: An autosomal recessive inheritance suggests congenital adrenal hyperplasia caused by 11β-hydroxylase or 17α-hydroxylase deficiency whereas an autosomal dominant pattern might suggest a phaeochromocytoma associated with a multiple endocrine neoplasia syndrome.

• Virilization in a girl might suggest congenital adrenal hyperplasia.

• Clinical signs of Cushing's syndrome (see Chapter 8).

• The presence of cutaneous signs suggestive of neurofibromatosis, or of mucosal neuromas which are associated with von Hippel–Lindau disease, may suggest the presence of an associated phaeochromocytoma.

Investigations

The following preliminary investigations should be considered if an endocrine cause of hypertension is suspected:

• Serum electrolytes and creatinine
• Three 24-hour urinary-free cortisol collections
• Urinary steroid metabolite profiling
• Urinary catecholamine metabolites
• Abdominal ultrasound

If Cushing's syndrome seems likely, additional investigations to confirm the diagnosis and treatment are described (see Chapter 8). If the urinary excretion of catecholamine metabolites is increased, then a blood sample should be taken for the measurement of catecholamines. Two-thirds of phaeochromocytomas are located in the adrenal medulla but may also be found anywhere in the sympathetic chain, most commonly close to the renal hilum or aortic bifurcation. Abdominal imaging with magnetic resonance imaging (MRI), computerized tomography (CT), ^{123}I-metaiodobenzylguanidine (MIBG) scanning and, possibly, selective venous catecholamine sampling by catheterization may be necessary to locate the site(s).

Diagnosis

The various causes of endocrine hypertension are shown in Table 9.4. Hypertension in 11β-hydroxylase- and 17α-hydroxylase-deficient congenital adrenal hyperplasia results from accumulation of the potent mineralocorticoid deoxycorticosterone, resulting in sodium and water retention with suppression of renin and aldosterone. 11β-hydroxylase deficiency is also associated with excess androgen production and virilization whereas 17α-hydroxylase deficiency causes androgen deficiency with inadequate masculinization of the male.

Primary aldosteronism is associated with hypernatraemia, increased plasma volume and hyporeninaemia. Hypertension is common in childhood Cushing's syndrome. The syndrome of apparent mineralocorticoid excess is characterized by low plasma renin and aldosterone concentrations and is associated with a deficiency of 11β-hydroxysteroid dehydrogenase 2 which is responsible for metabolizing cortisol to cortisone to prevent high concentrations of cortisol from binding to the mineralocorticoid receptor.

Liddle's syndrome arises from an abnormality of renal tubular transport caused by an activating mutation of the amiloride-sensitive sodium channel, resulting in increased sodium reabsorption and potassium loss with a biochemical and clinical picture similar to that

Table 9.5 Causes of hypernatraemia.

Mechanism	Examples
Gastrointestinal fluid loss with relatively more water loss than salt loss	Gastroenteritis with hypertonic dehydration
Decreased water intake	Water deprivation
	Impaired thirst
	• Congenital adipsia and hypodipsia
	• Acquired osmoreceptor damage
Excessive salt intake	Salt poisoning
Vasopressin deficiency (central diabetes insipidus)	
1 Congenital causes	Autosomal dominant vasopressin deficiency
• Familial gene disorder	Septo-optic dsyplasia, holoprosencephaly
2 Acquired causes	Craniopharyngioma, germinoma
• Tumours	Histiocytosis, sarcoidosis
• Inflammatory	Head injury, neurosurgery
• Trauma	Autoimmune, narcotic agonists
• Other	
• Brain malformation	
Vasopressin resistance (nephrogenic diabetes insipidus)	
1 Primary defect in vasopressin/aquaporin responsiveness	V2 receptor or *aquaporin 2* gene defect
	Nephrocalcinosis, nephronophthisis polycystic kidney
2 Secondary causes	disease
• Renal parenchymal disease	Urethral valves
• Obstructive uropathy	Hypercalcaemia, hypokalaemia
• Electrolyte disturbances	Lithium, demeclocycline, tolvaptan
• Drugs	
• Other	

of apparent mineralocorticoid excess. Glucocorticoid-suppressible hyperaldosteronism is a rare disorder in which primary aldosteronism is regulated by ACTH rather than renin–angiotensin because of fusion of regulatory sequences of the 11β-hydroxylase gene to coding sequences of the aldosterone synthase gene.

Treatment

In 11β-hydroxylase- and 17α-hydroxylase-deficient congenital adrenal hyperplasia, hypertension responds to glucocorticoid therapy which suppresses ACTH secretion and thus deoxycorticosterone production. The treatment of Cushing's syndrome is discussed in detail in Chapter 8.

A phaeochromocytoma requires surgical removal in an experienced specialist centre with skilled anaesthetic support. Pre- and perioperative control of blood pressure must be achieved by the use of adequate beta blockade using phenoxybenzamine. As this is achieved, salt intake may need to be increased to assist in extracellu-

lar fluid expansion. Beta blockers may also be necessary to treat alpha-blocker-induced tachycardia. When a neuroblastoma causes catecholamine-induced hypertension, similar medical management will be necessary in the preoperative period.

Hypernatraemia

The mechanisms of hypernatraemia are shown in Table 9.5 and include gastrointestinal fluid loss in which relatively more water is lost than salt, excessive salt intake (e.g. due to deliberate poisoning), decreased water intake through impaired thirst, and excessive renal water losses, including diabetes insipidus. It is important to recognize that some patients with neurological disability may have a combination of impaired thirst and central diabetes insipidus. Rarely, congenital adipsia/hypodipsia may be seen in the context of a mid-line defect with single central incisor. Unexplained episodic hypernatraemia should raise the possibility of factitious illness caused by the deliberate administration of salt by the child's parent or carer.

Diabetes insipidus

Aetiology

Diabetes insipidus may occur either as a result of inadequate secretion of AVP (cranial diabetes insipidus) or when there is resistance to the antidiuretic effect of AVP (nephrogenic diabetes insipidus). Cranial diabetes insipidus may be congenital due to a familial gene defect or to one of the cerebral malformations (e.g. septo-optic dysplasia, holoprosencephaly); or caused by acquired disease (e.g. craniopharyngioma, histiocytosis or surgery) of the hypothalamo–pituitary axis (Table 9.5). Autosomal dominant cranial diabetes insipidus may be caused by a mutation of the AVP–neurophysin II gene which leads to impaired processing of the AVP hormone precursor causing progressive damage to the neurosecretory neurones of the hypothalamus and the development of increasingly severe symptoms of diabetes insipidus with increasing age. Nephrogenic diabetes insipidus may occur as a consequence of mutations affecting the V2 receptor gene (X-linked) or aquaporin 2 gene (autosomal recessive) or because of disorders of the kidney which impair other components of the urinary concentrating mechanism (Table 9.5).

History and examination

The cardinal symptoms of diabetes insipidus are polyuria and polydipsia. Other causes of these symptoms must be considered – osmotic diuresis from glycosuria in diabetes mellitus and reduced nephron mass in chronic renal failure; excessive intake in habit drinking; and impaired renal tubular function in hypercalcaemia and hypokalaemia. Additional clinical features of diabetes insipidus include constipation, fever, vomiting, loss of weight, failure to thrive and dehydration.

The following points should be highlighted in the history and clinical examination:
• The nature and severity of the polyuria and polydipsia. Excess consumption of flavoured liquids only as opposed to water suggests habitual excess drinking. Drinking from unusual places, such as from the toilet or bath, or unusual fluids, such as shampoo, suggests severe thirst due to an underlying organic disorder.
• Whether the symptoms were present from birth, suggesting a congenital abnormality, or developed later in life, suggesting an acquired disorder.

• Associated neurological symptoms (e.g. blindness, neurodevelopmental delay, headache) and signs (e.g. optic atrophy) or history of a recent neurological disorder suggesting risk factors for hypothalamo–pituitary dysfunction.
• Past medical history of renal disease.
• Symptoms suggestive of diabetes mellitus (weight loss and hyperphagia within the past 6 weeks) or hypercalcaemia (anorexia, abdominal pain, constipation).
• Medication.
• Family history of similarly affected cases.
• Congenital abnormalities especially in the mid-line of the brain and face.
• Blood pressure or presence of enlarged kidneys.
• Growth status – short stature suggestive of associated growth hormone (GH) deficiency.

Investigations

Habitual excess drinking is common in toddlers and preschool children, and if often part of a wider management problem including a poor sleeping pattern. The child is otherwise healthy and the problem can usually be both diagnosed and cured by asking parents to stop flavoured fluids but allow the child unrestricted access to water. If symptoms persist, the child should be admitted for observation and the severity of the polyuria and polydipsia be confirmed by measurement of the 24-hour fluid intake and urinary losses. A fasting blood sample should be taken for the measurement of plasma glucose and serum sodium, potassium, calcium and creatinine concentrations. Urine should be tested for glycosuria and proteinuria.

In a significantly symptomatic individual, an early morning blood and urine sample should be taken for the measurement of serum electrolytes and osmolality and urinary osmolality. Diabetes insipidus may be confirmed by the presence of a hyperosmolar state (i.e. serum osmolality >295 mOsm/kg) with inappropriately dilute urine (urine <750 mOsm/kg) and the plasma or urine sample should then be sent for the measurement of AVP to confirm whether the cause is cranial or nephrogenic. In these circumstances, a water deprivation test would be dangerous and is contraindicated. Furthermore, a water deprivation test is not required when there is a clear history of polydipsia and polyuria in the context of underlying disease or treatment (e.g. craniopharyngioma, histiocytosis, and postoperative phase of craniopharyngioma) which is known to cause cranial diabetes insipidus.

Water deprivation test

This test is time consuming for staff and unpleasant for the child and family. It can usually be avoided, being either unnecessary (young child with habit drinking), unsafe (e.g. postoperative craniopharyngioma) or both. It should only be carried out after consultation with an experienced physician and must be undertaken with particular care in young children. The following protocol can be used:

1 Allow the child to consume their normal overnight fluid intake.

2 Weigh child at 8.00 a.m. at start of the fluid deprivation and measure plasma and urinary osmolalities.

3 Repeat weight, blood and urine samples every 2 hours and monitor the child carefully to prevent fluid intake.

4 For most children, an 8-hour fast is adequate and the test should be discontinued before then if more than 5% of body weight is lost or the thirst cannot be tolerated longer.

5 At the end of the fluid deprivation, administer desmopressin [DDAVP] either as an injection of 0.3 mg (subcutaneously, intramuscularly or intravenously) or 5 μg by the intranasal route and collect simultaneous urine and blood samples for osmolality measurements about 4 hours later. During the 4 hours following DDAVP, the child can be allowed to drink up to 1.5 times the volume of any urine voided.

Hypertonic saline infusion test

In children in whom the water deprivation test has given equivocal results and who are old enough to tolerate two IV cannulae with adequate blood samples for AVP measurements, a hypertonic saline infusion test may clarify the diagnosis. This requires the infusion of 0.05 mL/kg/min of 5% saline for 2 hours, or less if a plasma osmolality >300 mOsm/kg is achieved before then. Blood samples should be taken every 30 minutes from 30 minutes before the start of the test for the measurement of plasma osmolality and AVP concentrations which can be interpreted from Figure 9.1. Urine samples should be collected from before the start of the test and approximately every hour thereafter for the measurement of sodium and osmolality. Thirst and blood pressure should be documented every 30 minutes.

Central nervous system testing and other investigations

If a diagnosis of cranial diabetes insipidus is made, MRI of the hypothalamo–pituitary axis should be performed as there may be a pituitary tumour or stalk abnormality. The serum tumour markers β-hCG and α-foetoprotein

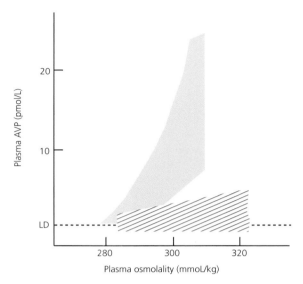

Fig. 9.1 The interrelationship between plasma osmolality and AVP concentration. Measurements which fall within the grey area suggest normal osmoregulation. Values which plot above and to the left of this area suggest nephrogenic diabetes insipidus whereas values below and to the right (in the striped area) are suggestive of cranial diabetes insipidus.

should also be measured. If the MRI demonstrates thickening of the pituitary stalk, repeat scans should be organized over the next few years to monitor the development of infiltrative disorders such as histiocytosis X or a germinoma, especially if symptoms such as headache or additional pituitary hormone deficiencies develop.

Tests of anterior pituitary function may also be indicated. Diabetes insipidus may be masked by concurrent adrenal insufficiency. If adrenal failure is present, glucocorticoid treatment should be instituted before diagnostic tests for diabetes insipidus are performed.

Diagnosis

If during the water deprivation test, the plasma osmolality remains between 282 and 295 mOsm/kg and the urine osmolality increases to >750 mOsm/kg, the patient does not have diabetes insipidus and the possibility of primary polydipsia because of abnormal drinking habits should be considered.

A diagnosis of cranial diabetes insipidus is suggested by the development of increased plasma osmolality >295 mOsm/kg in the presence of a urine osmolality <300 mOsm/kg which is then increased to >750 mOsm/kg following the administration of DDAVP. Failure of the urine to respond to DDAVP is indicative of nephrogenic diabetes insipidus. A partial urinary response (300–750 mOsm/kg) to water deprivation or DDAVP suggests partial cranial or nephrogenic diabetes insipidus. In these circumstances, the plasma AVP response to the hypertonic saline infusion test should clarify the diagnosis (see Figure 9.1).

Treatment

Cranial diabetes insipidus

This should be treated with the long-acting AVP analogue DDAVP and the following preparations are available:

• DDAVP subcutaneous injection containing 4 μg/mL. This should only be given in hospital and is not administered on a regular basis.
• DDAVP nasal solution containing 100 μg/mL and given via an intranasal catheter. This preparation is suitable for giving doses of 0.05 mL = 5 μg. For very young children, the pharmacy may need to dilute the solution to 25 μg/mL so that doses of 1.25 μg can be given.
• DDAVP nasal spray (Desmospray) delivering a fixed dose of 10 μg/spray. A low dose DDAVP delivers 2.5 μg/spray.
• DDAVP tablets (Desmotabs) 200 μg which are scored.
• DDAVP sublingual tablets (Desmomelt) 120 or 240 μg.

Widely varying dose regimens may be required, usually in two or three divided doses. The complete replacement dose of intranasal DDAVP is around 15 μg/m^2 per day and 10 μg of nasal DDAVP is roughly equivalent to 100 μg of oral DDAVP and to 60 μg of sublingual DDAVP. In those individuals taking DDAVP by the nasal route, an increase in the dosage of medication may be required during upper respiratory tract illnesses which may cause congestion of the nasal mucosa and impaired drug absorption. For this reason there has been a shift from nasal to oral DDAVP and, in recent years, a further move towards the sublingual preparation.

Patients with cranial diabetes insipidus fall into three broad categories: postoperative craniopharyngioma patients who require very careful monitoring; cranial diabetes insipidus with intact thirst; and cranial diabetes insipidus with impaired thirst.

1 *Postoperative craniopharyngioma patients:*
These patients show a triphasic pattern with initial diabetes insipidus for up to 24 hours, followed by a period of vasopressin excess for 2–4 days as the necrosing posterior pituitary gland releases this hormone, followed by permanent diabetes insipidus. DDAVP should not be given regularly during the first phase, will not be required during the second phase, but will be needed regularly thereafter.

2 *Cranial diabetes insipidus with intact thirst:*
Since patients may be very sensitive to DDAVP, treatment should start with small doses and gradually increase according to the clinical and biochemical responses. The initial response to therapy should be monitored closely by measurement of the serum electrolytes and osmolality every few days at the start of therapy. Over-treatment may be recognized by an abnormally low serum sodium concentration and osmolality. Once stabilized on treatment, patients should be reviewed in clinic at least 3-monthly as seasonal changes in temperature may alter their requirements for DDAVP. Patients who are experienced in the management of their diabetes insipidus may be allowed to adjust their own doses if they detect recurrence of polyuria. However, it is advisable to allow a short period of diuresis during the day to allow the patient to excrete any excess water load which may have occurred after excess fluid intake.

3 *Cranial diabetes insipidus with impaired thirst:*
This is seen in some children with neurodisability who have impaired osmoreceptor but normal barometric responses so that they will produce inadequate vasopressin until they become hypovolaemic. It is also seen in some craniopharyngioma patients who have sustained hypothalamic osmoreceptor damage either from the tumour or from surgery. Correction of any hypernatraemia, which may be of long standing, should be gradual in these patients to avoid seizures. A small dose of DDAVP is given initially together with a fixed daily volume of water, for example 1500 ml/1.73 m^2.

Nephrogenic diabetes insipidus

This should be managed by treatment of any underlying metabolic cause. In the absence of this, treatment with indomethacin (0.5–1.0 mg/kg twice daily) and/or a thiazide diuretic (e.g. hydrochlorothiazide 0.5–1.0 mg/kg twice daily from birth to 12 years of age, or 12.5–25 mg twice daily in older children) together with a potassium-sparing diuretic such as amiloride (5–10 mg/1.73 m^2 twice daily) can be tried. Unfortunately, patients with nephrogenic diabetes insipidus often respond poorly to treatment and must be allowed adequate access to liberal amounts of fluid intake as required.

When to involve a specialist centre

• If the investigation and diagnosis of individuals with disturbances of their salt and water balance is proving difficult (e.g. in determining whether hyponatraemia is caused by salt loss or water retention, whether diabetes insipidus is cranial or nephrogenic or in cases of suspected diabetes insipidus in infants).

- When a water deprivation test is contemplated.
- Endocrine causes of hypertension which usually require specialist investigations and expertise (e.g. endocrine surgeons).
- Diabetes insipidus, particularly when associated with impaired thirst sensation which can be difficult to manage.
- If patients fail to thrive following the introduction of apparently appropriate treatment for salt or water loss.
- Patients with oncological causes of their salt and water imbalance.
- Multiple hormone dysfunction.

Future developments

- The management of nephrogenic diabetes insipidus remains difficult and further research is required to understand the mechanisms more clearly so that more effective treatments can be developed.
- Excessive urine output and natriuresis leading to hyponatraemia is a recognized complication of a serious central nervous system insult (so-called 'cerebral salt wasting') which is distinct from SIADH. Clarification of whether this is a consequence of inappropriate atrial natriuretic peptide secretion and appropriate treatment options are required.
- Recent research has suggested that the endocrine control of blood pressure in foetal and early postnatal life may be responsible for the 'programming' of blood pressure in adult life. This hypothesis requires further examination.

Controversial points

- Should intranasal DDAVP be replaced by oral and sublingual DDAVP in most patients?
- To what extent should the hypertonic saline infusion test replace the water deprivation test as the investigation of first choice in patients with possible diabetes insipidus?
- What is the most appropriate treatment for nephrogenic diabetes insipidus?

Potential pitfalls

- Failure to recognize the tri-phasic pattern of vasopressin problems following craniopharyngioma surgery, resulting in hypernatraemia in the initial postoperative phase followed by hyponatraemia 2–4 days later due to the syndrome of inappropriate ADH secretion.
- Inappropriate and potentially life-threatening management of hyponatraemia due to failure to undertake a sufficiently careful history and clinical examination to distinguish between causes due to salt loss and those due to water retention.
- An inconclusive water deprivation test result due to inadequate supervision of the patient who surreptitiously obtained water to drink (e.g. from the tap in the toilet while producing a urine sample for measurement of osmolality) or failure to extend the test for a sufficient length of time.
- Symptomatic hyponatraemia following administration of DDAVP at the end of the water deprivation test due to failure to prevent the thirsty child consuming excess water.
- Symptomatic hyponatraemia in a child with cranial diabetes insipidus receiving regular DDAVP due to failure to allow a short period of diuresis each day to excrete any excess fluid intake or due to inadequately frequent outpatient review and adjustment of DDAVP dose to take into account changing fluid requirements through the seasons.
- Failure to plan and frequently adjust the fluid intake in a child with cranial diabetes insipidus and adipsia.
- Inadequately aggressive management of nephrogenic diabetes insipidus leading to failure to thrive.
- Inadequate cortisol replacement in hypopituitary states resulting in poor control of DI; this relates to the role of cortisol in facilitating water excretion.

Emergencies

- Hypernatraemic dehydration with impairment of consciousness, particularly if accompanied by convulsions, is an indication for admission to a high dependency unit for careful fluid input and output balance, twice daily weight, and cardiovascular monitoring. Shock (capillary refill >2 seconds +/– hypotension) is treated with 20 mL/kg boluses of 0.9% saline, otherwise the estimated fluid deficit is replaced slowly (over 48–72 hours), checking the plasma sodium at least 6-hourly in the first instance.

N.B.: If severe hypernatraemia is long-standing, as seen in adipsic and hypodipsic patients, slow oral rehydration over several days is carried out in preference to IV fluids.
• Severe hyponatraemia due to sodium loss is managed with 20 mL/kg boluses of 0.9% saline to correct shock, and replacement of the remaining deficit over 24–36 hours.
• Salt and water management can be particularly difficult in patients with hypopituitarism and diabetes insipidus who are on hormone replacement. Such patients may present to the emergency department with illnesses accompanied by vomiting and/or diarrhoea. In this situation, there may be uncertainty as to their cortisol status. In the context of cortisol deficiency DDAVP may be ineffective resulting in dehydration, while the cortisol deficiency itself may cause water retention since cortisol is required to enable water excretion. In the latter situation, a relative excess of DDAVP may lead to water intoxication, dilutional hyponatraemia and possible convulsions and neurological injury. Where doubt exists about the patient's cortisol status it is safer to provide the correct dose of cortisol, stop the DDAVP and monitor the input/output balance with regular paired plasma and urine electrolytes and osmolality, which may need to be done hourly initially. High fluid volumes may be required but, provided that water and salt balance are monitored meticulously, this will be safe.

Case histories

Case 9.1

A 2-week-old boy was admitted with hyponatraemia following an 11-day history of vomiting, constipation and failure to regain his birth weight. On examination, he appeared underweight, with no other abnormal signs. The mother's brother was known to have developed a similar problem in infancy and was receiving long-term treatment for this. Initial investigations demonstrated the following:

Sodium 114 mmol/L
Potassium 8.1 mmol/L
Cortisol 241nmol/L [8.7 μg/dL]
17-hydroxy progesterone 5.4 nmol/L [179 mg/dL]

Questions

1 What is the most likely diagnosis?
2 What additional investigations are indicated?
3 What treatment should the baby be given?

Answers

1 In the context of severe hyponatraemia, the cortisol is inappropriately low. The low 17-hydroxy progesterone excludes 21-hydroxylase-deficient congenital adrenal hyperplasia and the family history suggests a likely diagnosis of X-linked congenital adrenal hypoplasia.
2 A blood sample for the measurement of plasma glucose, renin, aldosterone, ACTH, luteinizing hormone (LH), follicle stimulating hormone (FSH), testosterone and glycerol (gonadotrophin and glycerol kinase deficiencies are associated with X-linked congenital adrenal hypoplasia). A urine sample for the measurement of steroid metabolites or a Synacthen stimulation test will help confirm the diagnosis if there is any doubt.
3 Once the initial blood sample for investigations has been taken, the baby should be treated with IV fluids containing 0.9% saline with additional dextrose to provide a concentration of 10% dextrose. He requires IV hydrocortisone at a dosage of approximately 60 mg/m^2 per day subdivided 8-hourly which can be reduced to 10–15 mg/m^2 per day orally once the patient has recovered from the presenting illness (see Chapter 8). Once the vomiting has ceased, oral fludrocortisone can be added at a dosage of 150 mg/m^2 per day.

Case 9.2

An 11-year-old boy presented with an 8-week history of polyuria and polydipsia. He was otherwise well apart from recent headaches. Investigations in clinic demonstrated the following:

Serum sodium 142 mmol/L
Serum potassium 3.7 mmol/L
Serum urea 2.3 mmol/L [6.5 mg/dL]
Serum creatinine 52 μmol/L [0.6 mg/dL]
Plasma osmolality 305 mOsm/kg
Plasma glucose 6.2 mmol/L
Urine sodium 16 mmol/L [112 mg/dL]
Urine osmolality 78 mOsm/kg

Questions

1 What further investigation is required to clarify the diagnosis?
2 What additional investigations are then required?

Answers

1 Given that this child is spontaneously hyperosmolar, a formal water deprivation test is contraindicated. However, it is not clear whether this child has cranial or nephrogenic diabetes insipidus and the response to DDAVP needs evaluating. His urinary osmolality increased from 75 to 530 mOsm/kg and there was a dramatic reduction in his urine output suggesting that he has cranial diabetes insipidus.

2 Given a diagnosis of cranial diabetes insipidus and a history of headaches, a full assessment of pituitary function and cranial imaging are indicated. His hypothalamo–pituitary axis was normal on MRI. A basal blood sample demonstrated normal thyroid function and cortisol concentrations. However, after 6 months he demonstrated poor growth despite a dramatic resolution of his symptoms with regular DDAVP. In response to insulin-induced hypoglycaemia, his maximum serum growth hormone concentration was 4.7 mU/L (normal >20). Repeat MRI demonstrated the presence of a tumour which was shown to be a germinoma.

Case 9.3

A 13-week-old baby girl is admitted for assessment with poor feeding. She was born at 41 weeks' gestation weighing 3.4 kg to a mother aged 29 years. She became hypoglycaemic during the first 24 hours, and required phototherapy for jaundice. She was not fixing or following by 6 weeks and was found at 10 weeks to have small optic discs and absent electroretinogram response to light by the ophthalmology department. On examination she is a pale, still infant weighing 5.36 kg (−1.05 SD), length 60.5 cm (0.12 SD), head circumference 40.7 cm (0.17 SD). She is hypotonic and has roving nystagmus.

Questions

1 What is the most likely diagnosis?
2 What further assessment is indicated?

Answers

1 The finding of roving nystagmus and failure to fix and follow with small optic discs in the context of neonatal hypoglycaemia and jaundice is strongly suggestive of septo-optic dysplasia (SOD) with optic nerve hypoplasia and hypopituitarism (including cortisol and thyroxine deficiency).

2 Cranial ultrasound to look for absence of the septum pellucidum, and blood for thyroxine (T4), TSH, random cortisol, and electrolytes are required.

Serum sodium is 163 mmol/L, chloride 124 mmol/L, urea 3.3 mmol/L, creatinine 50 μmol/L. Urine osmolality is low at 132 mOsm/kg. Random cortisol is 220 nmol/L, peak cortisol response to a standard dose of synthetic ACTH (250 μg) is 1269 nmol/L, free T4 is 13.9 pmol/L with TSH 3.8, 26 and 33 mU/L at 0, 30 and 60 minutes after TRH stimulation. Peak GH after arginine stimulation is low/normal at 8 μg/L (24 mU/L).

Questions

1 What do these results indicate?
2 What treatment should be given?

Answers

1 The baby is one of the unfortunate minority of subjects with SOD who have diabetes insipidus. She has incipient hypothalamic hypothyroidism but, surprisingly, no evidence of cortisol deficiency on a standard Synacthen test.

2 She clearly requires treatment with DDAVP, given as 25 μg daily initially, adding in T4 25 μg daily when the free T4 falls to 8.9 pmol/L at 5 months of age.

At 7 months the infant is admitted acutely unwell with poor perfusion, mottled and cold peripheries and capillary glucose only 1.3 mmol/L. Sodium is elevated at 167 mmol/L and glucose 2.2 mmol/L. She is given IV fluids and her DDAVP dose is adjusted, but her diabetes insipidus is very hard to control, with sodium fluctuating between 130 and 156 mmol/L.

Question

How can the unsatisfactory progress of this infant be explained?

Answer

Clinically the child is ACTH deficient, and diabetes insipidus cannot be properly controlled in the context of cortisol deficiency since the latter is required for water excretion. The peak cortisol level after Synacthen stimulation was achieved using a standard rather than low dose. Random cortisol levels during illness were 200–300 nmol/L, and never >500 nmol/L, and the child was accordingly started on hydrocortisone. Only when a full replacement dose of hydrocortisone was given did her diabetes insipidus stabilize. The height remained on the 10th centile until 5 years of age when it fell to the 3rd centile, with IGF-I low at 35 µg/L after which GH therapy was started.

Comment
This case demonstrates the difficulty of diagnosing central adrenal insufficiency, the important role of cortisol in water balance, and the evolving pattern of GHD in SOD, with normal GH levels often found during infancy.

Case 9.4
A male infant is referred to the ophthalmology department because it was noted at 12-week check that he was not fixing and following. He was born at 38 weeks' gestation weighing 2.95 kg and smiled late, with delayed gross motor development. Ophthalmic assessment showed visual inattention with nystagmus, normal optic discs and electroretinogram but reduced visual-evoked potentials consistent with a visual pathway abnormality. In the course of investigations for developmental delay aged 10 months, he was found to have a very high serum sodium of 160 mmol/L, chloride also high at 120 mmol/L, bicarbonate high/normal at 26 mmol/L, urea 5.9 mmol/L and creatinine 41 µmol/L. Urine specific gravity is l010, confirming a urine concentration defect. On direct questioning his parents say that he does not appear particularly thirsty but that his nappies are quite wet. The infant is referred to the endocrine team for further assessment.

Questions
1 What is the most likely diagnosis, based on the information given so far?
2 How should the child be managed initially?

Answers
1 It appears that this child has a central nervous disorder (CNS) disorder affecting neurodevelopment including vision and the hypothalamus with a combination of reduced thirst

and diabetes insipidus – hypodipsic DI. In this situation osmoreceptor function is impaired so that vasopressin response to hypernatraemia is reduced, but baroreceptor function is preserved so that vasopressin will be produced in response to low blood pressure. The high/normal bicarbonate probably reflects volume contraction, with enhanced bicarbonate absorption at the proximal tubule, while the normal urea and creatinine show that the baby is not markedly dehydrated.
2 The hypernatraemia will be long standing in nature, and abrupt attempts to correct it will result in convulsions. The child is thoroughly examined and found to have dysmorphic features including mid-line crease in the nose, sloping forehead, low set posteriorly rotated ears and prominent metopic suture. He is hypotonic, visually inattentive, and has poor peripheral perfusion with doughy texture to the subcutaneous tissues, heart rate 120/min and blood pressure 115/75 (crying). Weight is 14.2 kg (>99.6th centile), length 74 cm (50th centile), head circumference 47.2 cm (50th centile).

Hypodipsic DI in a child with an unclassified dysmorphic syndrome is diagnosed on the basis of the clinical and biochemical findings. A nasogastric tube is passed initially and 1000 mL per day of diluted milk (800 mL milk and 200 mL water) is given together with oral DDAVP 25 µg daily. The sodium normalizes on this regime and is 144 mmol/L 18 days after it was started, by which time the child has been at home for 2 weeks and managing to take the target volume of fluid orally.

Questions
1 What further investigations are indicated?
2 What approach to management should be adopted?

Answers
1 Further hypothalamic assessment is required, together with a genetic opinion and DNA analysis. The MRI of brain shows absence of the pituitary bright spot but is otherwise unremarkable. Combined pituitary function testing aged 13 month shows a peak GH of 1.9 µg/L (5.7 mU/L) in response to arginine stimulation but IGF-I is normal for age at 33 µg/L; free T4 is 10 pmol/L with a sustained,

exaggerated TSH response to TRH (6, 52 and 69 mU/L at 0, 30 and 60 minutes, respectively) indicating compensated hypothalamic hypothyroidism. Peak cortisol response to low dose Synacthen (500 ng/1.73 m^2) is borderline low at 411 nmol/L. FSH and LH responses to luteinizing hormone releasing hormone (LHRH) are normal for age. These results indicated hypothalamic hypopituitarism with GH and ACTH deficiency, and incipient hypothyroidism.

The child is started on thyroxine 25 μg daily, and hydrocortisone 2.5 mg twice daily in addition to oral DDAVP. Genetic studies show normal chromosomes and multiplex ligation-dependant probe amplification (MLPA) screening is negative. A further DNA sample is sent for array comparative genomic hybridization (CGH).

2 The management approach towards this severely disabled child must be multidisciplinary, involving ophthalmology, audiology, neurodevelopmental, community and social work professionals. A case discussion is held to ensure good communication between the various disciplines and to devise an integrated care plan.

Useful information for parents

Diabetes insipidus – patient's average guide Series No. 12. Website:
http://www.eurospe.org/patient/english/average/diabetes%20insipidus%20average%20readability.pdf

Further reading

Baylis, P.H. & Cheetham, T. (1998) Diabetes insipidus. *Archives of Disease in Childhood* **79**, 84–89.

Deal, J.E., Sever, P.S., Barratt, T.M. *et al.* (1990) Phaeochromocytoma: investigation and management of 10 cases. *Archives of Disease in Childhood* **65**, 269–274.

Gruskin, A.B. & Sarnaik, A. (1992) Hyponatraemia: pathophysiology and treatment, a paediatric perspective. *Paediatric Nephrology* **6**, 280–286.

Ishikawa, S. & Schrier, R.W. (2003) Pathophysiological roles of arginine vasopressin and aquaporin-2 in impaired water excretion. *Clinical Endocrinology* **58**, 1–17.

Maghnie, M., Cosi, G., Genovese, E. *et al.* (2003) Central diabetes insipidus in children and young adults. *New England Journal of Medicine* **343**, 998–1007.

Mohn, A., Acerini, C.L., Cheetham, T.D. *et al.* (1998) Hypertonic saline test for the investigation of posterior pituitary function. *Archives of Disease in Childhood* **79**, 431–434.

Sakarcan, A. & Bocchini, J. (1998) The role of fludrocortisone in a child with cerebral salt wasting. *Paediatric Nephrology* **12**, 769–771.

Schrier, R.W., Gross, P., Gheorghiade, M., *et al.* (2006) Tolvaptan, a selective oral vasopressin V2-receptor antagonist, for hyponatremia, *N Engl J Med* **355** (20), 2099–112.

10 Calcium and Bone

Physiology

Introduction

About 99% of the total body calcium is found in the skeleton bound to phosphate and hydroxyl ions in the form of hydroxyapatite. The normal total serum calcium concentration at all ages ranges from 2.2 to 2.6 mmol/L and consists of physiologically active ionized calcium (about 50%), with the remainder being either bound to albumin or globulins (about 40%) or circulating complexed to citrate, phosphate or other constituents in the serum (about 10%). Calcium in intracellular and extracellular fluid is involved in many metabolic processes, including many enzymatic reactions, hormone secretion and blood coagulation. Serum calcium concentrations are influenced by:

- intestinal calcium absorption;
- calcium deposition in bone and mobilization of calcium following bone resorption; and
- renal tubular calcium reabsorption.

Approximately 85% of body phosphate is contained within bone hydroxyapatite. Many cellular reactions require either organic or inorganic phosphate. Normal inorganic serum phosphate concentrations drop from 1.3–2.3 mmol/L in infancy to 0.8–1.5 mmol/L at the end of puberty. About 15% of circulating phosphate is protein bound. Free phosphate is required together with ionized calcium for normal bone mineralization. Calcium metabolism is regulated primarily by vitamin D, parathyroid hormone (PTH) and calcitonin.

Vitamin D

Vitamin D is either ingested in the diet or synthesized in the skin following ultraviolet irradiation from sunlight. Circulating vitamin D (Figure 10.1) is metabolized in the liver to 25-hydroxyvitamin D and then in the kidneys to either a metabolically active form (1,25-dihydroxyvitamin D) or an inactive form (24,25-dihydroxyvitamin D). 1,25-dihydroxyvitamin D synthesis is stimulated by hypocalcaemia, PTH and hypophosphataemia.

Circulating vitamin D exerts its target organ effect by binding to an intracellular vitamin D receptor. Vitamin D stimulates the activity of osteoclast-like cells but suppresses that of osteoblast-like cells and, in the presence of PTH, mobilizes calcium from bone. 1,25-dihydroxyvitamin D stimulates intestinal calcium absorption but whether it influences renal handling of calcium and phosphate is less clear. Vitamin D receptors have been located in many other tissues in the body, suggesting a wider role for vitamin D than just regulation of calcium metabolism.

Parathyroid hormone

The PTH gene has been localized to the short arm of chromosome 11. PTH is synthesized as a pre-pro-hormone in the four parathyroid glands. Pre-pro-PTH is converted

Practical Endocrinology and Diabetes in Children, Third Edition. Joseph E. Raine, Malcolm D.C. Donaldson, John W. Gregory, Guy Van Vliet.
© 2011 Blackwell Publishing Ltd. Published 2011 by Blackwell Publishing Ltd.

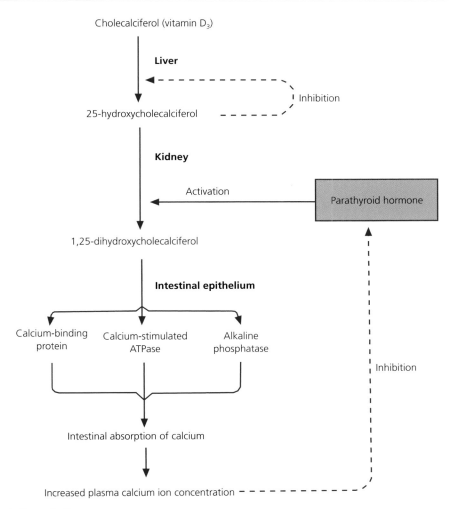

Fig. 10.1 Vitamin D metabolism.

to pro-PTH as it is transported across the rough endo-plasmic reticulum and is stored in secretory granules in the form of the mature 84 amino-acid peptide PTH. PTH release is stimulated by hypocalcaemia and inhibited by hypercalcaemia acting through a specific calcium-sensing receptor on the plasma membrane of the parathyroid cell.

The primary function of PTH is to prevent hypocal-caemia. Within minutes, changes in PTH secretion affect renal tubular function, increasing calcium absorption and phosphate excretion, and osteoclastic bone resorption. Over a period of 1–2 days, by stimulating the synthesis of 1,25-dihydroxyvitamin D, PTH also increases intestinal calcium absorption.

PTH produces its target cell effect by binding to a membrane-bound receptor which stimulates guanine nucleotide-binding protein (G protein) mediated produc-tion of cyclic adenosine monophosphate (cAMP) from adenosine triphosphate (ATP). This, in turn, stimulates activation of protein kinase A and phosphorylation of intracellular enzymes leading to the physiological action of PTH.

Calcitonin

Calcitonin is produced in the 'C' or parafollicular cells of the thyroid gland. Calcitonin is encoded by a gene also located on the short arm of chromosome 11 and is synthesized in the form of a large precursor molecule.

Tissue-specific processing may lead to an alternative calcitonin gene product, calcitonin gene-related peptide, which is a potent vasodilator.

Calcitonin secretion is stimulated by calcium and some gastrointestinal hormones (gastrin, cholecystokinin and glucagon). The primary function of calcitonin is unclear as it appears to have a relatively minor role in calcium metabolism. It reduces serum calcium concentrations by direct inhibition of PTH and 1,25-dihydroxyvitamin D mediated osteoclastic bone resorption. Calcitonin also increases the urinary excretion of calcium and phosphate but facilitates the absorption of nutrition-derived calcium into blood.

Bone metabolism

Bone has two main functions – (1) forming the rigid skeleton and (2) having a central role in calcium and phosphate homeostasis. Macroscopically, there are two types of bone:

1 *Trabecular (cancellous, spongy) bone* is found in the metaphyseal areas of long bones, vertebrae and most flat bones. It accounts for about 20% of the skeleton and is metabolically very active, having an important role in calcium and phosphate metabolism.

2 *Cortical bone* is found in the diaphyses of the long bones and is relatively metabolically inactive.

Bone consists of:
- an organic matrix – mostly collagen;
- an inorganic mineral phase – hydroxyapatite;
- osteoblasts which synthesize and mineralize the organic bone matrix;
- osteoclasts which resorb bone and are then replaced by osteoblasts which produce new bone; and
- osteocytes which are osteoblasts which have become embedded within mineralized bone and which may play a part in sensing mechanical strain or controlling rapid mineral exchange between bone and serum without bone matrix degradation.

Bone growth and reshaping takes place throughout childhood and adolescence. Longitudinal growth of the long bones occurs by enchondral bone formation (Figure 10.2). In this process, cartilage cells (chondrocytes) proliferate in columns and undergo hypertrophic differentiation within the growth plate. Chondrocyte proliferation is regulated locally by the interaction of fibroblast growth factor with the fibroblast growth factor receptor-3 (FGFR3). Activating mutations of the *FGFR3* are responsible for achondroplasia and hypochondroplasia. Hypertrophic differentiation of the chondrocyte is regulated by a negative feedback loop involving the cytokine parathyroid hormone-related peptide (PTHrP) and signalling molecule known as 'Indian hedgehog'. The hypertrophic chondrocytes become surrounded by

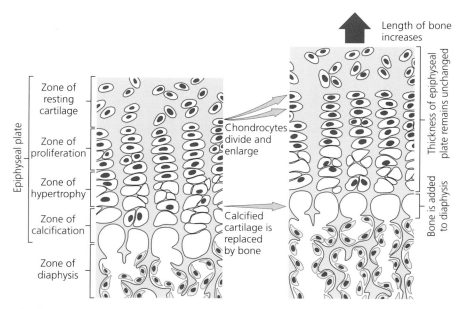

Fig. 10.2 Longitudinal growth of the long bones by enchondral bone formation.

Table 10.1 Factors which influence peak bone mass.

Influence	Increased bone mass	Decreased bone mass
Genetic	Afro-Caribbeans	Caucasians
		Orientals
Hormones	Calcitonin	Parathyroid hormone
	Oestrogen	Vitamin D
	Growth hormone	Glucocorticoids
Cytokines	Transforming	Interleukin 1
	growth factor β	Tumour necrosis factor α
Nutrition	Calcium	Anorexia
	Obesity	Malabsorption
Mechanical	Exercise	Inactivity

Table 10.2 Causes of hypocalcaemia.

Infancy	Childhood
Prematurity	Vitamin D deficiency
Asphyxia	Vitamin D-dependent
Gestational diabetes	rickets (types 1 and 2)
Transient or permanent	Chronic renal failure
hypoparathyroidism	Hypoparathyroidism
High milk phosphate load	Pseudohypoparathyroidism
Hypomagnesaemia	
Parenteral nutrition	
Exchange transfusion	
Chronic alkalosis or	
bicarbonate therapy	
Maternal	
hyperparathyroidism	

a matrix in which calcium is laid down. Newly calcified cartilage then condenses to become surrounded by osteoblasts which produce calcified osteoid. This calcified tissue is resorbed and replaced by bone trabeculae. By contrast, growth in width and thickness occurs by the process of intramembraneous bone formation. This process occurs at the periosteal surface, without a cartilage matrix and with bone resorption taking place at the endosteal surface.

By contrast, bone remodelling is the lifelong process by which skeletal tissue is being continuously resorbed and replaced to maintain skeletal integrity, shape and mass. In healthy individuals, the balance between bone formation and bone resorption is finely tuned. Bone mass increases progressively through childhood and adolescence until the maximum is attained in young adult life (so-called 'peak bone mass') during the third decade. Thereafter, a net loss of bone mass occurs as bone resorption exceeds the synthesis of new bone in later life. The amount of peak bone mass is a major risk factor for fractures in old age and is influenced by genetic factors, hormones, nutrition and mechanical strain (Table 10.1).

Hypocalcaemia

Aetiology

The causes of hypocalcaemia may be subdivided into those which present in infancy and those which present in older children as shown in Table 10.2. PTH-deficient hypoparathyroidism may be familial (autosomal dominant, recessive or X-linked recessive) and associated with other abnormalities, such as Addison's disease or deafness.

Non-familial PTH-deficient hypoparathyroidism may present in infancy and be transient or persistent (e.g. in association with DiGeorge's syndrome). In older children, it may be idiopathic or secondary (e.g. following surgical removal of the parathyroids or hypomagnesaemia).

Pseudohypoparathyroidism is caused by resistance to the action of PTH. This is known as Albright's hereditary osteodystrophy (AHO) when associated with the dysmorphic features described in Table 11.5 and Figure 11.4. The PTH resistance of AHO is most commonly associated with decreased G-protein activity in cell membranes (type 1a), which may also affect other G-protein coupled receptors (e.g. adrenocorticotrophic hormone (ACTH), thyroid stimulating hormone (TSH), luteinising hormone (LH), follicle stimulating hormone (FSH) and glucagon).

History and examination

When assessing a child with hypocalcaemia, the following points should be highlighted in the clinical history:
- Symptoms suggestive of hypocalcaemia (e.g. paraesthesia, muscle cramps or tetany, seizures and diarrhoea).
- Predisposing risk factors (e.g. intestinal or renal tubular disease) for hypomagnesaemia.
- Evidence of endocrine disease affecting other G-protein coupled receptors (e.g. previous thyroxine treatment for a low normal serum T4 concentration with mildly elevated serum TSH concentration).
- Symptoms of autoimmune disease.
- Previous surgical risk factors (e.g. thyroidectomy or parathyroidectomy).
- A family history of hypoparathyroidism.

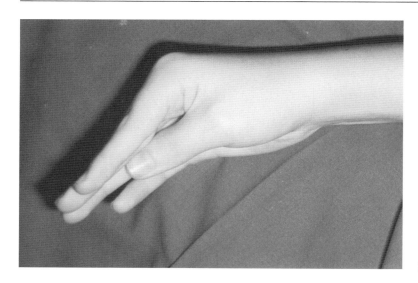

Fig. 10.3 Trousseau's sign.

If an older child is suspected to have hypocalcaemia, latent tetany may be detected from positive Chvostek's sign (facial twitching in response to tapping of the facial nerve in front of the ear) and Trousseau's sign (carpal spasm within 3 minutes of inflating a blood pressure cuff above systolic blood pressure; Figure 10.3) or stridor. Extrapyramidal signs from basal ganglia calcification, cataracts, papilloedema, dry skin, coarse hair, brittle nails and enamel hypoplasia with dental caries are signs suggestive of chronic hypocalcaemia. In contrast with the older child, hypocalcaemia in infancy is associated with relatively non-specific symptoms including tremor, apnoea, cyanosis and lethargy. Clinical signs suggestive of autoimmune hypoparathyroidism and pseudohypoparathyroidism are shown in Table 10.3 with details of the dysmorphic features of pseudohypoparathyroidism shown in Table 11.5 and Figure 11.4.

Investigations

If hypocalcaemia is suspected, a blood sample should be taken for the measurement of:

- calcium;
- phosphate;
- alkaline phosphatase;
- PTH;
- 25-hydroxyvitamin D; and
- a sample stored for possible measurement of 1,25-dihydroxyvitamin D concentration later, should this be indicated.

The differential diagnosis of biochemical abnormalities of calcium metabolism is shown in Table 10.4.

Treatment

Emergency management of acute hypocalcaemia complicated by tetany or a seizure

1 Take initial diagnostic blood sample.
2 Slow intravenous (IV) injection over 5–10 minutes of 0.11 mmol (0.5 mL)/kg body weight of 10% calcium gluconate.
3 Maintain IV infusion of 10% calcium gluconate:
   a *Neonates:* 0.5 mmol/kg per day (may be necessary for a few days).
   b *Children aged 1 month to 2 years:* 1 mmol/kg per day (usual maximum 8.8 mmol).
   c *Children aged 2–18 years:* 8.8 mmol over 24 hours.
4 Once acute symptoms are resolved, treatment should be changed to oral preparations and adjusted according to response:
   a *Neonates:* 0.25 mmol/kg four times daily.
   b *Children aged 1 month to 4 years:* 0.25 mmol/kg four times daily.
   c *Children aged 5–12 years:* 0.2 mmol/kg four times daily.
   d *Children aged 12–18 years:* 10 mmol four times daily.

Care must be taken when IV calcium is administered as extravasation of calcium into subcutaneous tissues around the injection site can lead to tissue necrosis. Long-term maintenance treatment of hypocalcaemia requires vitamin D given as alfacalcidol (neonates 50–100 ng/kg daily, children aged 1 month to 12 years 25–50 ng/kg daily and

Table 10.3 Clinical signs to look for on examination.

Clinical sign	Possible diagnosis

Candidiasis
Dental enamel and
  nail dystrophy
Alopecia
Vitiligo
Signs of Addison's disease or
  hypothyroidism
	Autoimmune
	  hypoparathyroidism
	  (polyglandular
	  autoimmune
	  disease type 1)

Short stature Subcutaneous calcification Dysmorphic features	Pseudohypoparathyroidism

Swollen wrists
Prominent costochondral
  junctions (rachitic rosary)
  and Harrison's sulci
Bow-leg or knock-knee
Craniotabes
Delayed dental eruption and
  enamel hypoplasia
Muscle weakness and tetany
	Vitamin D-deficient rickets

Poor growth Bowing of the legs	Hypophosphataemic rickets
Blue sclerae Abnormal dentition Hyperextensible joints Deafness	Osteogenesis imperfecta

Broad and prominent forehead
Short turned-up nose with flat
  nasal bridge
Overhanging upper lip
Late dental eruption
Supravalvular aortic stenosis
Peripheral pulmonary stenosis
Learning difficulties with
  emotional lability
Mild short stature
	Williams syndrome

children aged 12–18 years 1 µg daily) or calcitriol (children aged 1 month to 12 years initially 15 ng/kg daily, increased by 5 ng/kg daily to a maximum of 250 ng and children aged 12–18 years 250 ng daily increased by 5 ng/kg daily (maximum step 250 ng) every 2–4 weeks to a usual dose of 0.5–1.0 ìg daily). These preparations are recommended because of their short half-life and rapid cessation of action should toxicity occur. Vitamin D may need to be given in combination with calcium. Frequent monitoring of serum calcium concentrations is required shortly after starting treatment – weekly if there is concern about the response to therapy. Once the patient has demonstrated a satisfactory response, serum calcium concentration and the urinary calcium:creatinine ratio should be measured every 3 months thereafter with regular renal ultrasounds to monitor for calcification.

In children with hypoparathyroidism, the aim of therapy is to achieve low normal serum calcium concentrations (2.0–2.25 mmol/L) [8.0–9.0 mg/dL] while avoiding urinary calcium:creatinine ratios greater than 0.7 mmol/L [0.16 mg/dL]. In those with pseudohypoparathyroidism, the resistance to PTH primarily affects the proximal renal tubule. Therefore, to avoid adverse bone sequelae, treatment should suppress PTH levels to the normal range, which may require maintenance of serum calcium concentrations towards the upper end of the normal range (2.25–2.5 mmol/L) [9.0–10.0 mg/dL].

Rickets

Aetiology

Rickets is caused by delayed matrix mineralization at the growth plate resulting in excessive accumulation of uncalcified cartilage and bone (osteoid) matrix. The most common causes of rickets are those associated with vitamin D deficiency. They present most frequently at times of rapid growth which may occur in infancy or in puberty, particularly in Asian children. Vitamin D deficiency may be a result of dietary insufficiency, malabsorption (e.g. coeliac disease) or inadequate exposure to sunlight. There is a need for a greater clinical awareness of vitamin D-deficient rickets in Western industrialized societies as the current prevalence, particularly in infancy and adolescence, seems higher than is often appreciated even in relatively sunny countries. To prevent rickets, it is recommended that food be supplemented with 200 units of vitamin D daily for all infants under 6 months and 400 units daily for older children aged 6 months to 4 years and adolescents, particularly girls with darker skins. Rickets of prematurity is thought to be caused by calcium and/or phosphate deficiency rather than vitamin D deficiency.

Hypophosphataemic rickets is an X-linked dominant disorder which is associated with a failure of phosphate resorption in the proximal renal tubule. Vitamin D-dependent rickets is very rare and is caused either by deficiency of 1a-hydroxylation of 25-hydroxyvitamin D (type 1) or resistance to 1,25-dihydroxyvitamin D

Table 10.4 Differential diagnosis of disorders of vitamin D and parathyroid hormone (PTH) metabolism.

Diagnosis	Ca$_2$	PO$_4$	PTH	25-OHD	1,25-(OH)$_2$D
Vitamin D-deficient rickets	LN	L	H	L	L,N,H
Vitamin D-dependent rickets					
type 1 (deficiency of 1α-hydroxylation)	L	L	H	N,L	L
type 2 (resistance to 1,25-(OH)$_2$D)	L	L	H	N,L	N,H
X-linked hypophosphataemic rickets	N	L	N	N	L,N
Hypophosphataemic rickets with hypercalciuria	N	L	N	N	H
Tumour-induced rickets	N	L	N	N	L
Renal osteodystrophy	N,L	H	H		N,L
Primary hyperparathyroidism	H	L	H	N	N,H
Hypoparathyroidism	L	H	L	N	L,N
Pseudohypoparathyroidism	L	H	H	N	L,N
Vitamin D intoxication	H	N	L	H	N,H
Hypercalcaemia in granulomatous disorders	H	N	L	N	H

Abbreviations: Ca$_2$, calcium; PO$_4$, phosphate; 25-OHD, 25-hydroxyvitamin D; 1,25-(OH)$_2$D, 1,25-dihydroxyvitamin D; H, high; N, normal; L, low; LN, low–normal.

(type 2). The classification of the different forms of rickets and their biochemical characteristics are shown in Table 10.4.

In severe renal failure, 1,25-dihydroxyvitamin D synthesis is impaired which, in conjunction with increasing serum phosphate concentrations, leads to hypocalcaemia and secondary hyperparathyroidism with bone disease (renal osteodystrophy).

Both rickets and osteomalacia (defective mineralization of osteoid tissue) are common in the many causes of Fanconi's syndrome and type 2 renal tubular acidosis. The metabolic bone disease is caused by a combination of phosphaturia-induced hypophosphataemia, hypercalciuria, abnormal vitamin D metabolism and renal insufficiency.

History and examination

If a child presents with rickets, then the following details should be elicited:
- Symptoms suggestive of associated disease (e.g. renal failure, malabsorption).
- Dietary history of food intake, such as dairy products, which are rich in calcium and vitamin D.
- Risk factors for inadequate exposure to sunlight.
- Family history of rickets.

The child should undergo careful clinical examination, including documentation of growth and pubertal status. The clinical signs to look for on examination are shown in Table 10.3.

Investigations

Rickets causes abnormal bone mineralization which may be evident on X-ray. Additional radiological features commonly include a characteristic widening of the growth plate with cupping, splaying and fraying of an irregularly margined metaphysis (Figure 10.4). The characteristic clinical signs of vitamin D-deficient and hypophosphataemic rickets are detailed in Table 10.3 and Figures 10.5 and 10.6.

The lowered renal threshold for resorption of phosphate, which is associated with hypophosphataemic rickets, can be calculated from simultaneous serum and urinary biochemical measurements by reference to Kruse

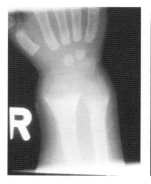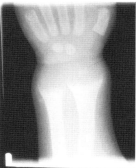

Fig. 10.4 X-ray of the wrist of a child with rickets caused by vitamin D deficiency.

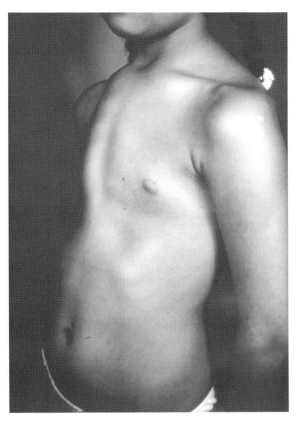

Fig. 10.5 Rachitic rosary.

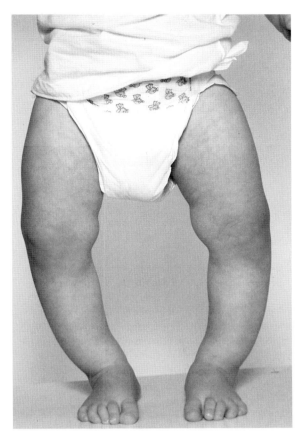

Fig. 10.6 Bowing of the legs in a child with hypophosphataemic rickets.

et al. (1982) or Shaw *et al.* (1990), which also contains details of age-appropriate reference ranges. The presence of glycosuria, amino-aciduria or a metabolic acidosis with inappropriately alkaline urine is suggestive of a wider defect of tubular function, such as Fanconi's syndrome or renal tubular acidosis.

Treatment

Depending on the cause of the rickets, different preparations of vitamin D are required for effective treatment as shown in Table 10.5. Where renal dysfunction is associated with metabolic bone disease, treatment of the wider systemic metabolic abnormality is required. Detailed guidance for this is beyond the scope of this volume and the reader is advised to consult appropriate textbooks on paediatric nephrology. Children with Fanconi's syndrome may require phosphate therapy whereas those with renal tubular acidosis require treatment with bicarbonate.

Osteoporosis

Aetiology

Unlike in adults, osteoporosis in childhood is not clearly defined but is caused by reduced bone mass per unit volume with a normal ratio of mineral to matrix. The possibility of osteoporosis should be considered in a child who presents with fractures following minimal trauma in whom there is also evidence of decreased bone mineral density (usually more than three standard deviations below the mean for age, size and puberty). This may occur as a result of an imbalance between bone formation and bone resorption because of a variety of reasons or as a result of abnormalities of type 1 collagen synthesis (e.g. osteogenesis imperfecta). The causes of decreased bone mineral density, which may predispose to osteoporosis and present in childhood, are shown in Table 10.6.

Table 10.5 Treatment of rickets.

Aetiology	Treatment
Vitamin D-deficient rickets	Calciferol 150,000 units by intramuscular injection, repeated at 1–2 months OR Cholecalciferol solution total dose of 150,000 units, preferably as a single dose orally or split over 3 days and repeated at 1–2 months
Rickets of prematurity as a result of phosphate deficiency	Phosphate 1 mmol/kg daily in 1–2 divided doses by mouth or as an IV infusion
Vitamin D-dependent rickets (type 1)	Calcitriol 0.25–2.0 μg per day
Vitamin D-dependent rickets (type 2)	Calcitriol, large doses (up to 50 μg per day) and long-term high-dose oral or IV calcium
Hypophosphataemic rickets	Phosphate, 2–3 mmol/kg daily in 2–4 divided doses orally (maximum dose 48 mmol in children aged 1 month to 5 years and 97 mmol in children aged 5–18 years) AND Calcitriol 15–20 ng/kg per day increased to 30–60 ng/kg per day subdivided into one or two daily doses orally.

History and examination

Osteoporosis may present with obvious signs of a long bone fracture following minimal trauma or with back pain and deformity because of underlying vertebral compression fractures (Figure 10.7). Clinical assessment and investigations should aim to exclude the causes of decreased bone mineral density shown in Table 10.6. If a child presents with osteopenia, then the following details should be elicited:

• Symptoms suggestive of associated disease (e.g. renal disease, malabsorption, inflammatory bowel disease).
• Features suggestive of growth failure or pubertal delay.
• Past medical history of fractures in the absence of significant underlying trauma.
• Medication (e.g. steroids).
• Family history of osteoporosis or fractures.

Clinical examination should include a careful assessment of growth, nutritional state, pubertal development and the clinical signs of osteogenesis imperfecta listed in Table 10.3. The presence of unexplained bone tenderness and pain, particularly in the spinal region, and in association with a spinal deformity, such as a kyphosis or scoliosis, might suggest previously unsuspected fractures. These may occur with severe osteoporosis or osteogenesis imperfecta.

Distinguishing between osteogenesis imperfecta and idiopathic juvenile osteoporosis may prove difficult. Osteogenesis imperfecta should be considered in the presence of the clinical signs listed in Table 10.3. A skull X-ray for the presence of wormian bones and a skin biopsy for fibroblast culture to assess abnormalities in the synthesis of type 1 collagen may assist in the diagnosis of osteogenesis imperfecta. Idiopathic juvenile osteoporosis may be suggested by X-ray evidence of metaphyseal compression fractures at the knee. Histomorphometric examination of bone biopsy material may also help distinguish between these two conditions.

Investigations

Bone mineral density may be measured by dual energy X-ray absorptiometry scanning of the lumbar spine or hip. This method involves minimal radiation exposure and is based on the measurement of the attenuation of X-rays of differing energy intensity as they pass through bone. However, these characteristics are influenced by the width of bone through which the X-rays pass which in children may vary as a consequence of age, body size or puberty in addition to illness. Interpretation of the data needs to take these factors into account. It is recommended that bone mineral density should only be measured in children with risk factors for low bone density associated with low trauma or recurrent fractures, back pain, spinal deformity or loss of height, change in mobility status or malnutrition.

Treatment

The following measures may help in the treatment of osteoporosis:

• Adequate analgesia for fractures.
• Physiotherapy, splints and orthopaedic intervention and occupational therapy where necessary.

Table 10.6 Causes of osteoporosis and other disorders which may lead to decreased bone mineral density.

Pathogenetic basis	Examples
Primary bone disease	Idiopathic juvenile osteoporosis
	Osteogenesis imperfecta
	Osteoporosis pseudoglioma syndrome
Inflammatory	Inflammatory bowel disease
	Rheumatoid arthritis
Endocrine	Cushing's syndrome
Drugs	Glucocorticoids
Others	Immobility
	Acute lymphoblastic leukaemia
	Thalassaemia
	Homocystinuria
	Post transplant
Causes of decreased bone mineral content (osteopenia) not necessarily severe enough to cause or osteoporosis	Anorexia
	Coeliac disease
	Hypopituitarism
	Hypogonadism (e.g. Turner's Klinefelter's syndromes)
	Hyperparathroidism
	Renal failure
	Chronic liver disease
	Thyrotoxicosis
	Burns
	Methotrexate

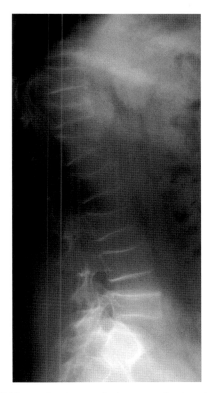

Fig. 10.7 X-rays showing vertebral compression in a child with osteoporosis.

- Optimal dietary calcium and vitamin D intake with supplements where necessary.
- Effective treatment of underlying disease.
- If osteoporosis is steroid induced, reduce daily glucocorticoid dosage as much as possible, consider alternate day therapy or use those with minimal side effects (e.g. deflazacort).
- Induction of puberty with low-dose testosterone or oestrogen if pubertal delay present (see Chapter 5).
- Calcitonin has been suggested in a few small studies to be beneficial in children with osteopenia.
- Bisphosphanates (e.g. pamidronate) have been used in childhood, mostly to treat osteogenesis imperfecta. Despite residual uncertainty about their very long-term safety, there is growing evidence that they benefit children by reducing the pain associated with fractures, increasing bone mineral density and facilitating physical rehabilitation and mobility. There seem to be few side effects in the short to medium term apart from a transient rise in body temperature, fever and influenza-like symptoms during the initial course of infusions. It is advised to optimize dietary calcium and vitamin D intake during therapy to reduce to a minimum the risks of developing hypocalcaemia. Furthermore, after prolonged use, consideration should be given to tapering the dose down gradually to avoid the development of an abrupt junction between bone formed whilst receiving bisphosphanate therapy and that formed thereafter, as this may represent a point of weakness at increased risk of fracture.

Hypercalcaemia

Aetiology

Hypercalcaemia occurs when the serum calcium concentration exceeds 2.65 mmol/L. The causes of hypercalcaemia are shown in Table 10.7.

Mild idiopathic hypercalcaemia of infancy presents with symptoms between the ages of 2 and 9 months,

Table 10.7 Causes of hypercalcaemia.

Gestational maternal hypocalcaemia
Idiopathic hypercalcaemia of infancy
Williams syndrome
Neonatal primary hyperparathyroidism
Preterm or intrauterine growth retarded-associated
    phosphate depletion
Vitamin D intoxication
Parathyroid adenoma
Isolated familial hyperparathyroidism
Multiple endocrine neoplasia type 1
Multiple endocrine neoplasia type 2A
Familial hypocalciuric hypercalcaemia
Hypercalcaemia in granulomatous disorders
Acute lymphoblastic leukaemia
Immobilization

but resolves spontaneously by the age of 4 years. When severe, it may present in the neonatal period in association with the dysmorphic features of Williams syndrome (Table 10.3 and Figure 10.8). Hypercalcaemia is associated with granulomatous disease (e.g. sarcoidosis and tuberculosis) as a result of the conversion of 25-hydroxyvitamin D to 1,25-dihydroxyvitamin D in granulomatous cells.

Neonatal hypercalcaemia

Neonatal primary hyperparathyroidism is a serious disorder of unknown aetiology which causes anorexia, hypotonia, chest deformities and respiratory distress. It is associated with a high mortality in the neonatal period and, to be successfully treated, requires urgent parathyroidectomy. This disorder is caused by homozygous mutations of the calcium-sensing receptor gene, the product of which regulates PTH secretion. Similar heterozygous mutations are responsible for autosomal dominant familial hypocalciuric hypercalcaemia.

Hypercalcaemia in childhood

Primary hyperparathyroidism may also occur in association with pituitary adenomas and gastrinomas or other pancreatic tumours (multiple endocrine neoplasia type 1) or in association with medullary thyroid cancer and phaeochromocytoma (multiple endocrine neoplasia type 2A). These two groups of disorders are inherited in an autosomal dominant fashion and all offspring of affected individuals should be screened for these endocrinopathies. The presence of elevated serum concentrations of PTH will distinguish hyperparathyroidism

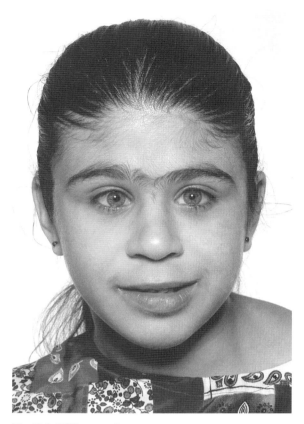

Fig. 10.8 Williams syndrome.

from hypercalcaemia caused by vitamin D intoxication, idiopathic infantile hypercalcaemia, granulomatous disease and malignancy.

History and examination

When assessing a child with possible hypercalcaemia, the following points should be highlighted in the clinical history:
- Symptoms suggestive of hypercalcaemia (e.g. weakness, anorexia, nausea and vomiting, constipation, polyuria and polydipsia).
- Symptoms suggestive of tuberculosis or sarcoidosis.
- Vitamin D therapy.
- A family history of multiple endocrine neoplasia.

Investigations

If hypercalcaemia is suspected, a blood sample should be taken for the measurement of:
- calcium;
- phosphate;

- PTH;
- 25-hydroxyvitamin D; and
- a sample stored for possible measurement of 1,25-dihydroxyvitamin D concentration later, should this be indicated.

The differential diagnosis of biochemical abnormalities of calcium metabolism is shown in Table 10.4.

Treatment

The treatment of hypercalcaemia involves promoting a low-calcium diet and where relevant, stopping vitamin D, calcium supplements and other drugs, such as thiazides, which increase calcium concentrations. Patients should be encouraged to drink plenty of fluids. If significant dehydration is present, this should be corrected with IV 0.9% saline. Prednisolone may be helpful if hypercalcaemia is secondary to sarcoidosis or vitamin D intoxication. If hypercalcaemia persists, bisphosphanate therapy may help by inhibiting mobilization of calcium from the skeleton. A parathyroid adenoma may be located by careful ultrasound examination and treated by surgical removal of the affected gland. Hyperparathyroidism caused by diffuse hyperplasia requires surgical removal of all four glands.

When to involve a specialist centre

- Hypoparathyroidism.
- Hypophosphataemic rickets.
- Osteoporosis which is of sufficient severity that treatment with bisphosphanates is to be considered.
- Osteoporosis secondary to other underlying disorders (e.g. inflammatory bowel disease, rheumatoid arthritis or Cushing's syndrome) should have the treatment of their underlying disease discussed with the relevant specialists.
- Hyperparathyroidism.

Transition

Many causes of hypocalcaemia, rickets and hypercalcaemia are transient and resolve in childhood without the need for referral onto adult services. However, where the underlying cause has potential implications into adult life (e.g. hypoparathyroidism or pseudohypoparathyroidism), then referral through local transition arrangements should be organized. Of note, even if well and currently asymptomatic, children known to be at risk of multiple endocrine neoplasia require referral into adult

services for organization of ongoing monitoring. Where there is an underlying genetic cause for a disorder of bone or calcium biochemistry which may have implications for future offspring, organization of genetic counselling may be particularly important.

Given the importance of bone mineral accretion into the third decade of life, teenagers undergoing monitoring for osteopenia should also be referred. Discussion may need to take place between paediatric and adult specialists regarding the interpretation of successive bone mineral density scan reports given that paediatric practice involves interpreting data for body size whereas the tendency in adult practice is to interpret data relative to peak bone mass (T scores).

Future developments

- Administration of sufficiently high doses of phosphate to children with hypophosphataemic rickets remains problematical and alternative therapeutic strategies are required to prevent the development of bone deformity in these children.
- The cause of idiopathic juvenile osteoporosis remains to be established. A diagnostic test for both this and osteogenesis imperfecta is much needed to assist clinicians in the investigation and management of children presenting with fractures associated with severe osteoporosis.
- More information is required about the long-term safety of bisphosphanate treatment and on alternative strategies for the treatment of severe childhood osteoporosis.
- Clarification of the molecular basis of primary hyperparathyroidism will enable earlier detection of this disorder and of multiple endocrine neoplasia type 1. The discovery of the calcium-sensing receptor offers the promise of alternative therapeutic strategies for the treatment of hyperparathyroidism.

Controversial points

- Does the severity of osteopenia in the growing child predict the future fracture risk as in postmenopausal women?
- Do girls with Turner's syndrome have an increased risk of osteopenia over and above that caused by inadequately treated hypogonadism?
- Do androgens have a direct effect on bone mineralization which is independent of their conversion to oestrogens?

• Is bisphosphanate treatment indicated for the treatment of osteopenia in the absence of fractures?
• Is bisphosphanate treatment in young children without risk to future bone health?
• What are the frequency and aetiology of fractures in infancy not due to non-accidental injury?

Potential pitfalls

• *Diagnostic confusion between vitamin D deficiency and hypoparathyroidism as the cause of hypocalcaemia in infancy:* Careful interpretation of serum concentrations of phosphate, PTH and vitamin D should help distinguish between the two conditions.
• Overaggressive treatment of hypoparathyroidism increasing the risks of nephrocalcinosis.
• Unnecessary measurement of bone mineral density in a child at relatively low risk of developing osteoporosis.

• Incorrect diagnosis of osteoporosis based only on X-ray findings reportedly suggestive of osteopenia or from failure to take into account a child's small size when interpreting a dual energy X-ray measurement of bone mineral density.
• Failure clinically to suspect vertebral compression fractures. These should be considered in any child with osteoporosis who complains of backache or stiffness or who has evidence of even relatively minor spinal shape deformity.
• *Diagnostic confusion between osteogenesis imperfecta and non-accidental injury as the cause of fractures in a young child:* Where the diagnosis is unclear, these children should be referred for further evaluation by clinicians with expertise in child protection and bone disease.
• Failure to appreciate that most causes of hypercalcaemia in infancy are benign, self-limiting and respond well to conservative management.

Case histories

Case 10.1

A 2-year-old boy was referred for further assessment of his increasingly bowed legs. His mother was known to have hypophosphataemic rickets. X-rays show bowing of the femoral shafts but no radiological evidence of rickets. The following blood measurements were obtained:

Calcium 2.37 mmol/L [9.50 mg/dL]
Phosphate 1.13 mmol/L [3.50 mg/dL]
Alkaline phosphatase 805 IU/L (reference range 100–400 IU/L)
PTH 1.3 pmol/L [12.35 pg/mL] (reference range 0.9–5.5 pmol/L)

Questions

1 Is this child likely to have X-linked hypophosphataemic rickets?
2 What additional investigations may clarify the diagnosis?

Answers

1 This boy has a 50% chance of inheriting rickets from his mother. With an X-linked dominant disorder, he would be expected to be more severely affected than his mother. In the presence of his bone deformity, the absence of biochemical evidence of hypophosphataemia is surprising.
2 A simultaneous blood and urine sample should be obtained for the measurement of phosphate and creatinine so that the renal threshold phosphate concentration can be calculated (Kruse *et al.* 1982; Shaw *et al.* 1990). In this patient, the diagnosis of X-linked hypophosphataemic rickets was confirmed by the demonstration of a markedly decreased tubular reabsorption of phosphate (55%) and a renal threshold phosphate concentration of 1.4 mmol/L.

Case 10.2

A 9-year-old girl was admitted with severe back pain after she had fallen over her dog. She had sustained a previous fracture of her wrist following significant trauma. Her weight was above the 99th centile, height on the 50th centile and she had early breast development.

X-rays demonstrated multiple wedge collapse fractures of several thoracic and lumbar vertebrae and widespread osteopenia. Initial investigations demonstrated the following:

 Calcium 2.45 mmol/L [9.82 mg/dL]
 Phosphate 1.32 mmol/L [4.10 mg/dL]
 Alkaline phosphatase 264 IU/L (reference range 100–400 IU/L)
 PTH 4.2 pmol/L [40 pg/mL] (reference range 0.9–5.5 pmol/L)
 25-hydroxyvitamin D 12.4 ng/mL [39.9 pg/mL] (reference range 8–50 ng/mL)
 C-reactive protein <1 mg/L
 Normal renal, liver and thyroid function tests, and antiendomysial antibody concentrations

Questions
1 What further clinical observations would be of interest?
2 What additional investigations are required?
3 What is the differential diagnosis?

Answers
1 It would be helpful to know if she had evidence of blue-coloured sclerae, joint hyperextensibility or abnormal hearing which might suggest osteogenesis imperfecta. Given her obesity, it might also be important to assess for other signs suggestive of Cushing's syndrome.
2 A dual energy X-ray absorptiometry scan confirmed the severity of the osteopenia with a lumbar spine bone mineral content of −112.79SD and femoral neck −3.65SD. Three 24-hour urine collections demonstrated normal cortisol excretion rates which excluded Cushing's syndrome.
3 This girl is most likely to have either idiopathic juvenile osteoporosis or, possibly, osteogenesis imperfecta.

Case 10.3
A 3-month-old boy presented to a peripheral unit with cyanosis during feeding. No abnormalities were found on clinical examination and these episodes did not reoccur thereafter. Investigations at presentation showed the following:
 Serum calcium 2.72 mmol/L [10.9 mg/dL]

 Serum phosphate 1.73 mmol/L [5.37 mg/dL]
 Urinary calcium:creatinine ratio 0.91 mmol/mmol creatinine (normal <0.7 mmol/mmol creatinine)
Serial blood samples over the next 6 months continued to demonstrate mild hypercalcaemia. Although he remained clinically well, he was referred for further assessment.

Questions
1 What other investigations are indicated?
2 When and what treatment is worth considering?
3 Investigations following referral did not demonstrate any additional abnormal findings and the serum calcium concentration normalized at the age of 1 year. What is the likely diagnosis?

Answers
1 The infant should undergo measurement of PTH and vitamin D status. A renal ultrasound is useful to check for nephrocalcinosis. The parents should undergo measurement of their serum calcium, phosphate and PTH concentrations and if abnormalities are present, discussion with geneticists regarding mutational screening of genes involved in the calcium sensing receptor or PTH is indicated. The absence of any dysmorphic features makes a diagnosis of Williams syndrome relatively unlikely though this can be formally excluded by screening for mutations of the elastin gene.
2 In the presence of persistent hypercalcaemia, particularly when associated with symptoms, a calcium and vitamin D restricted diet should be offered.
3 The absence of any abnormal findings on investigation and spontaneous resolution of the hypercalcaemia would be consistent with a diagnosis of idiopathic infantile hypercalcaemia.

Case 10.4
A 2-year-old Pakistani girl was referred with bowing of her legs. She experiences no difficulties walking and is said to have a good diet with plenty of dairy products. Initial blood tests demonstrate the following:
 Calcium 2.43 mmol/L [9.7 mg/dL]
 Phosphate 1.66 mmol/L [5.15 mg/dL]

Alkaline phosphatase 330 IU/L (reference range 100–300 IU/L)

25-OH cholecalciferol <7.0 ng/ml (reference range (>30 ng/mL)

PTH 10.8 pmol/L (reference range 0.9–5.4 pmol/L)

Questions

1 What features in the clinical history should be explored?
2 What other investigations are indicated?
3 What treatment is required?

Answers

1 Enquiry should be made into how long this child was breast-fed and whether mother's vitamin D status is known. Also, the presence of symptoms of malabsorption should be explored. In this case, mother received treatment during pregnancy for vitamin D deficiency and breast-fed till 23 months with no recent assessment of her vitamin D status.
2 An X-ray of her legs is indicated to see if there are radiological signs of rickets.
3 She requires vitamin D treatment.

Case 10.5

A 4-month-old girl with a known ventriculo-septal defect and failure to thrive was admitted with diarrhoea after starting antibiotics for a chest infection. She was also receiving Amiloride and Frusemide. She was found to have hypocalcaemia and blood tests demonstrated the following:

Calcium 1.97 mmol/L [7.9 mg/dL]

Phosphate 2.61 mmol/L [8.1 mg/dL]

Alkaline phosphatase 270 IU/L (reference range 100–300 IU/L)

PTH 2.6 pmol/L (reference range 0.9–5.4 pmol/L)

Urine calcium:creatinine ratio 0.95 mmol/mmol creatinine

Questions

1 What other investigations does she require?
2 What is the likely diagnosis?
3 What treatment may be required?

Answers

1 She requires fluorescence *in situ* hybridization (FISH) studies for a microdeletion of chromosome 22q11 and given her clinical history, measurement of her T-cell subsets.
2 Despite the presence of normal T-cell subsets, a microdeletion of chromosome 22q11 was confirmed, consistent with a diagnosis of DiGeorge Syndrome.
3 She may require alfacalcidol therapy to maintain serum calcium around 2.0–2.2 mmol/L with ongoing monitoring of her urinary calcium losses to ensure that therapy does not put her at risk of nephrocalcinosis.

Key weblinks

www.nos.org.uk The National Osteoporosis Society is a UK-based charity dedicated to the diagnosis, prevention and treatment of osteoporosis.

Significant guidelines/consensus statements

Fewtrell, M.S., on behalf of the British Paediatric and Adolescent Bone Group (2003) Bone densitometry in children assessed by dual x ray absorptiometry: uses and pitfalls. *Archives of Disease in Childhood* **88**, 795–798.

Lewiecki, E.M., Gordon, C.M., Baim, S. *et al.* (2008) International Society for Clinical Densitometry 2007 adult and pediatric official positions. *Bone* **43**, 1115–1121.

Wagner, C.L., Greer, F.R., American Academy of Pediatrics Section on Breastfeeding & American Academy of Pediatrics Committee on Nutrition (2008) Prevention of rickets and vitamin D deficiency in infants, children, and adolescents. *Pediatrics* **122**, 1142–1152.

Useful information for patients and parents

National Osteoporosis Society, Camerton, Bath, BA2
0PJ, UK. Tel: 08454 500230. Website:
www.nos.org.uk. Contains useful information about
osteoporosis.
National Osteoporosis Foundation, 1232 22nd Street
NW, Washington DC 20037, USA. Tel: 1 (800) 231
4222. Website: www.nof.org. Contains helpful
information about bone health in adolescence.

Further reading

Al Zahrani, A. & Levine, M.A. (1997) Primary hyperparathyroidism. *Lancet* **349**, 1233–1238.
Kruse, K. (1992) Vitamin D and parathyroid. In: *Functional Endocrinologic Diagnostics in Children and Adolescents* (ed. M.B. Ranke), 1st edn., pp. 153–167. J & J Verlag., Mannheim.

Kruse, K., Kracht, U. & Göpfert, G. (1982) Renal threshold phosphate concentration (TmPO4/GFR). *Archives of Disease in Childhood* **57**, 217–223.
Marini, J.C. (2003) Do bisphosphanates make children's bones brittle or better? *New England Journal of Medicine* **349**, 423–426.
Reid, I.R. (ed.) (1997) *Baillière's Clinical Endocrinology and Metabolism: Metabolic Bone Disease.* Ballière Tindall, London.
Shaw, N.J., Wheeldon, J. & Brocklebank, J.T. (1990) Indices of intact serum parathyroid hormone and renal excretion of calcium, phosphate and magnesium. *Archives of Disease in Childhood* **65**, 1208–1211.
Singh, J., Moghal, N., Pearce, S.H.S. & Cheetham, T. (2003) The investigation of hypocalcaemia and rickets. *Archives of Disease in Childhood* **88**, 403–407.
Warner, J.T., Cowan, F.J., Dunstan, F.D.J. *et al.* (1998) Measured and predicted bone mineral content in healthy boys and girls aged 6–18 years: adjustment for body size and puberty. *Acta Paediatrica* **87**, 244–249.
Wharton, B. & Bishop, N. (2003) Rickets. *Lancet* **362**, 1389–1400.
Zipitis, C.S. & Akobeng, A.K. (2008) Vitamin D supplementation in early childhood and risk of type 1 diabetes: a systematic review and meta-analysis. *Archives of Disease in Childhood* **93**, 512–517.

11 Obesity

Physiology

Definition

In childhood, obesity may be assessed in different ways. Measurement of weight alone is inadequate given the influence of height on weight. Although obesity may be clinically obvious if the child's weight centile is greater than the height centile, the severity of obesity is better defined by the use of the body mass index (BMI) in which

$$BMI = weight(kg)/(height(m))^2$$

Alternatively, body fatness can be assessed from direct measurements of subcutaneous skinfold thickness using skinfold thickness calipers or from measurement of waist circumference. Given the normal variations of BMI, skinfold thickness and waist circumference through childhood, reference to centile charts is required for interpretation of the data. The utility of skinfold thickness and waist circumference measurements is limited by the practical difficulties of obtaining these measurements accurately and so measurement of BMI is currently the best clinical method for identifying and monitoring obesity in childhood.

There are no widely agreed definitions of obesity in childhood as there are few data correlating specific definitions with future health risks. In practice in the United Kingdom, children with a BMI above the age- and sex-specific 91st centile can be defined as overweight and those above the 98th centile as obese (see Appendix 2 for United Kingdom 1990 sex-specific BMI centile reference charts).

Throughout the industrialized world, there is clear evidence of a recent, rapid increase in the prevalence of obesity in children and adults, with older children more affected than infants. In the United States, more than 30% of children have a BMI that exceeds the 95th centile.

Aetiology

An increased risk of obesity is associated with genetic, environmental (Table 11.1) and pathological factors (Table 11.2). It is likely that a combination of an increasingly sedentary lifestyle combined with an excessive calorie intake for need is principally responsible for the rapid increase in prevalence of obesity noted over the last decade.

Obese children under 3 years of age without obese parents are at low risk of obesity in adulthood. However, in older children the presence of obesity becomes an increasingly important predictor of adult obesity, regardless of whether the parents are obese or not, with more than two-thirds of children who are obese aged 10 years or older becoming obese adults. Parental obesity more than doubles the risk of adult obesity in young children. Twin studies have suggested a heritability of fat mass of 40–70%.

Regulation of body fat

The normal amounts of body fat change through childhood, as can be seen from the BMI centile charts (Appendix 2). Infants gain fat, as a consequence of increasing adipose cell size, relatively rapidly until the age of 1 year, but then slim down until the age of approximately

Table 11.1 Non-pathological risk factors for obesity.

Risk factor	Examples
Genetic	Obesity in either or both parents
	Early adiposity rebound
Environmental	Socioeconomic deprivation
	Single child
	Single parent
Diet-related	Bottle-fed in infancy
	High fat diet
	Disorganized eating patterns
Activity-related	Physical inactivity
	Increased television watching
	Short sleep duration

6 years as adipose cells reduce in size. From this point onwards, there is a steady increase in body fat into young adult life (the so-called 'adiposity rebound') associated with increases in adipose cell numbers. There is little difference in the amount of body fat in infant girls and boys.

Table 11.2 Pathological causes of obesity.

Cause	Examples
Syndromes	Laurence–Moon–Biedl syndrome
	Down's syndrome
	Prader–Willi syndrome (Fig. 11.2)
Single gene mutations	*Melanocortin-4 receptor*
	Proopiomelanocortin
	Leptin
	Leptin receptor
	Pseudohypoparathyroidism
Hypothalamic damage	Trauma
	Tumours, e.g. craniopharyngioma
	Post encephalitis
Endocrine abnormalities	Growth hormone deficiency
	Hypothyroidism
	Cushing's syndrome
	Hyperinsulinism
Immobility	Spina bifida
	Cerebral palsy
Impaired skeletal growth	Achondroplasia
Drugs	Insulin
	Steroids
	Antithyroid drugs
	Sodium valproate

However, after infancy subcutaneous fat increases more rapidly in girls, particularly during puberty when males demonstrate greater centralization of body fat stores.

Obesity occurs when energy intake chronically exceeds energy expenditure. In obese children there are wide variations in energy intake and not all obese children eat excessively. The high calorie density and fat content of the modern diet is associated with an increased risk of obesity.

The hypothalamus has a central role in the regulation of energy balance, integrating neuronal, hormonal and nutrient messages from within the body and transmitting signals which lead to the sensations of hunger or satiety (Figure 11.1). The hypothalamus also influences energy expenditure via autonomic nerve function and the regulation of pituitary hormone release. Many hypothalamic neurotransmitters have been shown to influence energy intake (Table 11.3).

Energy expenditure consists of the following three components:

1 Resting metabolic rate is the energy expended at rest for the maintenance of basic cellular activities, excluding maintenance of body temperature, and it accounts for 60–70% of total energy expenditure. Fat-free mass is metabolically more active than fat mass. Obese individuals have increased amounts of both body fat and fat-free mass and therefore most obese individuals have increases in their **absolute** resting metabolic rates because of their increased fat-free mass.

2 Thermogenesis is the energy expended in response to digestion and absorption of food, temperature changes, emotional influences or drugs which influence the physiological responses to such stimuli. It accounts for about 10% of total energy expenditure. It is unlikely that variations in thermogenesis are clinically important in the energy balance of the obese individual.

3 Energy expended in physical activity in children varies widely both on an individual daily basis and between individuals and accounts for 20–30% of total energy expenditure. Although obese children may be relatively physically inactive, they have an increase in the energy cost of weight-bearing activities and therefore do not demonstrate marked reductions in this component of energy expenditure when compared to normal-weight children.

As a consequence of these influences on energy expenditure, in most obese children, **absolute** total energy expenditure is increased. However, there is evidence that a low **relative** metabolic rate (i.e. adjusted for body size) predisposes to weight gain.

Complex interactions exist between signalling pathways that control energy intake and satiety and those that

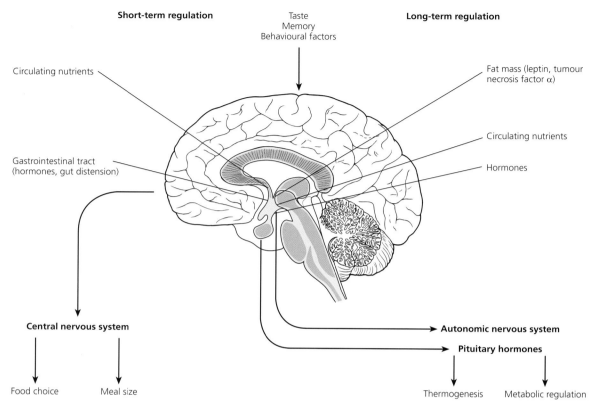

Fig. 11.1 Influences on the hypothalamic control of satiety.

regulate fat mass. Adipose tissue may influence the hypothalamic regulation of energy balance through the secretion of leptin, a hormone which crosses the blood–brain barrier and suppresses the production of neuropeptide Y within the hypothalamus leading to reduced appetite and increased energy expenditure. However, most obese children have increased leptin concentrations in proportion to their increased body fat. Disorders of leptin synthesis or action are very rare and account for few cases of obesity.

Preliminary examination and investigation

History

Most children with obesity do not have an underlying pathological cause and have so-called 'simple obesity'. Such children usually demonstrate rapid growth and physical development. By contrast, children who are obese, short and growing slowly are much more likely to have an endocrine abnormality or, if associated with dysmorphic features and intellectual impairment, a syndromic cause to their obesity. A careful history and examination is required to distinguish the few children with significant underlying pathology causing their obesity from those who have 'simple obesity'. The history should include the following details:

• *Birth weight:* If increased this suggests an underlying mechanism, such as hyperinsulinism, which may have started *in utero.*

• Age of onset of obesity, as early onset of obesity (before the age of 2 years) or while exclusively breast-fed is more suggestive of a genetic or syndromic cause.

• Presence of congenital abnormalities or symptoms suggestive of a syndrome (e. g. initial feeding problems requiring nasogastric tube feeds and hypotonia with certain dysmorphic features might suggest Prader–Willi syndrome; see Figure 11.2).

• *Detailed feeding and dietary history:* It is often useful to go through a typical day's diet.

Table 11.3 Factors which influence the hypothalamic regulation of energy intake.

Factors which increase food intake	Factors which decrease food intake
Noradrenaline	Serotonin
Opioids	Dopamine
Ghrelin	Cholecystokinin
Galanin	Corticotrophin-releasing factor
Neuropeptide Y	Neurotensin
Melanin-concentrating hormone	Bombesin
Agouti-related peptide	Calcitonin gene-related peptide
	Amylin
	Adrenomedullin
	Peptide YY$^{3-36}$
	Leptin
	Glucagon
	Glucagon-like peptide 1
	α-Melanocyte stimulating hormone
	Cocaine- and amphetamine-related peptide

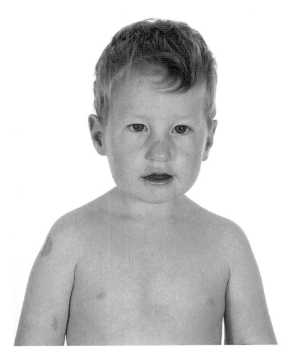

Fig. 11.2 Prader–Willi syndrome.

- Information about levels of physical activity.
- The extent to which the obesity may be having adverse effects — particularly psychosocial or related to school — on the child, the desire of the child and parents for the child to lose weight and the extent and success of previous interventions to achieve weight control.
- Medication.
- Symptoms of hypothalamo–pituitary pathology (e.g. headache, visual symptoms or previous history of trauma or encephalitis).
- Symptoms suggestive of endocrine abnormality (Table 11.2).
- Presence of polydipsia and polyuria (indicative of type 2 diabetes).
- Family history of obesity.

Examination

On examination, the child should undergo an accurate assessment of height and weight with measurements plotted on height, weight and BMI centile charts. Height measurements should be compared with the target height range derived from the mid-parental height centile as those who are relatively short for their genetic background are more likely to have a syndromic or endocrine cause for their obesity, whereas those who are relatively tall are more likely to suffer from simple obesity. Further assessment of the severity of the obesity can be made from the measurement of waist circumference or triceps and subscapular skinfold thickness although these measurement techniques require training and are difficult to perform in very obese individuals. Not all pathological causes of obesity will be self-evident and careful clinical examination is required to identify signs suggestive of certain disorders or complications of obesity. It is particularly important to note the presence of acanthosis nigricans (Plate 1) most commonly seen in the axillae or neck as this may indicate evolving insulin resistance and an increased risk of developing type 2 diabetes. Key signs to note on clinical examination are shown in Table 11.4. The clinical features of syndromes, which may present with obesity, are summarized in Table 11.5.

Complications

The main adverse effects of obesity are summarized in Table 11.6. In childhood, acute medical complications of

Table 11.4 Clinical signs to look for on examination.

Clinical sign	Possible diagnosis
Acanthosis nigricans (Plate 1)	Type 2 diabetes (insulin resistance)
Hypertension	Syndrome X
Dysmorphic features (see Table 11.5)	Laurence–Moon–Biedl syndrome (Fig. 11.3)
	Prader–Willi syndrome (Fig. 11.2)
	Pseudohypoparathyroidism (Fig. 11.4)
	Beckwith–Wiedemann syndrome
Impaired visual fields	Intracranial tumour,
Papilloedema or optic atrophy	e.g. craniopharyngioma
Tall stature or increased height velocity	Simple obesity Hyperinsulinism
Short stature or decreased height velocity	Growth hormone deficiency Hypothyroidism Laurence–Moon–Biedl syndrome Prader–Willi syndrome Pseudohypoparathyroidism
Cranial midline defects (e.g. cleft lip and palate)	Growth hormone deficiency
Truncal obesity Goitre Prolonged ankle tendon reflexes	Hypothyroidism
Proximal myopathy Hypertension Truncal obesity	Cushing's syndrome
Abnormal gait	Spina bifida Cerebral palsy

simple obesity are usually few and minor. The combination of insulin resistance, hypertension, hypertriglyceridaemia and a low concentration of high-density lipoprotein cholesterol (so-called 'Syndrome X' or the 'multimetabolic syndrome') used to be rarely seen in childhood though in the United States, 'one in four' overweight children in the age group 6–12 years now has impaired glucose tolerance and 60% of these have at least one risk factor for heart disease. There are particular concerns about the increased prevalence of obesity and its metabolic complications in ethnic minority groups in both the United Kingdom and USA. Furthermore, being overweight in childhood has recently been shown to be a major risk fac-

tor for the development of the multimetabolic syndrome in adult life. More commonly, obese children are tall for their age and have advanced skeletal development with an advanced bone age. A few may undergo precocious puberty with potentially adverse consequences for their final adult height. Why excess body fat has this effect is unclear. Obese children may also have an impaired self-image and for boys this may be complicated by a marked suprapubic fat pad leading to the penis being buried in fat and, as a result, appearing very small.

Investigations

The following investigations should be considered in those in whom there is clinical concern regarding an underlying pathological cause or a possible metabolic complication of obesity:

• An assessment of glucose tolerance, for example urinalysis for glycosuria, fasting blood glucose or, occasionally, an oral glucose tolerance test.
• Increased fasting serum insulin and decreased sex-hormone-binding globulin concentrations may confirm the presence of insulin resistance.
• Lipid profile.
• Thyroid function tests (TFTs) (serum T4 and TSH concentrations).
• Liver function tests.
• Three 24-hour urinary cortisol estimations.
• Bone age.
• Serum LH, FSH, oestradiol, 17-hydroxy progesterone, androstenedione and testosterone concentrations and a pelvic ultrasound in a girl with hirsuitism or menstrual irregularity thought to be at risk of having polycystic ovarian disease. The need for additional investigations will depend on the level of clinical concern.
• In cases of suspected or proven hypothyroidism, Cushing's syndrome, hyperinsulinism or growth hormone (GH) deficiency, consult the relevant chapter for further investigations.
• If Laurence–Moon–Biedl syndrome is suspected, referral to a geneticist may be of help in identifying the relevant dysmorphic features and referral to an ophthalmologist for detailed retinal examination including electroretinography is important.
• Children with Prader–Willi syndrome caused by a deletion of chromosome 15(q11–13) or unimaternal disomy may be diagnosed by a combination of fluorescent in situ hybridisation (FISH) probing and DNA testing.
• If pseudohypoparathyroidism is suspected, measure serum calcium, phosphate and parathyroid hormone (PTH) concentrations. In the case of a low serum calcium

Table 11.5 Clinical features of common syndromic causes of obesity (Figs 11.2, 11.3 and 11.4).

System	Prader–Willi syndrome	Laurence–Moon–Biedl syndrome	Pseudohypo-parathyroidism
Facial	Narrow forehead Olive-shaped eyes Antimongoloid slant Epicanthic folds Squint Carp mouth Micrognathia Abnormal ear lobes	Squint	Round facies Short neck
Skeletal	Short stature Small hands and feet Clinodactyly Syndactyly Scoliosis Dislocated hips	Short stature Polydactyly Clinodactyly	Short stature Shortened fourth metacarpals and metatarsals
Neuromuscular	↓ IQ Hypotonia and feeding problems in infancy Insatiable appetite Uncontrollable rage	↓ IQ Retinitis pigmentosa	↓ IQ
Endocrine	Hypogonadotrophic hypogonadism Type 2 diabetes	Hypogonadotrophic hypogonadism Diabetes insipidus	PTH-resistant hypocalcaemia
Other		Renal anomalies	Subcutaneous calcifications

and elevated phosphate and PTH, the diagnosis may be confirmed by demonstration of deactivating mutations of the gene encoding the G protein stimulatory, a subunit which is located on the long arm of chromosome 20.

• In syndromes associated with hypogonadism, investigation of the pituitary–gonadal axis should be considered in those who have genital hypoplasia, markedly delayed puberty or inadequate development of secondary sex characteristics (see Chapter 5).

Treatment

Young infants frequently appear obese and a spontaneous reduction in body fat occurs as part of the normal changes in body composition with increasing age. In general, therefore, it is rare that a slimming regimen needs to be considered in the young child. However, investigations to exclude a pathological cause of obesity should be undertaken in all infants with severe, early onset obesity. If calorie restriction is deemed necessary in infancy, the aim should be maintenance of body weight rather than weight loss, as the latter may lead to specific dietary (e. g. vitamin) deficiencies or growth failure.

For many obese children, weight loss down to an 'ideal body weight for height' is probably unrealistic. Nevertheless, more modest weight reduction, or even prevention of further weight gain, may produce significant longer term health benefits. Such goals, which are more likely to be achievable, should be considered when planning individual therapeutic regimens. Unfortunately, there is almost no published evidence for any effective treatment for childhood obesity.

Older children with simple obesity should be encouraged to try and control their weight gain by:

• educating about the nature of obesity and its longer term consequences;

• realistic assessment of the ease and likely benefits of slimming regimens;

• healthy eating (e. g. regular family meal times, avoidance of excessive 'snacking', fried foods, added fats and sugars and high energy drinks while encouraging foods with high fibre content) with modest calorie restriction and advice from a dietitian where necessary;

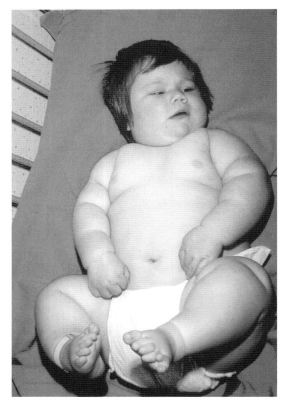

Fig. 11.3 Polydactyly in a child with Laurence–Moon–Biedl syndrome.

Table 11.6 Complications of simple obesity.

System	Adverse effect
Metabolic and endocrine	Hyperinsulinaemia
	Impaired glucose tolerance
	Type 2 diabetes
	Hyperlipidaemia
	Syndrome X (multimetabolic syndrome)
	Advanced pubertal development
	Polycystic ovarian disease
	Steatohepatitis
Cardiovascular	Hypertension
Respiratory	Breathless on exertion
	Obstructive sleep apnoea
	Pickwickian syndrome
Skeletal	Knock knee or bow legs
	Slipped capital femoral epiphysis
Psychological	Poor self-image
	Bullying
	Behavioural problems

• increasing habitual physical activity (e. g. walking rather than taking transport to school, participation in games or sports that the child enjoys, restricting television or computer games); and

• psychological support (e. g. regular attendance at a dedicated clinic with dietetic support, group therapy (e. g. Weight Watchers) with the emphasis on mutual support, promotion of positive self-esteem and enhancing motivation to change life-style factors).

Once a child has developed significant obesity, both weight loss and long-term maintenance of an improved body weight become difficult to achieve. Encouragement for children with simple obesity is best provided by

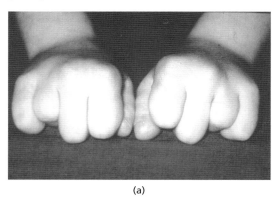

(a)

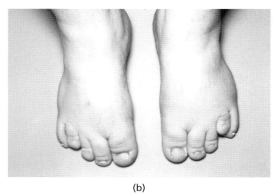

(b)

Fig. 11.4 Shortening of the fourth metacarpal (a) and metatarsal (b) in pseudohypoparathyroidism.

frequent visits (e. g. 3-monthly) by the patient to a clinic or support service with motivated and interested staff. Multidisciplinary services involving community paediatricians, general practitioners, dietitians, psychologists or psychiatrists may help to improve the outcome. However, there is no point in continuing to encourage attendance in obese patients who fail to adhere to suggested interventions and who fail to achieve significant weight loss, although intermittent clinical follow-up to monitor for early signs of the complications of obesity may still be necessary.

Although medical therapy, including inhibitors of nutrient absorption from the gut (e. g. acarbose, guar gum and pancreatic lipase inhibitors), appetite suppressants (e. g. amphetamine derivatives and serotoninergic agents) and agents which increase energy expenditure (e. g. thyroxine (T4) and adrenergic agonists), have been used in the treatment of obesity in adults there is little experience of their use and efficacy in childhood. Side effects may be problematical and their use is not currently recommended in children. There is increasing interest in the value of surgical interventions, such as laparoscopic gastric banding or the Roux-en-Y gastric bypass procedure in extremely obese children. When undertaken in children, dramatic amounts of weight loss can be achieved though such children will require careful monitoring for side effects in specialist clinical services.

Where obesity is the consequence of an underlying endocrinopathy, treatment of hormone deficiency with the relevant hormone replacement (e. g. GH or T4) should result in a decrease in body fat. There is evidence that Prader–Willi syndrome is associated with hypothalamic dysfunction, including impaired GH secretion. GH therapy (0.25 mg/kg per week to a maximum of 2.7 mg daily) is now indicated for the improvement of growth and body composition in children with Prader–Willi syndrome, providing there is no evidence of upper airway obstruction or severe obesity (weight exceeding 200% of ideal for height) and pre-treatment sleep studies do not demonstrate any evidence of sleep apnoea. Specific medical or surgical interventions for hyperinsulinism or Cushing's syndrome will also lead to significant weight loss.

When to involve a specialist centre

- Children with suspected hypothalamic tumours or endocrine causes of obesity should be managed in consultation with centres with expertise in the relevant neurosurgical investigations and paediatric endocrinology.

- Children with obesity of such severity that significant adverse cardio-respiratory consequences are suspected may need referral to a specialist unit for a detailed cardio-respiratory assessment, including sleep studies.
- Children with sufficiently severe obesity that drug treatment or surgery is to be considered should be referred to a specialist centre for further evaluation.

Future developments

- High-quality randomized controlled trials of lifestyle interventions which aim to prevent or treat obesity in childhood by altering eating behaviour or patterns of physical activity are required.
- A clarification of the role and benefits of pharmacological interventions in obese children.
- An evaluation of the risks and benefits of surgery to treat childhood obesity.
- Clarification of the value and ideal structure of an 'obesity service'.

Further research should clarify the role and relationship between the multiple neurotransmitters known to influence hypothalamic function in the hope that a compound will be discovered which may have a significant effect on satiety without adverse side effects.

Transition

Obese teenage patients who have significant co-morbidities such as type 2 diabetes or other metabolic abnormalities or those experiencing significant adverse effects on cardio-respiratory function will require referral to adult services in their mid- to late teenage years. Seeing these patients in a joint clinic staffed by both adult and paediatric specialists may be especially helpful to the paediatrician as it is likely that his adult colleagues will have much greater experience of a range of therapeutic interventions relevant to the management of the obese individual, some of which may be of value in the teenage age group.

Controversial points

- How extensively should tall, obese children with no dysmorphic features be investigated?
- How relatively important are genetic and environmental risk factors for obesity in childhood?

- What is the future risk of obesity in adult life for an obese young child?
- Is childhood-onset obesity a risk factor for adverse metabolic consequences in adult life, independent of the presence of obesity in adult life?
- Are children who become obese less active than those who do not?
- Do children from obese families, who are at increased risk of obesity, have an inherited decrease in their metabolic rates?

Potential pitfalls

- Failure to recognize the diagnostic importance of distinguishing between obese children who are relatively tall and those who are short.
- Excessive and unrealistic expectations of the likely success of interventions to treat childhood obesity, especially when both parents are already obese.
- Over-investigation for a non-existent pathological cause of obesity in an otherwise well, normally growing, relatively tall child.
- Encouraging obese children to achieve dramatic short-term weight loss is unlikely to be successful in achieving satisfactory regulation of longer term weight.
- Excessive weight loss may lead to impaired growth.
- Delayed diagnosis of type 2 diabetes or its misdiagnosis as type 1 diabetes in an obese child with minimal symptoms and absence of ketonuria when hyperglycaemia is finally documented.
- Failure to diagnose clinically significant disturbances of respiratory function during sleep.

Case histories

Case 11.1

A 12-year-old boy presented with obesity. He had been floppy and a poor feeder as an infant with recurrent fits until the age of 7 years. On examination, he had developmental delay and special educational needs. His height was on the 50th centile and weight well above the 97th centile. The following measurements were obtained on a basal blood sample:

   Calcium 1.95 mmol/L [7.82 mg/dL]
   Albumin 41 g/L [4.1 g/dL]
   Phosphate 1.90 mmol/L [5.9 mg/dL]
   Creatinine 78 μmol/L [0.9 mg/dL]

   Alkaline phosphatise 202 IU/L (reference range 100–400)
   PTH 14.5 pmol/L (reference range 0.9–5.5) [138 pg/mL (reference range 10–65)]
   25-OH-cholecalciferol 16.1 ng/mL (reference range 8–50)
   Free T4 11 pmol/L (reference range 9.8–23.1) [0.88 ng/dL (reference range 0.8–2.4)]
   TSH 5.7 mU/L (reference range 0.35–5.5)

Questions
1 What do these results demonstrate?
2 What is the most likely diagnosis?
3 What additional investigations may clarify the diagnosis?

Answers
1 Hypocalcaemia with hyperphosphataemia, raised PTH concentration and borderline TFT results.
2 Pseudohypoparathyroidism is the most likely diagnosis.
3 The presence of PTH resistance may be confirmed by demonstrating absence of a urinary cAMP response to an infusion of PTH. DNA analysis may confirm the underlying genetic defect. If hypothyroidism is suspected clinically, repeat thyroid function testing or a TRH stimulation test may be helpful to assess for possible associated TSH resistance.

Case 11.2

A 1-year-old girl was referred with massive obesity. She had been the product of a normal delivery at 41 weeks' gestation, birth weight 4.28 kg. She was noted to have polydactyly of both hands and a bifid left fifth toe. She was breast-fed from birth, with solids introduced at 9 months. There was no evidence of retinal pigmentation. Her general intelligence quotient (excluding locomotor skills) was 89. Initial serum biochemical investigations demonstrated the following:

   Urea, electrolytes and glucose normal
   Calcium 2.24 mmol/L [9.0 mg/dL]
   Phosphate 1.33 mmol/L [4.1 mg/dL]
   Free T4 14.9 pmol/L [1.2 ng/dL]
   TSH 1.82 mU/L
   IGF-I 5.7 nmol/L (reference range 5.0–33.6) [44 ng/mL (normal range (38–257)]

Questions

1 What is the most likely diagnosis?
2 What additional investigations may be of assistance?

Answers

1 Laurence–Moon–Biedl syndrome is the most likely diagnosis.
2 Further evaluation of her retinal function demonstrated no visual evoked potential or electroretinogram response to flash. An abdominal ultrasound examination did not demonstrate any associated renal abnormalities.

Case 11.3

A 10-year-old boy was referred for assessment of his overweight. His birth weight was 3.7 kg and after initial feeding difficulties he demonstrated early onset of excessive weight gain. He is progressing well in school and has no history of polydipsia or polyuria. At referral, he is tall (height + 2.6 SDS) with a BMI of 30.6 kg/m². He had no dysmorphic features and was pre-pubertal. Blood pressure was 126/70 mmHg and he had acanthosis nigricans on his neck and axillae.

Questions

1 What investigations are indicated?
2 What is the most likely diagnosis and prognosis?

Answers

1 The presence of acanthosis nigricans suggests he is developing insulin resistance and it would be advisable to measure fasting blood glucose and lipids to ensure he has not developed type 2 diabetes and other metabolic complications. Although his early feeding difficulties would raise the possibility of Prader–Willi syndrome, his lack of dysmorphic features and normal school progress make it unlikely that FISH probing and DNA testing would produce an abnormal result.
2 Given his tall stature and lack of dysmorphic findings, the most likely diagnosis is 'simple obesity'. He should be supported in efforts to lose weight as he is likely to be at high risk of developing type 2 diabetes in the future.

Case 11.4

A 15-year-old girl was referred with amenorrhoea of 2 years' duration following 1 year of a regular menstrual cycle. In recent years, she had encountered increasing problems of excess weight gain. Her height was on the 50th centile and weight 5 kg above the 99.6th centile. Since menarche, she had been troubled with acne and excessive body and facial hair. Initial blood tests demonstrated the following:

LH 6.7 U/L
FSH 4.7 U/L
Oestradiol 214 pmol/L
Testosterone 3.1 nmol/L
Free T4 14.7 pmol/L (reference range 9.8–23.1)
TSH 1.86 mU/L (reference range 0.35–5.5)
Prolactin 154 mU/L
Sex hormone binding globulin 24.8 nmol/L (reference range 19.8–122 nmol/L)
DHEAS 3.7 μmol/L (reference range 1.8–10.0)
17-OH-progesterone 6.3 nmol/L (reference range 2.0–6.0)
Androstenedione 18.0 nmol/L (reference range <3.6)

Questions

1 What is the most likely diagnosis?
2 What additional investigations may be of assistance?
3 What treatment may be advised?

Answers

1 The development of secondary amenorrhoea in the context of obesity, acne and hisuitism makes a diagnosis of polycystic ovarian syndrome likely. Although an elevated androstenedione concentration raises the possibility of congenital adrenal hyperplasia, the minimally raised 17-OH-progesterone and normal testosterone concentrations make this unlikely.
2 A pelvic ultrasound examination should be undertaken to assess the presence of ovarian cysts consistent with a diagnosis of polycystic ovarian syndrome, which was confirmed in this case. If there is uncertainty about the presence of congenital adrenal hyperplasia, then examination of a urinary steroid metabolite profile should exclude this differential diagnosis.
3 This girl should be advised to lose weight if at all possible. In the longer term, this may lead to reduced hirsuitism though in the short term, local cosmetic approaches will be required. The use of combined oral contraceptives containing the anti-androgen cyproterone acetate may help reduce

hair growth and acne and there has been much interest in the possibility that metformin may be beneficial in this condition though this remains unlicensed for this indication in the United Kingdom at present.

Case 11.5

A 7-year-old girl of Pakistani origin was referred with obesity (BMI 27.9 kg/m²) and acanthosis nigricans affecting her neck and axillae. A fasting blood sample demonstrated a plasma glucose of 4.3 mmol/L, although 2 hours following an oral glucose tolerance test, she had a plasma glucose of 7.6 mmol/L. Despite dietetic and lifestyle advice she continued to gain weight and on examination has developed hepatomegaly. One year later, a fasting blood sample demonstrates the following:

HbA1 c 7.1%

Triglyceride 1.4 mmol/L (reference range 0.4–1.6)

Cholesterol 4.1 mmol/L (reference range 2.5–5.2)

HDL-cholesterol 0.8 mmol/L (reference range 0.9–2.0)

Aspartate transaminase 47 IU/L (reference range 5–45)

Questions

1 What is the interpretation of these data?

2 What additional investigations may be of assistance?

3 What treatment should be advised?

Answers

1 The rising HbA1 c concentration suggests that this girl has now developed type 2 diabetes. A suppressed HDL-cholesterol concentration suggests she is also at risk of developing wider features of the multimetabolic syndrome. The presence of hepatomegaly and a rising aspartate transaminase concentration suggests she may also be showing evidence of non-alcoholic steatohepatitis.

2 A hepatic ultrasound is indicated. This confirmed the presence of an enlarged, echogenic liver in keeping with fatty infiltration.

3 The failure of dietary advice to help her control her weight gain and the development of evidence of type 2 diabetes are indications for a trial of metformin treatment. If this fails to improve matters then sulphonylurea or insulin therapy may be required.

Key weblinks

www.healthforallchildren. co.uk Source of the UK-WHO 2009 growth charts and body mass index centile charts.

www.mendprogramme.org MEND (Mind, Exercise, Nutrition. . .Do it!) is a childhood family-based obesity programme developed at Great Ormond Street Hospital in London dedicated to reducing global childhood and family overweight and obesity levels through the provision of free healthy living programmes.

Significant guidelines/consensus statements

Caprio, S., Daniels, S.R., Drewnowski, A. et al. (2008) Influence of race, ethnicity, and culture on childhood obesity: implications for prevention and treatment: a consensus statement of Shaping America's Health and the Obesity Society. *Diabetes Care* **31**, 2211–2221.

Daniels, S.R., Greer, F.R. & Committee on Nutrition (2008) Lipid screening and cardiovascular health in childhood. *Pediatrics* **122**, 198–208.

Daniels, S.R., Jacobson, M. S., McCrindle, B. W. et al. (2009) American Heart Association Childhood Obesity Research Summit: executive summary. *Circulation* **119**, 2114–2123.

Speiser, P. W., Rudolf, M. C., Anhalt, H. et al. (2005) Childhood obesity. *Journal of Clinical Endocrinology and Metabolism* **90**, 1871–1887.

Useful information for patients and parents

www.bsped.org.uk/patients/nick/OVRWEGHT.htm gives some limited background information endorsed by the British Society for Paediatric Endocrinology. The Child Growth Foundation is a UK-based charity relating to children's growth including the prevention of obesity. Website: www.childgrowthfoundation.org The National Obesity Forum is an independent UK-charity working to improve the prevention and management of obesity. Website: www.nationalobesityforum.org.uk www.healthiergeneration.org/parents.aspx?gclid= CLDLxpyYyp8CFWlr4wodtye20 A is a page on an Alliance Healthcare Initiative website with useful advice for parents.

Further reading

Gortmaker, S.L., Must, A., Perrin, J.M. *et al.* (1993) Social and economic consequences of overweight in adolescence and young adulthood. *New England Journal of Medicine* **329**, 1008–1012.

Livingstone, M.B., McCaffrey, T.A. & Rennie, K.L. (2006) Childhood obesity prevention studies: lessons learned and to be learned. *Public Health Nutrition* **9**, 1121–1129.

Mattsson, N., Rönnemaa, T., Juonala, M. *et al.* (2007) The prevalence of the metabolic syndrome in young adults. The cardiovascular risk in young Finns study. *Journal of Internal Medicine.* **261**, 159–169.

Miller, J., Rosenbloom, A. & Silverstein, J. (2004) Childhood obesity. *Journal of Clinical Endocrinology & Metabolism* **89**, 4211–4218.

Oude Luttikhuis, H., Baur, L., Jansen, H. *et al.* (2009) Interventions for treating obesity in children. *Cochrane Database of Systematic Reviews* **21**, CD001872.

Scottish Intercollegiate Guidelines Network (SIGN) (2003) Management of obesity in children and young people. Edinburgh: *SIGN.*

12 Endocrine Effects of Cancer Treatment

Pathophysiology

There has been a remarkable increase in the survival rates of children with most malignancies during the past 40 years. This improvement has resulted from the use of sophisticated regimens of multi-agent chemotherapy, frequently combined with radiotherapy and surgery. Treatment of childhood cancer is intensive and associated with effects on a number of organs, of which the endocrine system is particularly vulnerable. The risk of late endocrine effects in survivors is related more to the treatment received than to the nature of the underlying malignancy. Organs related to endocrine function or growth which are susceptible to the effects of cancer treatment are shown in Table 12.1.

Chemotherapy

Cytotoxic chemotherapy may damage normal developing cells and the damage is dependent on the type and dose of chemotherapeutic agent used. The germinal epithelium in the testis is highly susceptible to alkylating agents, such as cyclophosphamide. Similarly, the potential for normal ovarian function may be impaired with intensive chemotherapy. Direct damage to the growth plate is currently being studied as a mechanism of chemotherapy-induced growth impairment.

Radiotherapy

Radiotherapy, used either alone or in combination with chemotherapy or surgery, is effective in treating a number of childhood cancers. However, there is frequently a cost in terms of endocrine function and growth. The potential for damage is related to the dose of radiotherapy delivered, the protocol of delivery and the site of the primary lesion. Damage to the hypothalamo–pituitary axis is relatively common following irradiation of tumours of the brain, face, orbit and adjacent areas. The thyroid is susceptible to head and neck irradiation and the growing spine is vulnerable to direct or indirect radiotherapy. Similarly, the pre-pubertal testis — often the site of relapse in leukaemia — is susceptible to direct treatment.

Surgery

Surgery may represent an additional risk factor for these children. Any neurosurgery in the area of the hypothalamo–pituitary axis may impair signalling between these glands which may present relatively acutely but transiently (e. g. postoperative diabetes insipidus) or in the longer term (e. g. 'hypothalamic' obesity). Self-evidently, surgery which involves removal of substantial proportions of a gland may also place the child at risk of subsequent endocrine gland dysfunction.

Practical Endocrinology and Diabetes in Children, Third Edition. Joseph E. Raine, Malcolm D.C. Donaldson, John W. Gregory, Guy Van Vliet.
© 2011 Blackwell Publishing Ltd. Published 2011 by Blackwell Publishing Ltd.

Table 12.1 Organs related to endocrine function or growth which are susceptible to damage from cancer treatment.

Hypothalamic–pituitary axis
   Growth hormone
   Adrenocorticotrophic hormone
   Luteinizing hormone/follicle-stimulating hormone
   Thyroid-stimulating hormone
Thyroid
Testis
Ovary
Spine
Long bones
Growth plate
Breast tissue
Fat mass

Investigation and management of late endocrine effects

The combined oncology–endocrine clinic

The establishment of a combined oncology–endocrine clinic, or alternatively an oncology 'late effects' clinic with an endocrinologist in attendance, has been shown to be of benefit to patient management (Figure 12.1). Paediatricians and paediatric endocrinologists should be encouraged to work closely with oncologists to establish a joint clinic aimed at identification, investigation and management of late endocrine effects. The principal aim of the oncologist is to treat and monitor the status of the patient's primary disorder. The endocrinologist can support this process by contributing knowledge and experience of potential and actual endocrine and growth dysfunctions. Auxological monitoring is an essential function of this clinic.

Referral to the oncology–endocrine clinic

Late referral to this clinic can lead to considerable delay in diagnosis of treatable endocrine effects. Consequently, **all patients** who have received radiotherapy in childhood **to any organ** should be referred 1 year after completion of treatment. In this way auxological monitoring can identify early growth failure and potential abnormalities of puberty can be monitored. Patients treated with chemotherapy, which can cause potential endocrine dysfunction, should also be referred. Any oncology patient with concerns about growth, puberty or changes in body composition, for example obesity, can benefit from early referral to this clinic.

Investigation and monitoring of patients

Procedures which may be undertaken either in or associated with the joint clinic are shown in Table 12.2.

Specific endocrine and growth abnormalities associated with cancer treatment

Cancer treatment may affect the function of a number of specific endocrine organs and tissues related to growth. Frequently, several organ systems are affected in the same

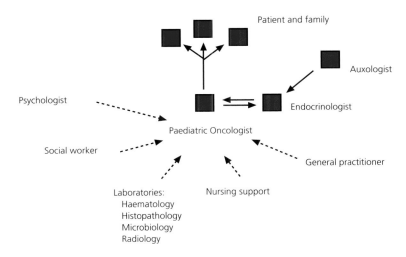

Fig. 12.1 Suggested model for a joint paediatric oncology–endocrinology clinic.

Table 12.2 Procedures in or associated with the joint oncology-endocrine clinic.

Clinic attendance — every 4–6 months
Auxology monitoring
　Height
　Height velocity
　Sitting height
　Weight
　Bone age
　Body mass index
Puberty development staging (including testicular volume)
Hormone measurements
　Basal levels
　T4, TSH, cortisol, testosterone, oestradiol, LH, FSH, prolactin, IGF-I
　Dynamic tests
　Growth hormone (and ACTH) stimulation, e.g. glucagon, insulin, clonidine tests, overnight growth hormone profile
　LHRH test
　TRH test
　hCG stimulation
Thyroid ultrasound
Pelvic ultrasound
DEXA scan for bone mineral density and body composition

Abbreviations: ACTH, adrenocorticotrophic hormone; FSH, follicle-stimulating hormone; hCG, human chorionic gonadotrophin; IGF-I, insulin-like growth factor I; LH, luteinizing hormone; LHRH, LH-releasing hormone; T4, thyroxine; TRH, thyrotrophin-releasing hormone; TSH, thyroid-stimulating hormone.

patient. The major endocrine organs at risk and growth abnormalities are described individually.

Abnormal linear growth

Growth can be impaired by:
• direct effect of radiotherapy on the spine;
• damage to the hypothalamo–pituitary axis with resulting growth hormone (GH) deficiency;
• gonadal damage with sex steroid deficiency, resulting in impaired pubertal growth; and
• effect of radiotherapy and chemotherapy on growth plates.

Spinal irradiation

Spinal irradiation, as given for conditions such as medulloblastoma (Figure 12.2) and germinoma, will seriously affect subsequent spinal growth. The effect is particularly severe in early childhood. Spinal growth is an essential component of the adolescent growth spurt. Consequently, short stature with disproportion because of shortness of the trunk is frequently seen in these patients.

GH deficiency

Damage to the hypothalamo–pituitary axis resulting in GH deficiency can occur following radiotherapy given in:
• high doses (>3000 cGy) as curative therapy for brain, orbit or adjacent tissue tumours;
• doses of 1800–2400 cGy as prophylaxis for central nervous system (CNS) leukaemia; and
• doses of 750–1600 cGy as total body irradiation.

The prevalence and severity of GH deficiency is related to the total dosage of radiotherapy and the fractionation schedule. The same total dosage given in a larger number of smaller fractions is likely to be less damaging. Radiotherapy regimens for brain tumours and tumours of the face and orbit, which deliver doses >3000 cGy to the hypothalamic–pituitary axis, will almost always result in GH deficiency. This is usually present by 2 years after treatment.

The frequency of GH deficiency following prophylactic CNS irradiation and after total body irradiation is variable. However, several studies have reported a prevalence of up to 50%. A more subtle form of GH deficiency may be seen where the GH response to pharmacological stimulation may be normal; however, physiological GH secretion and the normal increment in GH secretion occurring at puberty is impaired.

Diagnosis

A high index of suspicion is important when children at risk of GH deficiency are seen in the oncology–endocrine clinic. Children should undergo GH stimulation testing at the earliest suspicion of a subnormal height velocity. For interpretation of the results, see Chapter 3. The puberty status must always be assessed and considered when interpreting the auxological findings. Puberty will stimulate growth and, particularly when precocious, can mask coexistent underlying GH deficiency.

Treatment

The same principles apply to the treatment of irradiation-induced GH deficiency as with other aetiologies. There is no evidence that normal human growth hormone (hGH) therapy increases the risk of recurrence of malignancy after remission has been induced. Although it is recognized that in these patients the basic defect may

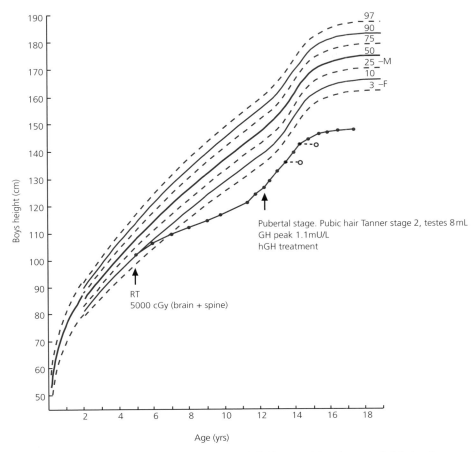

Fig. 12.2 Growth following radiotherapy to brain and spine for medulloblastoma. Note the severe height loss because of spinal irradiation, the rather early puberty and the severely restricted final height. RT, radiotherapy.

be in hypothalamic growth hormone releasing hormone (GHRH) secretion, therapy with hGH is indicated and, as always, early diagnosis will lead to the best long-term result.

Sex steroid deficiency and direct damage to growth plate and long bones

Radiotherapy is a well recognized cause of direct damage to gonads and bone. Sex steroid deficiency will be discussed in section 'Gonadal damage'. Growth failure in the absence of direct spinal irradiation or GH deficiency has also been described. The mechanism of this apparent effect of chemotherapy is not clear. It is possible that the growth plates in the spine and long bones are susceptible to damage from intensive chemotherapy.

Abnormal pituitary function

The GH axis is most vulnerable to damage by radiotherapy. Other anterior pituitary hormones are relatively resistant. Gonadotrophin and adrenocorticotrophic hormone (ACTH) deficiencies may occur at a longer interval of approximately 10 years after treatment, followed by thyroid stimulating hormone (TSH) deficiency, which appears to be even more infrequent.

Early puberty following cranial irradiation

This phenomenon was first reported in the 1980s and is now a recognized complication, particularly in girls. Children who received cranial irradiation, particularly at a young age, have a significantly earlier onset of puberty with respect to chronological age and bone age.

The combination of GH deficiency and early puberty severely reduces growth potential. In this situation, puberty should be suppressed using gonadotrophin-releasing hormone (GnRH) analogue therapy to allow maximum benefit from hGH replacement.

Gonadal damage

Gonadal damage in childhood can occur following chemotherapy or radiotherapy. There are specific differences affecting the testis and ovary, so each will be described separately.

The testis

Chemotherapy

The use of chemotherapeutic regimens which include alkylating agents, such as cyclophosphamide, chlorambucil and the nitrosureas, in addition to procarbazine, vinblastine, cytosine arabinoside and possibly *cis*-platinum, are likely to cause damage to germinal epithelium resulting in azoospermia and infertility in adult life. This has been reported particularly in leukaemia and Hodgkin's disease. With this established knowledge, chemotherapeutic regimens are now being modified with the aim of minimizing this complication. Elevation of basal follicle stimulating hormone (FSH) is a useful guide to damage of germinal epithelium. Testosterone production from Leydig cells is not generally affected.

Radiotherapy

The testis is vulnerable to radiation damage, which in turn depends on the total dosage and dose per fraction. Following total body irradiation (dose 1200–1500 cGy) to prepubertal children for leukaemia, Leydig cell function was not affected; however, azoospermia occurred. After direct testicular irradiation, testosterone production was severely reduced and infertility resulted.

Consequently, it is important to assess testicular size and function, by human chorionic gonadotrophin (hCG) stimulation if necessary and measurement of basal gonadotrophins, in order to define the need for testosterone replacement. Long-term androgen therapy may be indicated to ensure satisfactory pubertal development and normal testosterone levels in adult life.

The ovary

Chemotherapy

The ovary is apparently more resistant to damage than the testis. Normal fertility and endocrine function can be expected in adult survivors of childhood leukaemia

treatment. Intensive chemotherapeutic regimens for conditions such as Hodgkin's disease may confer more risk of ovarian dysfunction. Elevation of basal FSH may indicate ovarian damage.

Radiotherapy

The ovary is susceptible to damage from radiotherapy. Direct, or indirect radiotherapy as in total body irradiation, can cause ovarian failure with impairment of ovulation and possible subnormal sex steroid secretion. Vulnerable patients need to be carefully assessed by the endocrinologist and normal pubertal development ensured.

Thyroid abnormalities

Thyroid abnormalities are likely to occur after radiotherapy which has included the thyroid area. There are three main types of potential thyroid dysfunction: hypothyroidism, benign thyroid nodules and thyroid cancer. The children most at risk are those treated for Hodgkin's disease who received 3000–5000 cGy to the neck. In these patients, approximately 25% develop hypothyroidism during the first few years after treatment. The first sign is usually elevation of TSH, which should be promptly treated with thyroxine (T4) replacement. The frequency increases to >50% after 6 years.

Total body irradiation and cranial irradiation are also associated with hypothyroidism, which should be excluded by regular thyroid function tests (TFT) performed in the joint oncology–endocrine clinic. Thyroid nodules may develop after a longer interval. They can be detected clinically or on ultrasound.

Thyroid cancer is also usually a late complication of neck irradiation. Any suspected thyroid neoplasm should be investigated by ultrasound. Elevation of TSH for long periods of time is said to confer greater risk of malignancy in the irradiated gland.

Adrenal abnormalities

Abnormal adrenal function is rare in children treated for cancer. ACTH deficiency may be a late complication of high-dose (>3000 cGy) cranial irradiation and should be considered if other anterior pituitary hormones are deficient.

Abnormalities of body composition

It is being recognized that survivors of childhood leukaemia and brain tumours may become obese. Whilst surgery and radiotherapy in the hypothalamo–pituitary region may predispose to this finding due to direct adverse effects on hypothalamic functioning and GH deficiency, in many patients, there is currently no good explanation for this problem. In the longer term, obesity, impaired levels of physical activity and GH deficiency are being increasingly recognized as risk factors for the development of the 'metabolic syndrome' in adult life. Effective interventions to prevent this 'late effect' are being increasingly explored.

Impaired bone mineralization may also occur during childhood and can be demonstrated on dual energy X-ray absortiometry (DEXA) scanning. Chronic illness, reduced exercise, steroid therapy, direct effects of other chemotherapeutic agents on osteoblasts, GH deficiency and impaired sex steroid secretion at puberty are all potential factors contributing to this finding. The prompt and accurate diagnosis and treatment of endocrine deficiencies will help to normalize bone mineralization, hence diminishing the risk of osteoporosis in adult life.

When to involve a specialist centre

Many long-term survivors of childhood cancer who have received treatment known to place them at significant risk of endocrine 'late effects' will remain under follow-up review in a specialist oncology department. Where this risk is significant or there are concerns that the patient is developing signs suggestive of endocrine dysfunction, such as impaired growth or puberty, these patients should attend the joint oncology–endocrine follow-up clinic.

Future developments

- The challenge for oncologists is to develop future treatments which are effective for the treatment of the primary neoplasm but cause minimal 'late effects'.
- More specific and targeted radiotherapy techniques are being developed.
- Cryopreservation of gonadal tissue prior to cancer therapy is being explored within ethical limits.

Transition

Any patient who is receiving hormone replacement or is known to be at high risk of developing endocrine dysfunction such that they require regular endocrine testing should be seen in a clinical service that allows transition of care from a paediatrician to an adult physician with endocrine expertise. In addition, those demonstrat-

ing evidence of osteopenia or osteoporosis will require referral to an adult 'osteoporosis service'. It is also helpful for patients at risk of infertility to be seen (at least transiently) by adult specialists with expertise in infertility treatment, so that they are counselled about the options available to them should they choose, later in their adult lives.

Controversial points

- Ethical issues and practicalities of harvesting and cryopreservation of gametes prior to treatment causing gonadal damage.
- Possible protection of gonads from chemotherapeutic or radiotherapeutic damage by endocrine therapy, i.e. GnRH suppression of pituitary–gonadal axis.
- Management of prevention of menstruation in patients likely to develop heavy bleeding.

Potential pitfalls

- Failure to appreciate that a suboptimal growth response to GH in children with growth hormone deficiency (GHD) previously treated with cranio-spinal radiotherapy may reflect radiotherapy-induced growth plate damage.
- Importance of regular clinical staging of puberty to ensure that GHD coexistent with precocious puberty is not missed.
- Failure to appreciate, that absence of endocrine deficiency soon after radiotherapy does not mean that endocrine deficiency cannot evolve later. Hence the need for long-term follow-up in patients who received cranial irradiation in excess of 1800 or 2400 Gy.

Case histories

Case 12.1

A 3-year-old boy was diagnosed to have a rhabdomyosarcoma of the left maxillary antrum. He received radiotherapy to the tumour (5046 cGy) and chemotherapy. There has been no recurrence of the tumour. At the age of 5 years, his growth started to slow down. He was not referred to the joint oncology–endocrine clinic until the age of 7.4 years by which time his height was far below the 3rd centile and his height velocity was 3.6 cm per year.

Questions
1 What investigations are indicated?
2 What is the likely diagnosis and what tests would you do?
3 How do you interpret this test?
4 Does he have gonadotrophin deficiency in addition to his GH and TSH deficiencies?

Answers
1 Detailed auxology and basal hormone measurements were performed (Table 12.2). Biochemistry was normal. A dynamic GH stimulation test (glucagon 15 mg/kg intramuscularly) was performed and his peak GH level was 1.4 mU/L. He therefore had severe GH deficiency. He was started on GH therapy in a standard dosage of 4.9 mg/m² per week. His height velocity increased to 8.4 cm per year. At the age of 14 years, his T4 was 58 nmol/L (normal range 57–170) and his TSH was 1.6 mU/L (normal range 0.4–5.0). This is suggestive of central hypothyroidism.
2 The results suggest central hypothyrodism. A thyroid hormone releasing (TRH) test was performed with TRH 200 mg intravenously. The results were as shown in Table 12.3.

Table 12.3 Results of thyrotrophin-releasing hormone (TRH) test.

Time (min)	TSH (mU/L)
0	1.6
20	6.8
60	8.9

Abbreviation: TSH, thyroid-stimulating hormone.

3 This is an abnormal test. The 20-minute level should be higher than the 60-minute level. He has central hypothyroidism and was started on treatment with T4 100 µg per day. At the age of 15 years, he was still prepubertal.

4 This is very difficult to say and to diagnose at this age. No test is specific. The most important step is to treat his delayed puberty. He was started on testosterone enanthate 125 mg monthly. Overall diagnosis is multiple pituitary hormone deficiencies secondary to irradiation of a rhabdomyosarcoma in close proximity to the hypothalamic–pituitary axis.

Case 12.2
A 13.5-year-old boy previously treated for acute lymphoblastic leukaemia including testicular disease was referred for assessment because of concerns about his lack of puberty. He had received testicular radiotherapy 4 years earlier and had completed chemotherapy a year before referral. On clinical examination, he is prepubertal with 2 mL testes bilaterally. Blood tests showed the following:
FSH 23.1 mU/L
LH 5.8 mU/L
Testosterone <0.7 nmol/L (<18.9 ng/dL)

Questions
1 What prognosis for testicular function should he and his parents be given?
2 How should his puberty be managed?

Answers
1 Given his previous history of testicular irradiation, it is highly probable that testicular function will be significantly adversely affected. His elevated serum FSH concentration, despite his otherwise prepubertal state and small testicular volumes, suggest early evidence that his future fertility will be severely impaired. Although Leydig cells are more resistant to the adverse effects of radiotherapy, his rising serum LH concentration and undetectable testosterone level also begin to suggest evidence that Leydig cell function may be impaired which may prevent normal pubertal development.
2 Although not all boys will have entered puberty at the age of 13.5 years, given his past history and evidence of likely gonadal damage, induction of puberty with low doses of testosterone, steadily increased towards adult replacement levels over two to three years should there be no evidence of testicular growth, would be indicated. Once full

virilization has been completed, or earlier should he start to show signs of increasing testicular volumes, testosterone therapy should be temporarily discontinued to allow repeat biochemical evaluation of gonadal function to confirm that long-term testosterone therapy is required.

Case 12.3
A 15-year-old boy with Down's syndrome presents with increasing polyuria and polydipsia whilst receiving 6-mercaptopurine as maintenance chemotherapy for acute lymphoblastic leukaemia. Previously, he had experienced marked hyperglycaemia whilst receiving chemotherapy including dexamethasone and had required insulin therapy and metformin on several occasions though this had been discontinued between courses of glucocorticoids due to normalization of blood glucose levels. He is overweight and has acanthosis nigricans. His father has type 2 diabetes. His HbA1 c had increased from 6.2% to 7.0%.

Questions
1 What is his likely diagnosis and prognosis?
2 How should he be managed?

Answers
1 The previous history was strongly suggestive of steroid-induced diabetes. However, given his overweight, clinical signs of insulin resistance and family history, the recurrence of evidence of diabetes when not receiving steroid therapy suggests he is developing type 2 diabetes which is likely to persist and require longer term therapy.
2 The current picture strongly suggests insulin resistance to be the underlying problem. His urine or blood should be checked to confirm the lack of ketones and he should be started on metformin therapy. Should this fail to normalize his blood glucose concentrations, then additional oral hypoglycaemic or insulin therapy may need to be considered.

Case 12.4
A 6-year-old girl is referred with concerns about her growth following treatment 2 years earlier for a

metastatic pinealblastoma which included chemotherapy and craniospinal radiotherapy. On examination, her height is falling across the centiles and she has evidence of increased central adiposity. Blood testing in clinic demonstrated the following:
Free T4 13.5 pmol/L (1.05 ng/dL)
TSH 8.8 mU/L
Cortisol 234 nmol/L (8.48 µg/dL)
IGF-I 29.8 nmol/L (normal range 6.8–38.9)

Questions
1 What is the interpretation of these blood tests?
2 How should she be managed?

Answers
1 Although this girl is at risk of hypopituitarism, these initial results suggest the presence of primary hypothyroidism, presumably secondary to the effect of her spinal radiotherapy on the thyroid gland. The random serum cortisol is within the normal range for unstressed early morning samples. Her serum IGF-I concentration is also normal though it should be interpreted with caution in the context of obesity in which the effects of hyperinsulinism on IGF-I levels may mask evolving GHD.
2 She should be started on T4 treatment and doses adjusted at monthly intervals to suppress TSH levels to within the normal range. Significant growth failure and obesity are relatively unusual features of hypothyroidism, particularly when biochemically mild as in this case. The latter findings may be more suggestive of GHD and if they do not resolve following normalization of thyroid function, then formal GH-stimulation testing should be performed. In this case, a formal diagnosis of moderate GHD was confirmed less than a year later (maximum serum GH 8.4 mU/L and cortisol 721 nmol/L (26.1 µg/dL) in response to insulin-induced hypoglycaemia).

Case 12.5
An 8-year-old girl had been diagnosed with a medulloblastoma and spinal metastases aged 5 years. She was treated with chemotherapy and radiotherapy (40 Gy to the whole CNS, 15 Gy to the primary tumour site and 55 Gy boost to the spinal

metastases). A few months earlier, a diagnosis of primary hypothyroidism had been made and she was started on T4 treatment. On examination, she now has a height velocity of only 1.5 cm per year and is in mid-puberty with Tanner stage 3 breast development. Blood testing in clinic demonstrated the following:

Free T4 23.5 pmol/L (1.83 ng/dL)
TSH 0.07 mU/L
Cortisol 346 nmol/L (1.25 µg/dL)
IGF-I 6.8 nmol/L (normal range 12.9–64.0)

Questions

1 What is the interpretation of her growth pattern at present?
2 What investigations are indicated?
3 What treatment may be required?

Answers

1 Her present height velocity is extraordinarily low, particularly given her precocious pubertal development. It is likely that she has both GHD and impaired spinal growth due to the direct adverse effects of radiotherapy on the vertebrae.
2 Formal GH testing using insulin-induced hypoglycaemia confirmed the presence of severe GHD (maximum serum GH concentration 5.1 mU/L and cortisol 844.9 nmol/L (30.6 µg/dL) in response to a plasma glucose concentration of 1.9 mmol/L (34.2 mg/dL)).
3 hGH therapy is likely to significantly improve her height velocity though 'catch-up' growth may be limited by a poor spinal response due to local radiotherapy-induced damage to the vertebrae. Precocious puberty is not uncommon following a medulloblastoma and should be confirmed biochemically to be gonadotrophin-dependent. Further pubertal development can then be suppressed using luteinizing hormone releasing hormone (LHRH) analogue treatment to maximize final height in response to hGH therapy.

Key weblinks

www.childgrowthfoundation.org The Child Growth Foundation is a UK-based charity which supports children with growth and endocrine disorders and their families.

Significant guidelines/consensus statements

Skinner, R., Wallace, W. H.B. & Levitt, G. A. (2005) *Therapy Based Long Term Follow Up. Practice Statement.* www.ukccsg.org.uk/public/followup/Practice Statement/index.html
Children's Oncology Group (2008) Long-term follow-up guidelines for survivors of childhood, adolescent, and young adult cancers. www.survivorshipguidelines.org
NHS Improvement. Survivorship: living with and beyond cancer. www.improvement.nhs.uk/cancer/SurvivorshipLiving WithandBeyondCancer/tabid/65/Default.aspzx

Useful information for patients and parents

www.bsped.org.uk/patients/serono/index.htm and http://www.eurospe.org/patient/English/index.html are links providing downloadable booklets endorsed by the British Society for Paediatric Endocrinology and Diabetes and European Society for Paediatric Endocrinology, respectively, which provide information for children and their families about a range of endocrine problems encountered after treatment of childhood malignancies. www.lwpes.org/patientsFamilies/patientslinks.cfm contains a number of links to organizations suggested by the Lawson Wilkins Paediatric Endocrine Society. www.cclg.org.uk/families/booklet.php?bid=6&3id=31 &2id=9 lists several pages on the Children's Cancer and Leukaemia Group website which provide information about endocrine complications of childhood cancer treatment.

Further reading

Bath, L.E., Wallace, H.B. & Kelnar, C.J.H. (1998) Disorders of growth and development in the child treated for cancer. In: *Growth Disorders: Pathophysiology and Treatment* (eds C.J.H. Kelnar, M.O. Savage, H.F. Stirling & P. Saenger), pp. 640–641. Chapman & Hall Medical, London.

Wallace, H. & Green, D. (2004) *Late Effects of Childhood Cancer.* Arnold, London.

Wallace, W.H. & Thomson, A.B. (2003) Preservation of fertility in children treated for cancer. *Archives of Disease in Childhood* **88**, 493–496.

Wallace, W.H.B. & Kelnar, C.J.H. (2009) *Endocrinopathy after Childhood Cancer Treatment.* Karger, Basel.

APPENDIX

1 Growth and BMI Charts

Different growth and BMI charts exist in different countries with slight differences. The standard charts listed below are UK charts. The Down's chart is based on UK/Irish data, the Turner's chart on European data and the Noonan's and achondroplasia charts on North American data.

There also exist growth charts for less common disorders, such as height charts for the Silver–Russell syndrome, height charts for hypochondroplasia, and height and weight charts for the Prader–Willi syndrome.

In 2009, new UK-World Health Organisation (WHO) growth charts became available. These charts are based on the WHO child growth standards which describe the optimal growth of healthy breast-fed children. Previous UK charts were based on studies of both breast-fed and bottle-fed children and therefore did not reflect the normal weight fluctuations of breast-fed babies in the first few months of life. In these charts, the data is from breast-fed babies with the growth of breast-fed babies considered as the norm. These new charts combine UK90 and WHO data. They chart growth from birth to 4 years and include a low birth-weight chart from 23 weeks' gestation to 2 years. They include instructions on how to measure and plot readings and on how to interpret them. They also include a growth predictor that allows the prediction of the final adult height ($+/- 6$ cm) based on the height centile between 2 and 4 years of age. Also included are a body mass index (BMI) conversion chart and guidance on how to correct for gestational age. They should be used for both breast- and bottle-fed infants. They also incorporate length/height discontinuity at 2 years of age (length should be measured till 2 and then height subsequently) as a child's height is usually slightly less than their length. Existing charts should be used for children aged 4 years and over. The charts and instructions on their use are downloadable from www.growthcharts.rcpch.ac.uk

Practical Endocrinology and Diabetes in Children, Third Edition. Joseph E. Raine, Malcolm D.C. Donaldson, John W. Gregory, Guy Van Vliet.
© 2011 Blackwell Publishing Ltd. Published 2011 by Blackwell Publishing Ltd.

• Please place a sticker (if available) otherwise write in space provided.

Surname

First names

NHS no: Local no

G.P.   Code

H.V.   Code

GIRLS
GROWTH CHART
(BIRTH - 18 YEARS)

United Kingdom cross-sectional reference data : 1996/1

D.O.B. ...... : ...... : ...... WEEKS GESTATION ....

HOSPITAL COMPUTER No. ....

pre-term

for a girl born before 37 completed weeks, draw a vertical "pre-term" line at the appropriate week and plot measurements from this line for at least twelve months. For all later deliveries plot from the EDD (Estimated Delivery Date) line.

measurements

weight: an infant or toddler should always be weighed naked on a self-calibrating or regularly calibrated scale. An older child should be weighed with the minimum of clothing.

head circumference: head circumference measurements should be taken from midway between the eyebrows and the hairline at the front of the head and the occipital prominence at the back. Appropriate thin plastic or metal tape should be used: sewing tape or paper tape is not recommended for this purpose.

supine length: an infant:- a child up to approximately 18 months - should be measured supinely (on her back) by two people with equipment featuring both a headboard and moveable footboard. Whilst one person holds the head against the headboard, with the head facing upwards in the Frankfurt plane*, a second person measures the length by bringing the footboard up to the heels. The downward pressure on the child's knees to ensure that the legs are flat will not endanger hip dislocation.

standing height: standing height should be measured against an appropriate vertical measure, door or wall free from radiators, pipes or large skirting board. The feet should be together with the heels, buttocks and shoulder blades touching the vertical and the head positioned in the Frankfurt plane*. To ensure that the maximum height is taken, upward pressure to the mastoid processes should be considered.

*The Frankfurt plane is an imaginary line from the centre of the ear hole to the lower border of the eye socket.

guidelines for recording, plotting and referral

Record the measurement using the boxes on this chart immediately you have taken it. Enter the date, specify the measurement in the box with the asterisk (i.e. **H/C** = head circumference, **H** = height, **L** = length, **W** = weight) and name your entry. You might find it helpful to enter her current age in the appropriate column. Plot each measurement on the grid with a well defined dot. Trace the growth curve with a line but leave the dots clearly visible. A normal growth curve is one that always runs roughly on/parallel to one of the printed centile lines. If it doesn't, consider these guidelines:-

Refer a girl whose height falls above the 99.6th or below the 0.4th centile line or outside her Target Centile Range (TCR). Refer her also if, pre-school, her growth curve veers upwards/downwards over the period 12-18 months by the width of one centile band or, post school entry, by 2/3 of a band, If, prior to school entry, the curve veers by only 2/3 of a band or, subsequently, by 1/2 a band, flag the child for recall in 12 months and refer if the trend continues. Respond to parental concern about a child's growth, irrespective of the current centile, by monitoring height over a period of at least nine months and follow the criteria above. *(Source: BSPED September 1996)*

Date	Age	*	Measurement	Name
24 : 09 : 92	10/12	L	72 : 5 cm	Mary Brown
24 : 09 : 92	10/12	H/C	44 : 3 cm	Mary Brown
24 : 09 : 92	10/12	W	9 : kg	Mary Brown
: :	:		:	

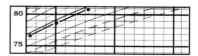

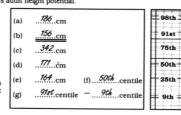

adult height potential

The table and illustrations below show how the adult height potential of a girl is calculated. They show that she is following her genetic pattern and that her growth curve should border the 50th centile to reach 164cm as an adult - **mid-parental height (MPH)**. The 50th centile is her **mid-parental centile (MPC)**, If the curve continuously follows a centile somewhere between the 91st-9th centiles (**MPH ± 8.5cm**) it will still be within her **target centile range (TCR)** and her growth will be considered normal. NB This calculation is not appropriate if either parent is not of normal stature.

Now use the box on the back page to calculate this girl's adult height potential.

Calculate (and complete on back page) as follows:-

(a) = father's height
(b) = mother's height
(c) = sum of (a) and (b)
(d) = (c) + 2
(e) = (d) - 7cm (**MPH**)
(f) = **MPC** - nearest centile to (e)
(g) = **TCR** (mid-parental height ± 8.5cm)

Arrow (h) the mid-parental height/centile and draw a vertical line above and below it to represent the target centile range.

(a) ...186..cm
(b) ...156..cm
(c) ...342..cm
(d) ...171..cm
(e) ...164..cm   (f) ...50th...centile
(g) ...91st..centile — ...9th...centile

98th	175	
91st	170	
75th		
50th	165	←(h)
25th	160	
9th	155	

references and acknowledgements

papers
1. Do growth chart centiles need a face lift? (TJ Cole) *BMJ 1994; 308: 641-2*
2. Cross-sectional stature and weight reference curves for the UK, 1990 (JV Freeman, TJ Cole, S Chinn, PRM Jones, EM White, MA Preece) *ARCH DIS CHILD 1995; 73: 17-24*
3. Growth Charts for ethnic populations in the UK (S Chinn, TJ Cole, MA Preece, R Rona) *The Lancet* March 23rd 1996; 347: 839-840
Compilation: Institute of Child Health, London (Freeman JV et al). *Data sources:* British Size Surveys, Loughborough Consultants Ltd (Jones PRM, Norgan NG, Hunt MJ, Hooper RH); National Study of Health and Growth (Chinn S, Rona RJ); ONS National Heights and Weight Survey, 1980 & National Diet and Nutrition Survey, 1995; Tayside Growth Study (White EM et al); MRC Dunn Nutrition Group, Cambridge (Lucas A, Paul AA, Whitehead RG); MRC Human Genetics Unit, Edinburgh (Ratcliffe SG, Butler GE); UCH, London, 1000 births 1987/88 (Colley NV, Hanson GL), Rosie Hospital, Cambridge (Glazebrock C, Rennie JM) & Northern RHA birth data (Wariyar UK); Chard 1976-1988 Normal Puberty Longitudinal Study (Dunger DB, Cameron N, Baines-Preece J, Cox L, Preece MA)

0191 +55 +236

Designed and Published by
© **CHILD GROWTH FOUNDATION 1996/1**
(Charity Reg. No 274325)
2 Mayfield Avenue,
London W4 1PW

Printed and Supplied by
HARLOW PRINTING LIMITED
Maxwell Street ◊ South Shields
Tyne & Wear ◊ NE33 4PU

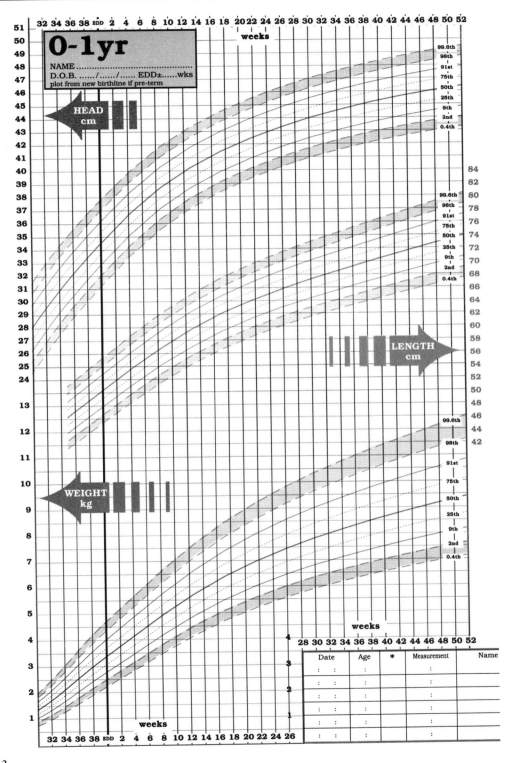

0-1yr

NAME ....

D.O.B. ....../....../...... EDD±......wks

plot from new birthline if pre-term

HEAD cm

LENGTH cm

WEIGHT kg

weeks

Date	Age	*	Measurement	Name
:	:	:	:	
: :	: :	:	:	
: :	: :	:	:	
: :	: :	:	:	
: :	: :	:	:	
: :	: :	:	:	

App. 1.2

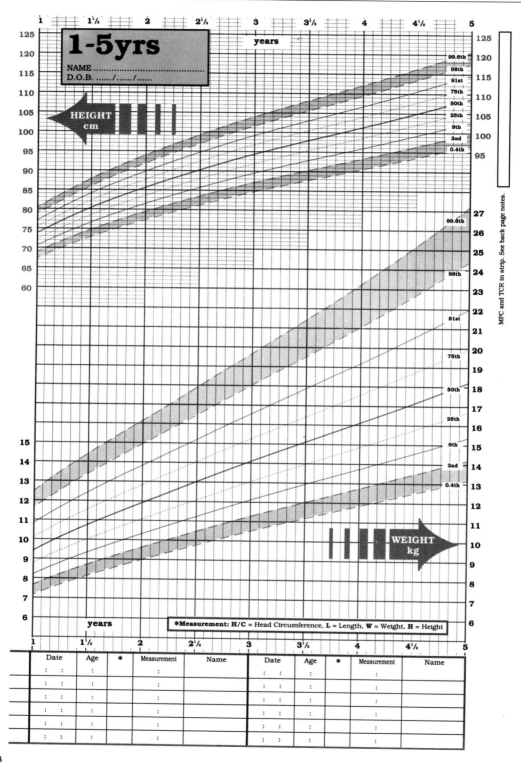

App. 1.3

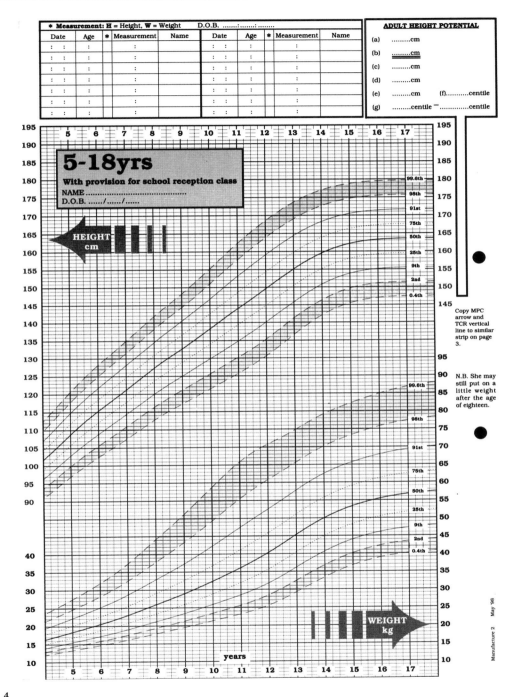

App. 1.4

• Please place a sticker (if available) otherwise write in space provided.

Surname

First names

NHS no: Local no

G.P.   Code

H.V.   Code

BOYS
GROWTH CHART
(BIRTH - 18 YEARS)
United Kingdom cross-sectional reference data : 1996/1

D.O.B. ...... : ...... : .....   WEEKS GESTATION ....

HOSPITAL COMPUTER No. ....

pre-term
for a boy born before 37 completed weeks, draw a vertical "pre-term" line at the appropriate week and plot measurements from this line for at least twelve months. For all later deliveries plot from the EDD (Estimated Delivery Date) line.

measurements
weight: an infant or toddler should always be weighed naked on a self-calibrating or regularly calibrated scale. An older child should be weighed with the minimum of clothing.

head circumference: head circumference measurements should be taken from midway between the eyebrows and the hairline at the front of the head and the occipital prominence at the back. Appropriate thin plastic or metal tape should be used: sewing tape or paper tape is not recommended for this purpose.

supine length: an infant:- a child up to approximately 18 months - should be measured supinely (on his back) by two people with equipment featuring both a headboard and moveable footboard. Whilst one person holds the head against the headboard, with the head facing upwards in the Frankfurt plane*, a second person measures the length by bringing the footboard up to the heels. The downward pressure on the child's knees to ensure that the legs are flat will not endanger hip dislocation.

standing height: standing height should be measured against an appropriate vertical measure, door or wall free from radiators, pipes or large skirting board. The feet should be together with the heels, buttocks and shoulder blades touching the vertical and the head positioned in the Frankfurt plane*. To ensure that the maximum height is taken, upward pressure to the mastoid processes should be considered.

*The Frankfurt plane is an imaginary line from the centre of the ear hole to the lower border of the eye socket.

guidelines for recording, plotting and referral
Record the measurement using the boxes on this chart immediately you have taken it. Enter the date, specify the measurement in the box with the asterisk (i.e. **H/C** = head circumference, **H** = height, **L** = length, **W** = weight) and name your entry. You might find it helpful to enter his current age in the appropriate column. Plot each measurement on the grid with a well defined dot. Trace the growth curve with a line but leave the dots clearly visible. A normal growth curve is one that always runs roughly on/parallel to one of the printed centile lines. If it doesn't, consider these guidelines:-

Refer a boy whose height falls above the 99.6th or below the 0.4th centile line or outside his Target Centile Range (TCR). Refer him also if, pre-school, his growth curve veers upwards/downwards over the period 12-18 months by the width of one centile band or, post school entry, by 2/3 of a band. If, prior to school entry, the curve veers by only 2/3 of a band or, subsequently, by 1/2 a band, flag the child for recall in 12 months and refer if the trend continues. Respond to parental concern about a child's growth, irrespective of the current centile, by monitoring height over a period of at least nine months and follow the criteria above. *(Source: BSPED September 1996)*

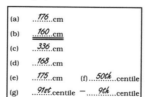

Date	Age	*	Measurement		Name
14 : 03 : 93	9/12	L	72 : 5 cm		John Smith
14 : 03 : 93	9/12	H/C	46 : cm		John Smith
14 : 03 : 93	9/12	W	9 : 3 kg		John Smith
: :			:		

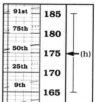

adult height potential
The table and illustrations below show how the adult height potential of a boy is calculated. They show that he is following his genetic pattern and that his growth curve should border the 50th centile to reach 175cm as an adult - **mid-parental height (MPH)**. The 50th centile is his **mid-parental centile (MPC)**. If the curve continuously occupies a centile somewhere between the 91st-9th centiles (MPH ± 10cm) it will still be within his **target centile range (TCR)** and his growth will be considered normal. NB This calculation is not appropriate if either parent is not of normal stature.
Now use the box on the back page to calculate this boy's adult height potential.

Calculate (and complete on back page) as follows:-

(a) = father's height
(b) = mother's height
(c) = sum of (a) and (b)
(d) = (c) ÷ 2
(e) = (d) + 7cm **(MPH)**
(f) = MPC - nearest centile to (e)
(g) = **TCR** (mid-parental height ± 10cm)

Arrow (h) the mid-parental height/centile and draw a vertical line above and below it to represent the target centile range.

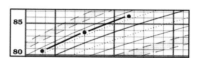

(a) .....*776*.....cm
(b) .....*160*.....cm
(c) .....*336*.....cm
(d) .....*168*.....cm
(e) .....*775*.....cm   (f) .....*50th*.....centile
(g) .....*91st*.....centile — .....*9th*.....centile

91st	185
75th	180
50th	175 ←(h)
25th	
	170
9th	165

references and acknowledgements
papers
1. Do growth chart centiles need a face lift? (TJ Cole) *BMJ* 1994; 308: 641-2
2. Cross-sectional stature and weight reference curves for the UK, 1990 (JV Freeman, TJ Cole, S Chinn, PRM Jones, EM White, MA Preece) *ARCH DIS CHILD* 1995; 73: 17-24
3. Growth Charts for ethnic minority populations in the UK (S Chinn, TJ Cole, MA Preece, R Rona) *The Lancet* March 23rd 1996; 347: 839-840
Compilation: Institute of Child Health, London (Freeman JV et al). *Data sources:* British Size Surveys, Loughborough Consultants Ltd (Jones PRM, Norgan NG, Hunt MJ, Hooper RH); National Study of Health and Growth (Chinn S, Rona RJ); ONS National Heights and Weight Survey, 1980 & National Diet and Nutrition Survey, 1995; Tayside Growth Study (White EM et al); MRC Dunn Nutrition Group, Cambridge (Lucas A, Paul AA, Whitehead RG); MRC Human Genetics Unit, Edinburgh (Ratcliffe SG, Butler GE); UCH, London, 1000 births 1987/88 (Colley NV, Hanson GL), Rosie Hospital, Cambridge (Glazebrook C, Rennie JM) & Northern RHA birth data (Wariyar UK); Chard 1976-1988 Normal Puberty Longitudinal Study (Dunger DB, Cameron N, Baines-Preece J, Cox L, Preece MA)

Designed and Published by
© **CHILD GROWTH FOUNDATION 1996/1**
(Charity Reg. No 274325)
2 Mayfield Avenue,
London W4 1PW

Printed and Supplied by
HARLOW PRINTING LIMITED
Maxwell Street ◊ South Shields
Tyne & Wear ◊ NE33 4PU

App. 1.5

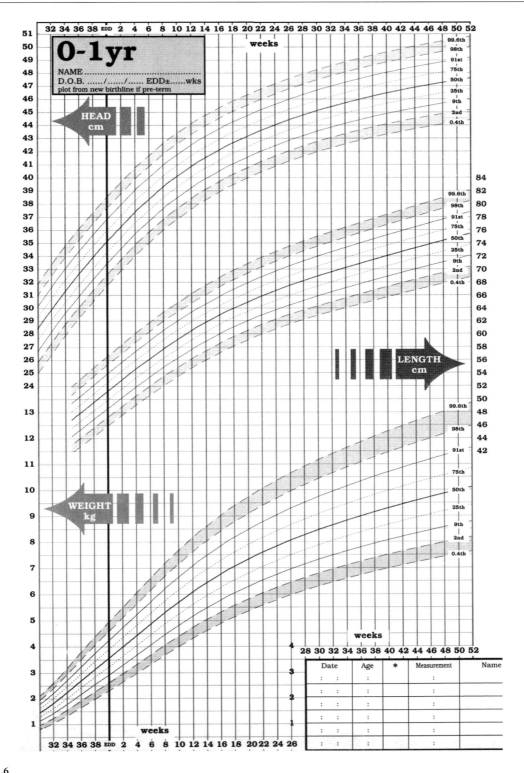

App. 1.6

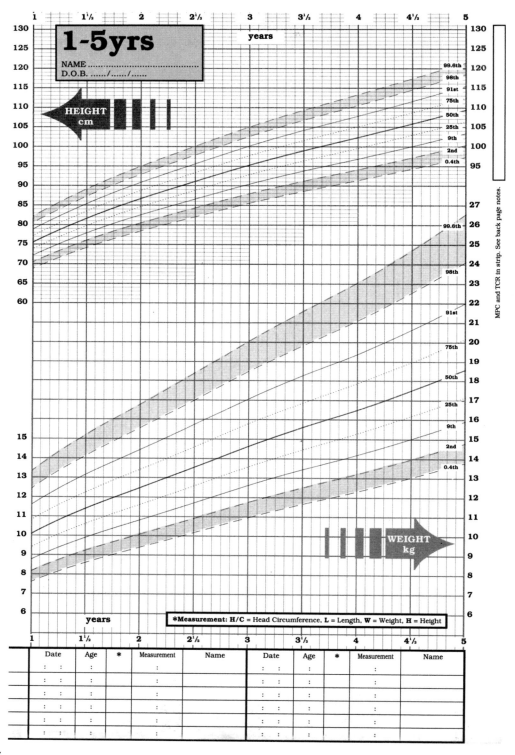

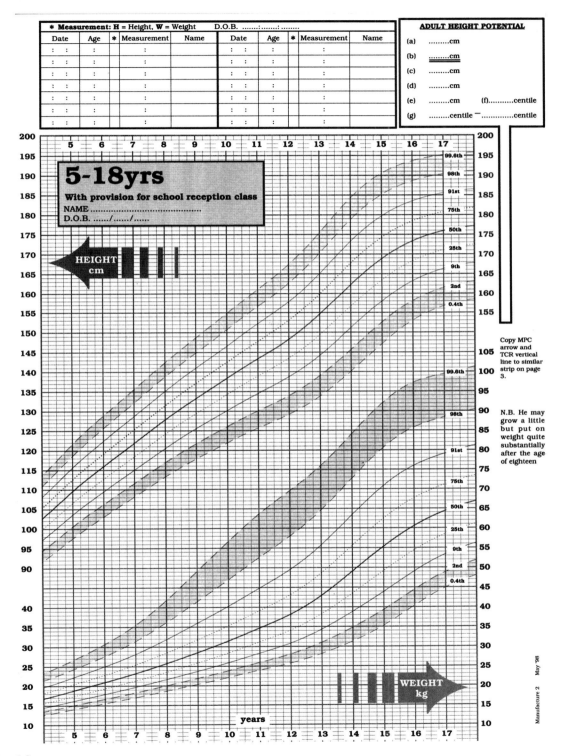

Referral guidelines

Consider referral for any girl whose BMI falls above the 99.6th centile/below the 0.4th centile as significantly over/underweight even on the basis of a single measurement. It is possible that a girl whose BMI falls in the tinted areas should also be referred. However, during infancy large but transient changes in centile may occur due to the shape of the charts, and these changes are normal. It should be remembered that the earlier the age of the second rise, the greater the risk of future obesity. Remember also that while BMI has a high correlation with relative fatness or leanness it is actually assessing the weight-to-height relationship: **this may give misleading results in girls who are very stocky and muscular who might appear obese on the BMI alone.**

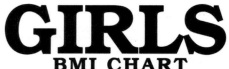

GIRLS
BMI CHART
(BIRTH – 20 YEARS)
United Kingdom cross-sectional reference data : 1995/1

Name...

NHS No.

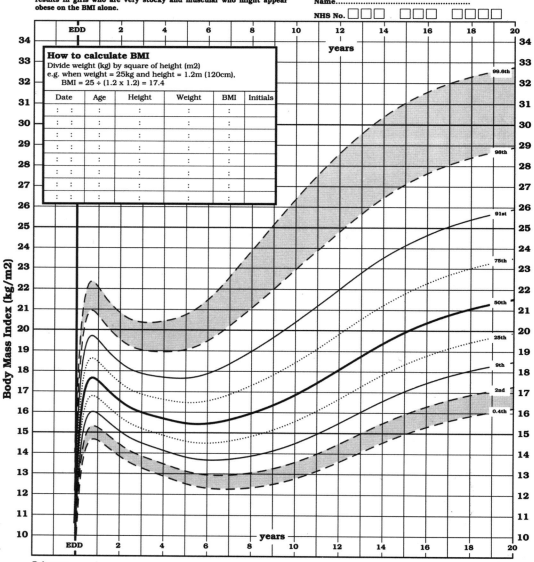

How to calculate BMI

Divide weight (kg) by square of height (m2)
e.g. when weight = 25kg and height = 1.2m (120cm),
   BMI = 25 ÷ (1.2 x 1.2) = 17.4

Date	Age	Height	Weight	BMI	Initials
: :	:	:	:	:	
: :	:	:	:	:	
: :	:	:	:	:	
: :	:	:	:	:	
: :	:	:	:	:	
: :	:	:	:	:	

Body Mass Index (kg/m2)

years

Reference

Body Mass Index reference curves for the UK, 1990 (TJ Cole, JV Freeman, MA Preece) *Arch Dis Child* 1995; **73**: 25-29

Designed and Published by
© CHILD GROWTH FOUNDATION 1995/1
(Charity Reg. No 274325)
2 Mayfield Avenue,
London W4 1PW

Printed by
HARLOW PRINTING LIMITED
Maxwell Street ◊ South Shields
Tyne & Wear ◊ NE33 4PU
Tel: 0191 455 4286 Fax: 0191 427 0195

App. 1.9

Referral guidelines

Consider referral for any boy whose BMI falls above the 99.6th centile/below the 0.4th centile as significantly over/underweight even on the basis of a single measurement. It is possible that a boy whose BMI falls in the tinted areas should also be referred. However, during infancy large but transient changes in centile may occur due to the shape of the charts, and these changes are normal. It should be remembered that the earlier the age of the second rise, the greater the risk of future obesity. Remember also that while BMI has a high correlation with relative fatness or leanness it is actually assessing the weight-to-height relationship: **this may give misleading results in boys who are very stocky and muscular who might appear obese on the BMI alone.**

BOYS
BMI CHART
(BIRTH - 20 YEARS)
United Kingdom cross-sectional reference data : 1995/1

Name...

NHS No.

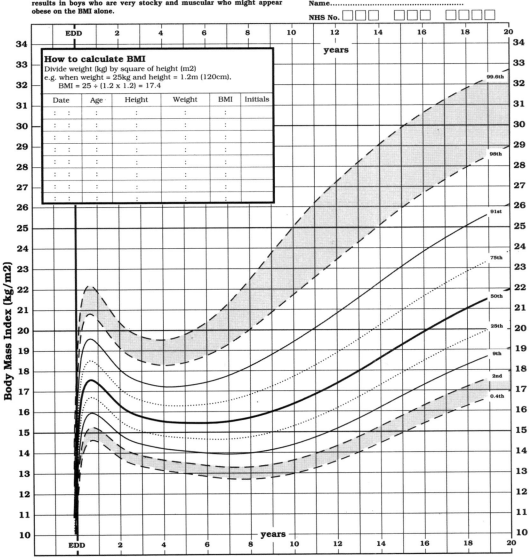

How to calculate BMI

Divide weight (kg) by square of height (m2)
e.g. when weight = 25kg and height = 1.2m (120cm),
  BMI = 25 ÷ (1.2 x 1.2) = 17.4

Date	Age	Height	Weight	BMI	Initials
: :	:	:	:	:	
: :	:	:	:	:	
: :	:	:	:	:	
: :	:	:	:	:	
: :	:	:	:	:	
: :	:	:	:	:	

Body Mass Index (kg/m2)

Reference
Body Mass Index reference curves for the UK, 1990 (TJ Cole, JV Freeman, MA Preece) *Arch Dis Child* 1995; **73**: 25-29

Designed and Published by
© CHILD GROWTH FOUNDATION 1995/1
(Charity Reg. No 274325)
2 Mayfield Avenue,
London W4 1PW

Printed by
HARLOW PRINTING LIMITED
Maxwell Street ◊ South Shields
Tyne & Wear ◊ NE33 4PU
Tel: 0191 455 4286 Fax: 0191 427 0195

App. 1.10

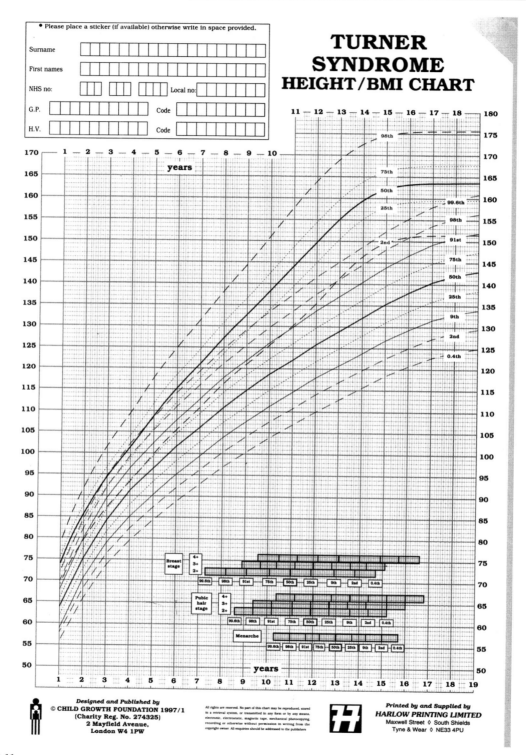

App. 1.11

DATA BOXES FOR INSERTION OF WEIGHT, HEAD CIRCUMFERENCE, LENGTH, HEIGHT AND BMI

Date	Age	Measurement	BMI	Name/Initials
: :	:	:	:	
: :	:	:	:	
: :	:	:	:	
: :	:	:	:	
: :	:	:	:	
: :	:	:	:	
: :	:	:	:	
: :	:	:	:	
: :	:	:	:	
: :	:	:	:	
: :	:	:	:	
: :	:	:	:	
: :	:	:	:	
: :	:	:	:	
: :	:	:	:	
: :	:	:	:	

Date	Age	Measurement	BMI	Name/Initials
: :	:	:	:	
: :	:	:	:	
: :	:	:	:	
: :	:	:	:	
: :	:	:	:	
: :	:	:	:	
: :	:	:	:	

How to calculate BMI

Divide weight (kg) by the square of length/height (m²)

example
weight = 25kg
length/height = 1.2m

equation
25 ÷ (1.2 x 1.2) = 17.4

Data: 1990

Manufacture 1 Apr '99

REFERENCES
Growth Curve for girls with Turner Syndrome (AJ Lyon, MA Preece, DB Grant) *ARCH DIS CHILD* 1985; 60: 932-935
Body Mass Index reference curves for the UK, 1990 (TJ Cole, JV Freeman, MA Preece) *Arch Dis Child* 1995; **73**: 25-29

App. 1.12

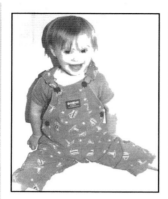

GIRLS
DOWN'S SYNDROME GROWTH CHART

UK/Republic of Ireland cross-sectional reference: 2000

STICKER

These charts are based on data from around 6000 measurements of 1100 children living throughout the UK and Republic of Ireland (Styles et al - in preparation). Growth can be charted from term to 18 years. Children with significant cardiac disease or other major pathology were excluded from the study population. In addition, data for those born before 37 completed weeks were excluded up to age two. The charts are therefore representative of healthy children with Down's syndrome growing in the U.K. and Republic of Ireland.

The charts were commissioned by the UK Down's Syndrome Medical Interest Group (DSMIG) and the data collected by Dr Mary Styles on DSMIG's behalf. The centiles were compiled under the guidance of Professor Michael Preece with statistical analysis provided by Professor Tim Cole, both of the Institute of Child Health, London. Data were analysed by Cole's LMS method. Dr Styles' data collection was funded by the Child Growth Foundation and remains the copyright of DSMIG.

PCHR - The charts are also available in A5 format for inclusion with the special PCHR Down's syndrome insert.

Preterm babies - We do not as yet have sufficient information to compile centiles for preterm babies with Down's syndrome. Measurements for those born before 37 completed weeks should not be plotted on the charts until the expected date of delivery (EDD) is reached. Thereafter they should be charted relative to EDD for at least a year. Those born at 38 weeks or later should be charted in the normal way from the EDD line.

More information about growth monitoring for children with Down's syndrome is included in the Medical Surveillance Guidelines for people with Down's Syndrome produced by the Down's Syndrome Medical Interest Group.

Overweight and underweight - Action guidelines:
Many older children with Down's syndrome are overweight and this is clearly reflected in this study population. Hence this reference data should not be used as a standard that children should aim to achieve. As with all children weight must be related to stature. Any child aged 5-18 years whose weight falls within the shaded area above the 75th centile should be charted on the BMI chart (see right). Those above the 98th centile on the BMI charts are significantly overweight and referral for further assessment and guidance should be considered.

Of those falling below the 2nd centile on the height and weight charts some will have major pathology, but some may be failing to thrive for other reasons - eg because of feeding difficulties. Again such children may need further assessment and guidance.

How to calculate BMI (Body Mass Index)
Divide weight (kg) by square of length/height (m²)
e.g. when weight = 25kg and length/height = 1.2m (120cm),
    BMI = 25 ÷ (1.2 x 1.2) = 17.4

Date	Age	Height	Ht²	Weight	BMI (Wt÷Ht²)	Initials
: :	:	:	:	:	:	
: :	:	:	:	:	:	
: :	:	:	:	:	:	
: :	:	:	:	:	:	
: :	:	:	:	:	:	
: :	:	:	:	:	:	
: :	:	:	:	:	:	

BMI CHART

Body Mass Index (kg/m²) plotted against years (6 to 20).

Printed and Supplied by
HARLOW PRINTING LIMITED
Maxwell Street ◊ South Shields
Tyne & Wear ◊ NE33 4PU

App. 1.13 Girls' Down's syndrome charts. Reprinted with permission from Jennifer Dennis and the Down's Syndrome Medical Interest Group.

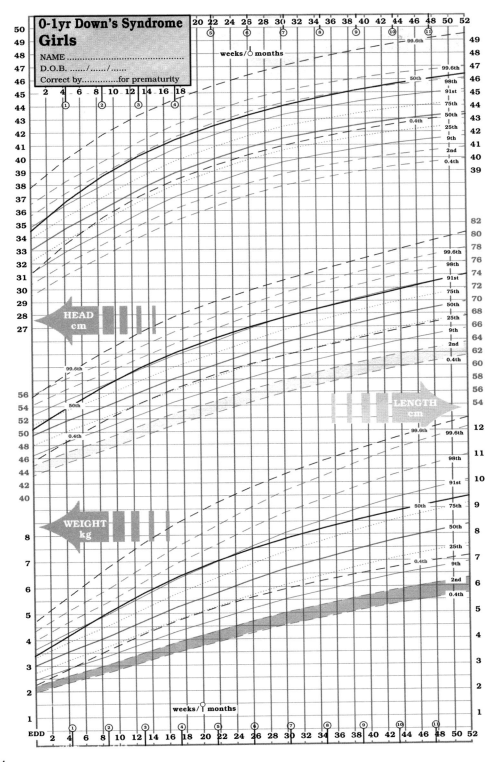

0-1yr Down's Syndrome Girls

NAME ....

D.O.B. ....../....../......

Correct by..............for prematurity

weeks/○ months

HEAD cm

LENGTH cm

WEIGHT kg

App. 1.14

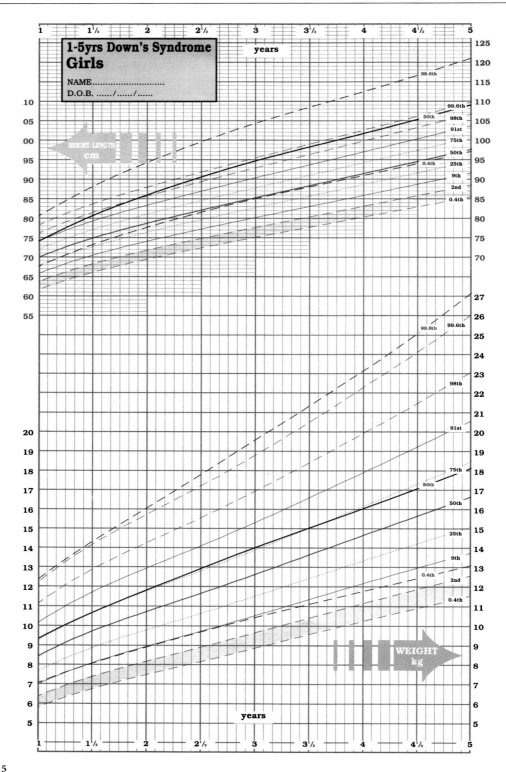

1-5yrs Down's Syndrome
Girls

NAME..............................
D.O.B. ....../....../......

years

HEIGHT/LENGTH cm

WEIGHT kg

App. 1.15

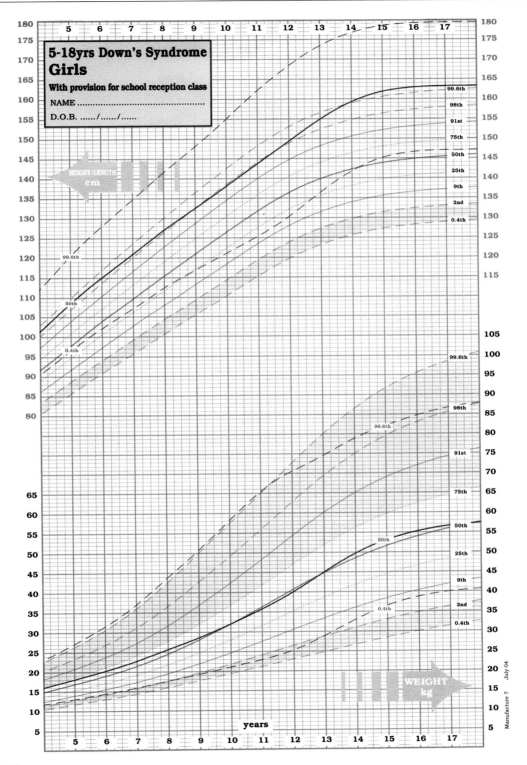

5-18yrs Down's Syndrome
Girls

With provision for school reception class

NAME ....

D.O.B. ....../....../......

HEIGHT/LENGTH cm

WEIGHT kg

years

App. 1.16

Manufacture 7   July 04

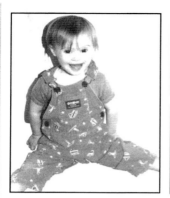

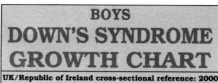

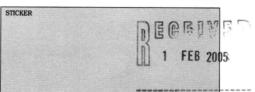

These charts are based on data from around 6000 measurements of 1100 children living throughout the UK and Republic of Ireland (Styles et al - in preparation). Growth can be charted from term to 18 years. Children with significant cardiac disease or other major pathology are excluded from the study population. In addition, data for those born before 37 completed weeks were excluded up to age two. The charts are therefore representative of healthy children with Down's syndrome growing in the U.K. and Republic of Ireland.

The charts were commissioned by the UK Down's Syndrome Medical Interest Group (DSMIG) and the data collected by Dr Mary Styles on DSMIG's behalf. The centiles were compiled under the guidance of Professor Michael Preece with statistical analysis provided by Professor Tim Cole, both of the Institute of Child Health, London. Data were analysed by Cole's LMS method. Dr Styles' data collection was funded by the Child Growth Foundation and remains the copyright of DSMIG.

PCHR - The charts are also available in A5 format for inclusion with the special PCHR Down's Syndrome insert.

Preterm babies - We do not as yet have sufficient information to compile centiles for preterm babies with Down's syndrome. Measurements for those born before 37 completed weeks should not be plotted on the charts until the expected date of delivery (EDD) is reached. Thereafter they should be charted relative to EDD for at least a year. Those born at 38 weeks or later should be charted in the normal way from the EDD line.

More information about growth monitoring for children with Down's syndrome is included in the Medical Surveillance Guidelines for people with Down's Syndrome produced by the Down's Syndrome Medical Interest Group. These are available from the address given below.

Overweight and underweight - Action guidelines:
Many older children with Down's syndrome are overweight and this is clearly reflected in this study population. Hence this reference data should not be used as a standard that children should aim to achieve. As with all children weight must be related to stature. Any child aged 5-18 years whose weight falls within the shaded area above the 75th centile should be charted on the BMI chart (see right). Those above the 98th centile on the BMI charts are significantly overweight and referral for further assessment and guidance should be considered.

Of those falling below the 2nd centile some will have major pathology, but some may be failing to thrive for other reasons - eg because of feeding difficulties. Again such children may need further assessment and guidance.

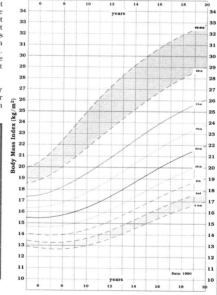

BMI CHART

How to calculate BMI (Body Mass Index)
Divide weight (kg) by square of length/height (m²)
e.g. when weight = 25kg and length/height = 1.2m (120cm),
BMI = 25 ÷ (1.2 x 1.2) = 17.4

Date	Age	Height	Ht²	Weight	BMI (Wt÷Ht²)	Initials
: :	: :	:	:	:	:	
: :	: :	:	:	:	:	
: :	: :	:	:	:	:	
: :	: :	:	:	:	:	
: :	: :	:	:	:	:	
: :	: :	:	:	:	:	
: :	: :	:	:	:	:	

© Down's Syndrome Medical Interest Group (DSMIG) 2000
Children's Centre City Hospital Campus
Nottingham
NG5 1PB

Printed and Supplied by
HARLOW PRINTING LIMITED
Maxwell Street ◊ South Shields
Tyne & Wear ◊ NE33 4PU

App. 1.17 Boys' Down's syndrome charts. Reprinted with permission from Jennifer Dennis and the Down's Syndrome Medical Interest Group.

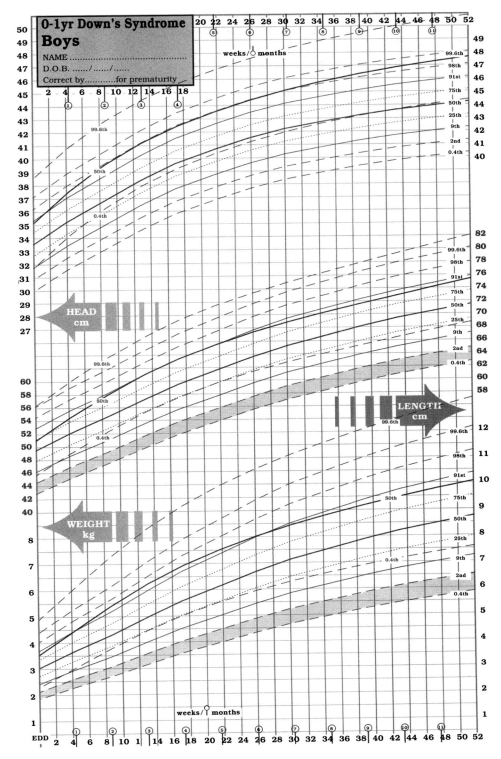

0-1yr Down's Syndrome Boys

NAME ....
D.O.B. ....../....../......
Correct by............for prematurity

weeks/○ months

HEAD cm

LENGTH cm

WEIGHT kg

weeks/○ months

EDD

App. 1.18

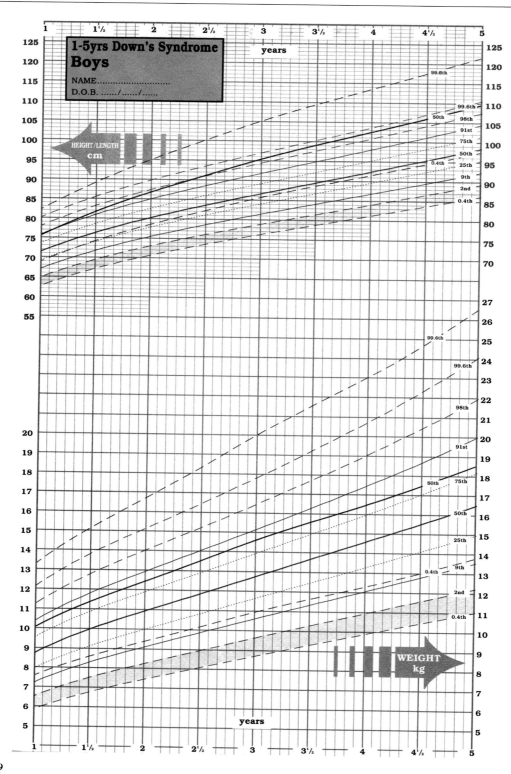

1-5yrs Down's Syndrome
Boys

NAME.............................
D.O.B. ..../......./......

years

HEIGHT/LENGTH
cm

WEIGHT
kg

years

App. 1.19

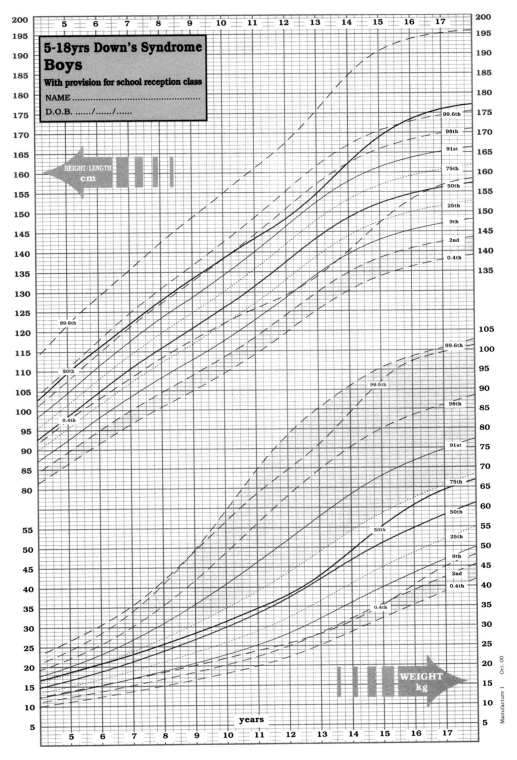

5-18yrs Down's Syndrome
Boys
With provision for school reception class
NAME ....
D.O.B. ..../......./.......

HEIGHT/LENGTH
cm

WEIGHT
kg

years

App. 1.20

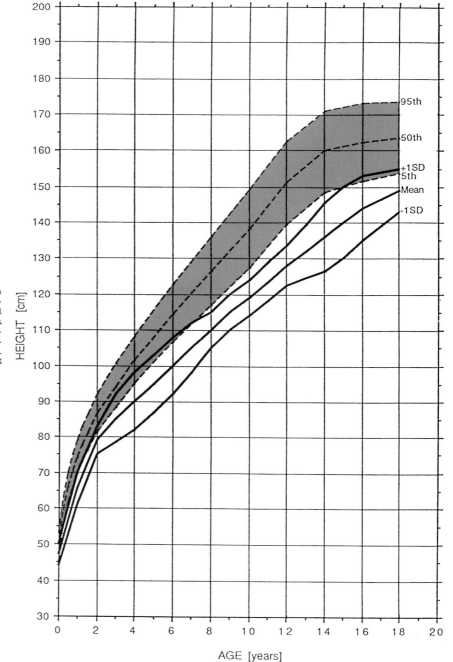

Growth curve for height in females with Noonan syndrome compared to normal values (dashed lines). Data obtained in 48 Noonan syndrome females from a collaborative retrospective review. Witt DR et al; Clin Genet 30:150, 1986.

App. 1.21 Girls' Noonan syndrome charts. Reprinted from Witt, D.R. *et al.* (1986) *Clinical Genetics* **30**, 150.

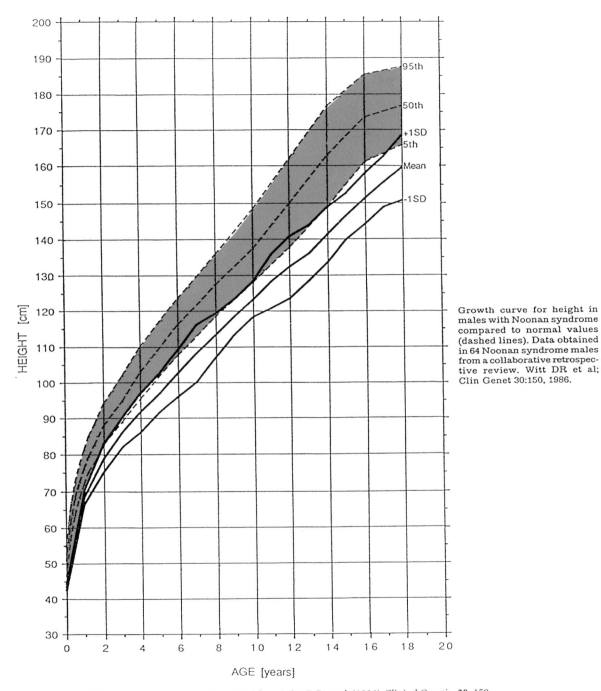

Growth curve for height in males with Noonan syndrome compared to normal values (dashed lines). Data obtained in 64 Noonan syndrome males from a collaborative retrospective review. Witt DR et al; Clin Genet 30:150, 1986.

App. 1.22 Boys' Noonan syndrome charts. Reprinted from Witt, D.R. *et al.* (1986) *Clinical Genetics* **30**, 150.

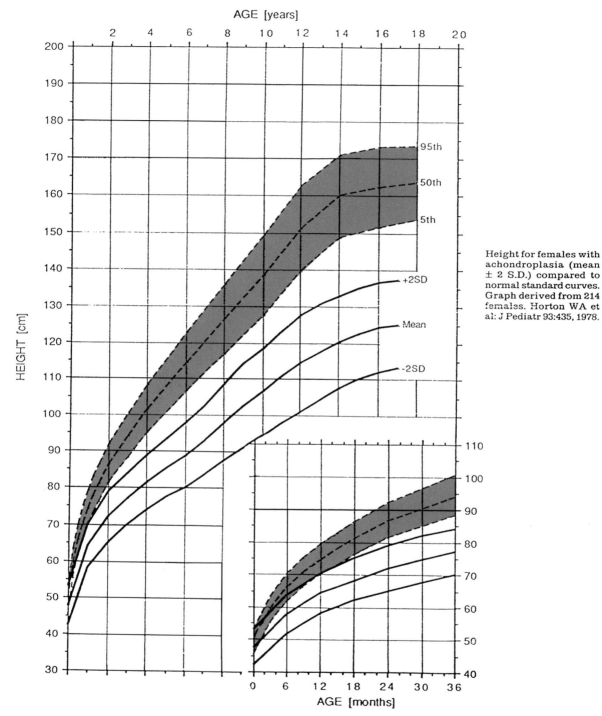

App. 1.23 Girls' achondroplasia charts. Reprinted from Horton, W. A. *et al.* (1978) Growth in achondroplasia. *Journal of Pediatrics* **93**, 435.

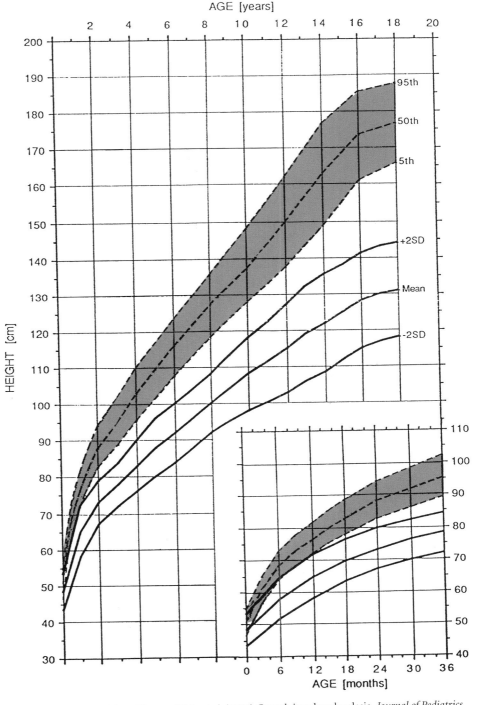

Height for males with achondroplasia (mean ± 2 S.D.) compared to normal standard curves. Graph derived from 189 males. Horton WA et al: J Pediatr 93:435, 1978.

App. 1.24 Boys' achondroplasia charts. Reprinted from Horton, W. A. *et al.* (1978) Growth in achondroplasia. *Journal of Pediatrics* **93**, 435.

2 CAH Therapy Card

NHS
Greater
Glasgow

CAH THERAPY CARD

The owner of this card has the condition
Congenital adrenal hyperplasia also known
as **CAH** or **Adrenogenital syndrome.**

Name ....

Address ....

....

DoB ....Hospital number ....

Hospital consultant: ....

Useful telephone numbers:

Hospital switchboard: ....
Ward ....
Dr A ....
Dr B ....
Endocrine Nurse ....
Endocrine Ward ....

GP's name / address / tel no ....

....

JCH/Med III 20556 / 41959 / 44656

Front and Back of Card

Instructions for Hospital Doctor

Dear Doctor,

If this child is brought to hospital by the parents as an emergency the following management is advised:

- Insert an I.V. cannula

- Take blood for U's and E's, glucose, and perform any other appropriate tests (e.g. urine culture)

- Check glucostix or dextrostix

- Give _____ mg hydrocortisone intravenously as bolus (unnecessary if parent has already given I.M. hydrocortisone)

- Commence I.V. infusion of 0.45% saline and 5% dextrose at maintenance rate (extra if child is dehydrated). Add potassium depending on electrolyte results.

- Commence hydrocortisone infusion (50mg hydrocortisone in 50ml normal saline via syringe pump) at _____ ml/hour

- **Important!** If blood glucose/glucostix is < 2.5mmol, give bolus of 2ml/kg of 10% dextrose

- If child is drowsy, hypotensive and peripherally shut down with poor capillary return give 20 ml/kg of normal saline stat.

Please contact named consultant at Yorkhill and inform of admission. *Thank you*

Current treatment

Fill in details of the drugs your child is taking, with the dates of any dose changes.

Date	Drug	Tablet size

Dose to be taken in

Morning	Afternoon	Evening

Inside of Card

What to do if your child is unwell

1. In the event of *mild to moderate illness*, e.g. cold, cough, sore throat, flu, tummy upset, double the total daily dose of hydrocortisone and give this doubled dose in 3 equal portions (morning, afternoon and evening) for the duration of the illness.

   The fludrocortisone dose should stay the same.

   i.e Hydrocortisone dose _____ x 3 per day

2. If your child
   - *does not get better* after you have increased the tablets, or
   - *feels drowsy*, or
   - *is unable to take the tablets orally* (e.g. due to continued vomiting),

   the hydrocortisone must be given by injection (intra-muscular).

   Please check that this is not past the expiry date

   The dose of hydrocortisone injection is _____

3. If your child continues to be ill and does not seem to be getting better, telephone the hospital and say that you are bringing him/her up for admission.

   Please bring this card with you and show it to the doctor.

Index